AN INTRODUCTION TO
NEUROSURGERY

BRYAN JENNETT
CBE MD FRCS

Emeritus Professor of Neurosurgery
The Institute of Neurological Sciences, Glasgow
and The University of Glasgow

KENNETH W. LINDSAY
PhD FRCS

Consultant Neurosurgeon
The Institute of Neurological Sciences, Glasgow

Fifth Edition

BUTTERWORTH
HEINEMANN

Butterworth-Heinemann Ltd
Linacre House, Jordan Hill, Oxford OX2 8DP

℞ A member of the Reed Elsevier group

OXFORD LONDON BOSTON
MUNICH NEW DELHI SINGAPORE SYDNEY
TOKYO TORONTO WELLINGTON

First published 1964
Second edition 1970
Reprinted 1973
Third edition 1977
Reprinted 1978
Reprinted 1981
Fourth edition 1983
Reprinted 1984
Fifth edition 1994

British Library Cataloguing in Publication Data

Jennett, Bryan
  Introduction to Neurosurgery. – 5Rev. ed
  I. Title II. Lindsay, Kenneth W.
  617.4

ISBN 0 7506 1580 X

Library of Congress Cataloguing in Publication Data

Jennett, Bryan.
  An introduction to neurosurgery/Bryan Jennett, Kenneth W.
  Lindsay. – 5th ed.
  p. cm.
  Includes bibliographical references and index.
  ISBN 0 7506 1580 X
  1. Nervous system – Surgery. I. Title.
  [DNLM: 1. Neurosurgery. Lindsay, Kenneth W.]
  RD593.J45 1993   93–31438
  617.4'8 – dc20   CIP

Printed and bound in Great Britain by Redwood Books, Trowbridge, Wilts

Contents

List of Illustrations

'Life is the art of drawing sufficient conclusions from insufficient premises.'

SAMUEL BUTLER
Notebooks, 1912

Preface to the Fifth Edition

Specialization in surgery has made it important to ensure that each specialty makes itself intelligible and accessible to others, in particular making it clear what it can achieve and which clinical situations need urgent attention and why. Too often neurosurgery has been regarded as dealing in desperate interventions of last resort. This book began 30 years ago in response to a *Lancet** editorial commenting on the delay in diagnosis and treatment of conditions requiring neurosurgery. It noted that this specialty might still lack the full confidence of the public and the profession. 'Or,' it went on, 'is the neurosurgeon right when he says that early symptoms and signs are not known by others as well as they might be?'

This book endeavours to dispel the mystery surrounding this specialty and to encourage those involved with neurosurgical patients to understand the principles of diagnosis and management. These include doctors, nurses and others not only in neurosurgical units but those who deal with neurosurgical patients before and after their episode of neurosurgery. Such a book cannot be comprehensive. Instead it deals at relative length with selected topics, emphasizing the principles rather than the details of operative procedures. For those who wish to know more there are suggestions for further reading, chosen for authority, scope and availability. These have been extensively updated since the last edition 9 years ago.

This new edition also sees some rearrangement and merging of chapters. The early chapters deal with intracranial lesions in general – their neurological localizing features, raised intracranial pressure, mental dysfunction, their investigation and the principles of surgical and other management. Chapters follow on intracranial tumours, vascular lesions and infections and with head injuries. Spinal and congenital conditions are then dealt with and lastly, functional neurosurgery and the treatment of pain. Many new illustrations appear in this edition, reflecting developments in computed tomographic (CT) scanning and magnetic resonance imaging (MRI), and for these we are grateful to Dr Evelyn Teasdale, Dr D. Hadley and Dr K. Grossart, neuroradiologists.

We are indebted to several other colleagues in the Institute in Glasgow for giving helpful advice on this edition, in particular Mr R. A. Johnston on spinal conditions, Mr T. A. Hide on congenital conditions and Mr P. Barlow on functional neurosurgery. The illustrations for the first edition were the work of Dr Robert Ollernshaw and Mr R. Neave in Manchester, and Mr Gabriel

*Lancet, 1961, ii, 917, 'Time in the Machine.'

Donald and Mr Hugh Gray in Glasgow. Permission to reproduce illustrations was kindly given as follows: Figures 1.3, 2.1, 12.1 and 16.2 from *Scientific Foundations of Surgery*, Heinemann: Figures 11.3 and 11.5 from *Operative Surgery* volume 14, Butterworths: Figure 12.2 from *MRS War Memorandum 7*, HMSO.

Madeleine Younger has coped patiently and skilfully with the irksome task of addenda, insertions and rewrites – so much more difficult than virgin text. Susan Devlin and Alison Duncan of Butterworth–Heinemann have dealt courteously and efficiently with the various problems that they must by now have come to expect from authors.

GLASGOW   B. J.
February, 1993   K. W. L.

Part I:

Intracranial Mass Lesions in General

Introduction

Much of the work of a neurosurgeon is taken up with the diagnosis and management of localized intracranial lesions – tumours, haematomas, ischaemia, contusions and lacerations. These often disclose their presence and whereabouts in the skull by focal neurological symptoms and signs, produced by effects on local structures. These may be the result of mechanical distortion, or of ischaemia or vascular congestion due to pressure on local blood vessels. Because they take up space in the only body cavity that is rigid and inelastic, many of these lesions sooner or later cause raised intracranial pressure (ICP) which is the means by which most masses eventually threaten life. The features of this may be the first sign of a mass, or may only later come to dominate the clinical picture. The recognition and management of raised ICP which may also result from non-focal pathology, are often a priority when dealing with intracranial lesions.

Because tumours usually grow relatively slowly it is easier in patients with them to recognize the phases in the evolution of focal and general pressure than in those with more acute conditions, when what takes months with a tumour may be telescoped into a few days or hours. The processes involved are the same, however, although their relative importance may vary. What follows applies both to tumours and other expanding lesions; the differential diagnosis usually depends on the duration of the history and on associated features (e.g. injury or infection).

The chapters in Part I cover these matters in the order in which a clinician usually works. Chapter 1 deals with where in the skull a lesion is likely to be, based on clinical evidence of focal dysfunction, Chapter 2 with the features of raised ICP and Chapter 3 with the variety of mental disorders that can occur – from personality change through dementia, confusion and coma to brain death. We next deal with investigation to refute or confirm clinical impressions (Chapter 4), and then with what can be done about intracranial mass lesions in general (Chapter 5). The three chapters in Part II deal with the commoner types of non-traumatic intracranial lesions in more detail – tumours (Chapter 6), vascular disorders (Chapter 7) and infections (Chapter 8).

Chapter 1

Localizing symptoms and signs

Limitations of localization

Anatomical classification of intracranial masses

Laterally placed supratentorial masses

    Epilepsy
    Dysphasia (language disorders)
    Parietal spatial disorders
    Frontal lobe – behavioural disorders
    Anosmia
    Homonymous hemianopia
    Sensorimotor hemiplegia

Centrally placed supratentorial masses

    Anterior part of third ventricle
    Sellar and parasellar masses

Infratentorial masses

Transtentorial masses

Limitations of localization

Effective and expeditious relief of brain compression depends on the surgeon's ability to recognize the site of the primary expanding lesion. There is no equivalent in neurosurgery of exploratory laparotomy; no means of opening the skull and passing a hand round the brain from lobe to lobe looking for lesions. Accurate localization rests on the interpretation of focal dysfunction in the nervous system and on the results of radiological and other studies.

Faith in the tendency of lesions to run true to physiopathological form, by producing only those disorders which would be anatomically anticipated, has been undermined by a better understanding of the organizational complexity of the nervous system and the subtleties of brain compression.

As stimulation and ablation studies in human subjects accumulate it has become apparent that concepts of localization of function in the brain have hitherto been too rigid. Owing to the complexity of neuronal connections, lesions in a single site may produce a wide range of phenomena in different individuals, whilst the same clinical syndrome can result from lesions in a variety of sites. The added effects of shifts and of pressure, and the part played by speed of development and spread of oedema, are difficult to allow for. 'Always' and 'never' are words seldom appropriate in describing the symptomatology of brain lesions; action must never be delayed until the completion of some syndrome, or relief denied a patient because of some apparent anomaly in the clinical picture.

However, the development of modern radiological techniques has added a new dimension to diagnosis in the nervous system. As a result the surgical neurologist now looks to the examination of the nervous system for a different order of accuracy in localization than was expected when he or she had to rely solely on clinical assessment to indicate where to operate.

But neuroradiological investigations are not diagnostic slot machines; choice must be made between different investigative techniques in respect of safety and the likelihood of their yielding the required information. Both for planning radiological and other studies, and for devising appropriate surgical measures when the situation is too urgent to wait for X-rays or when investigations have failed to pinpoint the lesion, the surgeon needs to know first and foremost which compartment of the skull is most likely to harbour the lesion.

Anatomical classification of intracranial masses

The tentorium is the most important divider in the cranium (Fig. 2.4, p. 25). Lesions above and below this structure produce distinctive syndromes, call for different methods of investigation, and carry their own perils. The chief concern is whether a mass is more likely to be above the tentorium or below, mainly central or lateral, and on the right side or the left (Fig. 1.1).

Tumours which grow through the tentorium laterally may produce features typical of disorder in both the main cranial compartments. By contrast, centrally situated tumours, in the posterior part of third ventricle or midbrain, may cause only internal hydrocephalus and midbrain signs, without any evidence of tumour either above or below the tentorium.

The clinical features characteristic of each location will now be described, but the possibility of large masses remaining neurologically silent and producing signs only of pressure must not be forgotten.

Laterally placed supratentorial masses

Epilepsy

Fits have already occurred in up to half the patients admitted with supratentorial masses, and in 80% of those with more than 2 years' history. In half the cases with epilepsy this was the initial symptom of the illness. Epilepsy is as likely to occur whether the lesion is extracerebral or intracerebral, but is three times more likely to complicate a frontoparietal than an occipital mass. Epilepsy is less common with ischaemic or haemorrhagic lesions, but more common with abscess (p. 174).

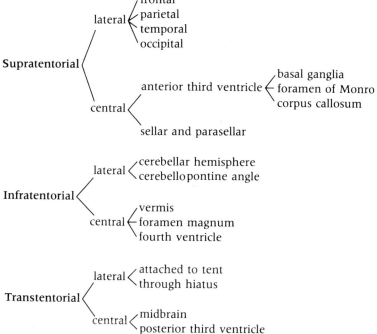

Fig. 1.1 Anatomical classification of intracranial lesion sites.

The variety of episodes now recognized as epileptic is enormous yet there is still a tendency to restrict the term to convulsions accompanied by tongue biting and incontinence of urine. No generally accepted classification of fits exists but it is most useful to distinguish between non-focal and focal (partial) seizures, accepting as focal any attack which suggests at any stage in its development activity confined to one area of the cerebral cortex, no matter how widely it subsequently spreads. Many patients suffer from more than one type of attack, but if any is focal this is of localizing significance.

Types of attack

In non-focal fits loss of consciousness is the primary event. Convulsions usually follow, affecting all four limbs, though one side may be more active than the other. Occasionally there is little or no convulsive activity, the patient falling unconscious and remaining limp throughout the attack. A focal fit which spreads until all the limbs are involved may mistakenly be regarded as non-focal if it is not observed from the beginning. With careful observation fewer and fewer attacks are regarded as non-focal. Petit mal is another form of non-focal epilepsy, but is rarely if ever due to a space-occupying lesion; the term is usually confined to very frequent and brief attacks in children, associated with a specific electroencephalogram (EEG) pattern (3 per second spike-and-wave).

Focal epilepsy takes many forms, best classified by the part of the brain which the paroxysm apparently first involves:

1. *Precentral gyrus* (motor strip) activity leads to twitching of one side of the body, which begins in one area and may remain localized or spread until the whole limb, the whole side of the body or all four limbs are involved. This is Jacksonian or focal motor epilepsy; the clue to localization is the first part to move, usually the thumb, foot or face, which have large cortical areas of representation. The part initially affected may be paralysed for a period of minutes or hours after the fit has finished (Todd's palsy); this may be valuable localizing evidence when the onset of the seizure has not been witnessed.

2. *The speech centre* in the left temporal lobe may be the focus of activity, recognized by sudden dysphasia, either an inability to speak or to understand the speech of others. Spread will usually be first to the face.

3. *The frontal eyefield* causes the head and eyes to turn towards the opposite side; consciousness is almost always lost before spread of activity to the limbs.

4. *The postcentral gyrus* gives sensory epilepsy, feelings of numbness, tingling or a sensation of movement in a limb (or part of it) which may be followed by twitching in the same distribution.

5. *The visual cortex* in the occipital lobe causes hallucinations of light and colours, not recognizable as objects or people, in the opposite visual field to the lesion.

6. *Temporal lobe epilepsy* (complex partial seizures) is now regarded as the explanation of many phenomena previously unexplained or ascribed to other causes. It is the commonest form of focal epilepsy, although frequently less dramatic and obvious than the focal motor form. All types of attack include an altered state of consciousness but additional features enable three main kinds of seizure to be recognized:

    (a) Momentary absences are pure lapses of consciousness during which contact is lost with the surroundings, the flow of speech broken, the thread of conversation lost. The patient does not fall and the episode may pass unnoticed by onlookers or may be mistaken for petit mal.

    (b) Psychic phenomena are experienced by the patient, often with little outward change in behaviour. Olfactory hallucinations, invariably unpleasant and usually unrecognizable, associated with a feeling of unreality or detachment from the surroundings constitute uncinate fits. Other sensations commonly reported are inexplicable fear, *déjà vu* – as though the situation and happenings occurring in reality around the patient had been lived through before – alterations or distortions of size and distance, and impressions of dissociation of body from soul. Some of these are transitorily experienced by normal people in the moments before falling asleep and when dozing after waking. If direct questions about these kind of phenomena are not asked, the patient seldom volunteers an account of them, fearing ridicule or the suspicion of mental illness.

    (c) Automatisms comprise complex and perfectly executed activities, essentially purposeless, for the duration of which the patient is subsequently amnesic. Often an attack consists of only simple automatic activity, usually stereotyped, such as closing a door, crossing a room, clapping hands, or uttering some stock phrase. But sometimes he or she may travel across a city to a place never visited before, driving a car or using public transport and seemingly in full possession of all faculties. The individual then suddenly regains full consciousness and is perplexed by where he or she is and at a loss to explain how he or she got there.

Is it epilepsy?

Unless an attack has been witnessed by an expert it may be impossible to decide its nature. In favour of epilepsy are altered consciousness with subsequent amnesia for the incident, cyanosis and frothing at the mouth, temporary bilateral pupillary dilatation, a bitten tongue or lip, incontinence of urine, injuries sustained during an attack, or Todd's palsy during recovery. None of these need accompany an epileptic attack, but if they do the presumption of epilepsy is high. Episodic disorders other than epilepsy may lead to confusion:

1. *Opisthotonus* in brief attacks usually occurs when the brainstem is compressed acutely, such as by foraminal impaction (p. 38). Arching of the neck and lower spine backwards is often accompanied by decerebrate rigidity of all four limbs (extensor or tonic spasms).
2. *Extensor posturing* (decerebrate attacks) are due to compression at a higher level in the midbrain, and more often result from tentorial coning (p. 36). Increased extensor tone causes straightening of the affected limbs with pronation of the forearm and plantar flexion of the foot. Often the limbs of only one side are affected, and sensory stimuli may set off a spasm which may be associated with respiratory overactivity (rather than the apnoea of epilepsy), and possibly by pupillary changes.
3. *Chalastic fits* are a contrasting type of disorder because they are characterized by limpness and atony. They occur when pressure is dangerously high from masses in either compartment of the skull, but particularly with tumours near the third ventricle. The knees suddenly give way and the patient falls to the ground without loss of consciousness, hence the term 'drop epilepsy'.
4. *Hydrocephalic attacks* (p. 17).
5. *Amblyopic attacks* (p. 34), though sometimes reported as blackouts, are purely visual phenomena.
6. *Hysterical fugues* closely resemble epileptic automatisms and the distinction will depend on the setting and background of the incident. If epileptic, the patient often suffers also from some attacks of a different nature which are more readily recognizable as epileptic.
7. *Internal carotid stenosis* can lead to episodic insufficiency of the circulation to one-half of the brain with transient hemiplegia, sometimes associated with transient loss of vision in the eye on the side of the stenosis. Such attacks may be indistinguishable from epilepsy except for the involvement of vision or their precipation by the sudden assumption of the upright position.
8. *Ménière's disease* causes episodic vertigo, almost always with vomiting, normally lasting several hours.
9. *Vasovagal attacks* result from peripheral vasodilatation causing transient reduction in cerebral blood flow. They usually develop in the upright position and are accompanied by pallor and sweating.

10. *Cardiac arrhythmias*, particularly heart block, can also cause transient global reduction of cerebral blood flow and 'fainting'.

Is the epilepsy symptomatic?

Epilepsy is a non-specific response of the brain to an injurious agent, be it mechanical, chemical, bacterial or metabolic. A large number of conditions can thus give rise to fits, and a space-occupying lesion is only one. Most often no overt cause is found and the diagnosis remains 'idiopathic' epilepsy, although there is probably an underlying structural abnormality in most cases, perhaps resulting from minor birth trauma.

Idiopathic epilepsy usually begins in childhood and it is when a patient suffers a first fit in adult life that suspicions are aroused regarding underlying organic disease. When fits are focal there is even greater likelihood of a local lesion. However, brain tumours more often cause non-focal attacks than focal, whilst focal attacks, especially of temporal lobe origin, are frequently found in idiopathic epilepsy.

There is nothing characteristic therefore about the epilepsy due to tumour to distinguish it from either idiopathic or other symptomatic epilepsy. In all forms the frequency of attacks varies widely, with long remissions, sometimes of years, sometimes occurring apparently as a response to anticonvulsant drugs. Attacks may be frequent for a few months and then disappear although the tumour continues to grow. Sometimes epilepsy persists but the pattern changes as the tumour grows into fresh areas of the brain.

Epilepsy first appearing in adult life is always suspicious of some acquired organic lesion, and a computed tomographic (CT) scan should always be carried out.

Other causes of symptomatic epilepsy are legion and would take too much space to list here. Perhaps the condition most often confused with tumour is cerebral arteriosclerosis, especially as dementia and hemiplegia may also occur.

A note on nomenclature

Epilepsy carries a stigma second only to that of mental illness, and it is especially feared because it precludes so many types of employment. Euphemisms are therefore often used by patients and may even be employed loosely by doctors, to their own confusion. Examples are convulsions, fits, attacks, blackouts, dysrythmic episodes and seizures.

The terms grand mal, generalized epilepsy and major fits are used to describe what have been described here under non-focal attacks. But the terms are imprecise; some contend that major means only that consciousness is lost, some that grand mal should be restricted to classical generalized convulsions with tongue biting and incontinence, whilst generalized does not specify whether the fit began in one area or was general from the start. Minor epilepsy is even more vague, whilst petit mal has a strictly limited application. Partial epilepsy is used by some to describe any attack which does not become generalized.

Status epilepticus refers to a succession of attacks of a generalized nature (though the onset may be focal) in which one attack follows another without return of consciousness between them. A dangerous state of affairs with an appreciable mortality, it may develop out of the very first fit a patient suffers, especially if the lesion is frontal; once it has happened it is liable to be repeated if that individual suffers further fits in the future, perhaps precipitated by sudden withdrawal of anticonvulsants. (For treatment see p. 227.)

Epilepsia partialis continuans is status epilepticus confined locally, usually to the face or fingers or foot. It may continue for hours or days without impairment of consciousness or any serious threat to life.

To summarize, epilepsy is a common manifestation of disease in the nervous system. The three important questions to answer are: Has the patient had an epileptic fit? Is there any indication of which part of the brain was primarily affected? Is there other evidence of brain damage?

Dysphasia (language disorders)

Language is largely dependent on the left temporal lobe in right-handed persons, and also in most who are left-handed. Dominance of either hemisphere appears to be less marked in true left-handers who may suffer dysphasia from lesions on either side, but they tend to recover more rapidly as the other side asserts itself. The right hemisphere is seldom dominant, but if the left brain is severely damaged in early childhood the right side of the brain seems able to assume responsibility for language function.

The various aspects of language function, speaking, reading, writing and listening are special cases of sensorimotor activity, with motor function represented anterior to sensory. Although mixed types of disorder are most common, predominantly motor or sensory defects can be recognized in many instances and are sometimes regarded as special varieties of apraxia or agnosia.

Motor (expressive) dysphasia is both the most frequent and the most obvious type, the patient being unable either to utter words which he or she has in mind, or to think of the correct words to express him or herself. Commonly only the names of certain objects or people are inaccessible whilst the patient is able to explain what an object is used for, indicating both that he or she has recognized it and has no difficulty in making sentence constructions using other words (nominal dysphasia). Indeed, purely nominal dysphasia may not be immediately obvious, particularly if the patient is not allowed to get beyond the exchange of clichés which is often the limit of daily contact with the doctor in hospital. These the patient may manage perfectly, but when asked to name a series of objects the defect is soon obvious, although he or she may name the first two or three correctly, mispronounce the next two names (paraphasia) and then be unable to name any more.

Perseveration is exhibited by many dysphasic patients: the name of one object correctly given is reproduced as the name for succeeding objects. It may be indicative of general mental clouding rather than of specific language disorder.

Dysgraphia is also a motor defect in language function, but is seldom the only one; more often the ability to write survives the loss of the spoken word. Wrong words, misspellings and perseveration all appear before the writing is reduced to a meaningless scribble.

Sensory (receptive) dysphasia comprises the inability to understand spoken or written words and commands. Reading aloud may still be possible but without comprehension. As with motor defects, this may be obvious only on direct testing, in the early stages, by giving a number of commands in rapid succession; perseveration of response may then be observed. If sensory dysphasia is present in addition to motor, the patient is unaware of mistakes when he or she speaks; this aggravates the motor disability and the almost speechless and largely inaccessible state which results is termed global aphasia. The words aphasia and dysphasia are loosely used in practice, without implying that aphasia means total inability to speak; likewise agraphia, dysgraphia; alexia, dyslexia.

The great value of dysphasia as a localizing sign makes its recognition important. Two conditions may stimulate it:

1. *Mental confusion* leads to inappropriate responses to questions and commands, and it may be impossible for even a skilled observer to decide whether language function is disturbed. The dysphasic patient will usually make a guess which is near the mark, or in some other way indicate that he or she has recognized but cannot name an object, thus giving the impression of trying to cooperate. It is curious that dysphasia seldom makes a person taciturn, and the prolix splutterings of the dysphasic patient making unnecessary conversation are characteristic.
2. *Dysarthia* due to bulbar palsy or cerebellar lesions causes slurred speech which may be difficult to understand, but a moment's thought will prevent this being mistaken for dysphasia. Confusion is less likely to arise if reference is made to disorders of *language* rather than of speech.

Parietal spatial disorders

The non-dominant, right parietal lobe is necessary for the correct appreciation of the image of a person's own body, and orientation in extrapersonal space. When this lobe is damaged a patient may neglect his or her limbs, in particular the left ones; he or she forgets where they are and allows them to lie in bizarre positions; even if the arms are not weak he or she fails to bring both into use for bimanual skills. If extrapersonal space is incorrectly perceived there will be difficulty in getting around even in familiar surroundings: wrong turnings taken in moving from room to room in a person's own house, an inability to recognize common landmarks or follow simple routes in the street. Asked to draw a map of the ward, or a clock, or to copy diagrams, he or she may be quite unable to do so, or else execute only a wobbly outline more fitting for a 4-year-old child.

The patient with a lesion in the left (dominant) parieto-temporal lobe may be unable to recognize parts of his or her own body, to distinguish between different fingers, between left and right limbs or even between his or her own limbs and those of the examiner. Inability to calculate, which involves the correct arrangement of serial symbols in space, is another sequel with left-sided lesions (dyscalculia).

The implications of these disorders of the mind and the insight they give into the way in which we relate to our surroundings are fascinating. But as a localizing sign they indicate no more than a lesion in the right parietal region, which will often be suspected already from the homonymous hemianopia usually accompanying these curious distortions of perception.

Frontal lobe – behavioural disorders

In spite of the reputed function of this part of the brain in controlling higher mental activity and the consistent effect produced by psychosurgery in this region, mental syndromes due to local disturbances are quite unusual. They are nothing like as common as those due to diffuse pathology, such as have been described above. Moreover a fairly extensive frontal lobectomy can be performed without any obvious impairment of mental functioning, but as soon as there is bilateral frontal damage, symptoms do become manifest. The most obvious syndrome produced is that commonly referred to as 'Witzelsucht syndrome', the nearest English translation being 'pathological joking'. The essential component is a lack of social restraint, the contribution of which to normal behaviour is clearly appreciated only when it is defective. There is incomplete awareness of the subtleties of social appropriateness; the patient may make tactless remarks and joke in unlikely situations, yet the superficial impression is of unusual liveliness and genuinely quick wit. The clue to this being more than natural exuberance lies in misjudgements of manners, an overstepping of good taste which is difficult to describe but easy to recognize. The euphoria of these patients, which is both enjoyable and contagious, usually precludes their having insight into their condition. When a frontal lesion affects primarily the corpus callosum, the effect is of a very profound dementia occurring as the primary clinical event.

Anosmia

Anterior fossa masses may damage the olfactory bulbs and tracts, giving anosmia on one or both sides. Unilateral loss is much more significant, but can be due to abnormalities in the nose, which must be excluded. Bilateral anosmia is a common and often permanent sequel of head injury which should be excluded before attributing anosmia to a local expanding lesion. Raised intracranial pressure over a long period may also impair olfactory function bilaterally.

Homonymous hemianopia

Interruption of the visual pathway anywhere from the optic tracts to the calcarine cortex will lead to complete or partial loss of the opposite visual field – homonymous hemianopia (Fig. 1.2). The temporal half of vision is lost in one eye and the nasal half in the other; whichever eye is used, the same half (either left or right) of the field will be lost. The projection is reversed, horizontally and vertically: right-sided lesions cause left hemianopia and a high lesion (parietal) gives loss of the lower quadrant, a low lesion (temporal) an upper quadrantic hemianopia. Most lesions involve the optic radiations which, being spread out over a wide area, are susceptible to damage from a wide range of lesions; these usually spare the macular part of the visual field. A lesion in the calcarine cortex itself, which is rare, involves the macular area; this is only likely to be appreciated if the fields are plotted on a perimeter or screen. Ischaemic lesions of the posterior circulation tend to spare the macula, probably due to rich collateral blood supply.

Confrontation can be used to test fields roughly: the patient fixes his or her eyes on those of the examiner, who brings in his or her fingers from the

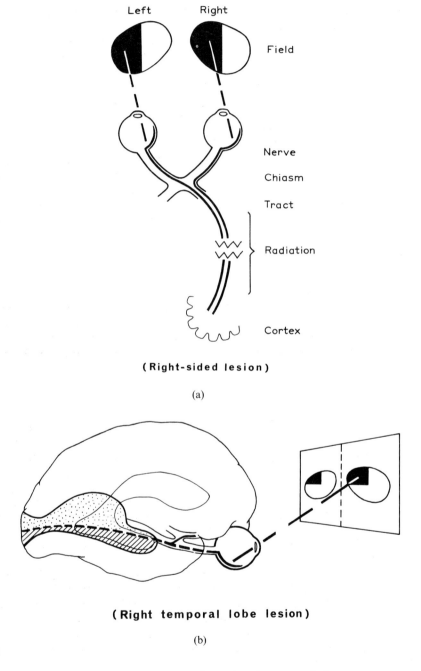

(Right temporal lobe lesion)

(b)

Fig. 1.2 Homonymous hemianopia. (a) Lesions of optic tract, radiation or cortex cause hemianopia on the opposite side. (b) Lesions affecting only the lower part of these pathways cause hemianopia in only the upper part of the affected field.

periphery of the fields. The examiner compares the patient's field with his or her own, whilst watching the patient's eyes for any failure to fix, which will falsify the result. If visual acuity is impaired a torch or waving white card or handkerchief may be used to plot a crude field which may none the less be invaluable; the inexperienced too readily accept the excuse that vision is too poor for field testing, or that the patient is too drowsy or uncooperative. In the latter event the reaction to menace from the two sides may be compared. Parietal lesions may give only an attention hemianopia – when objects are simultaneously presented in both right and left visual fields, only one is attended to; if the same stimulus is then applied again, in the defective field alone, it is immediately seen.

More accurate records of the visual fields in cooperative patients with adequate vision are obtained with a Goldmann *perimeter*. Small white objects, 1–5 mm in diameter, are moved into the field against a black background marked in degrees, and the field is mapped on a chart. Different isopters are drawn, expressed as object size over distance from the screen, and a defect which is not apparent with a large object may be obvious when a small one is used. The size of the blind spot and of any scotomata (islands of visual loss) can be charted in addition to the peripheral field; because the conditions are reproducible, serial examinations made over weeks or years can be accurately compared.

Like dysphasia, this is so important a localizing sign that no effort should be spared in the attempt to elicit it. Homonymous hemianopia is occasionally produced by parasellar lesions involving the optic tract, but there will usually be other signs of a lesion in this region. It may also be misleading when caused by posterior cerebral artery occlusion due to a tentorial cone or basilar artery thrombosis – again, conditions which normally declare themselves by obvious local signs.

Sensorimotor hemiplegia

This is less valuable as a localizing feature because it may be produced by a lesion anywhere on the pyramidal pathway from the cortex, through the internal capsule, cerebral peduncles and pons, to the medullary pyramids (Fig. 1.3). When due to a lesion of the cortex or the subcortical pathways, the paralysis seldom affects the whole of one side equally; only the face may be involved but more often both face and arm are weak, or the leg alone. Lower down in the pathway the fibres for face, arm and leg are so closely packed together that a lesion tends to produce a relatively total hemiplegia. Concomitant dysphasia, hemianopia or focal epilepsy indicate that the lesion is above the tentorium.

The severity of hemiplegia ranges from complete paralysis to mild increase in tone, first noticed in the forearm pronators and reflected in tendon hyperreflexia; there is an extensor plantar reflex (Babinski response). Weakness due to a hemisphere lesion usually affects fine peripheral movements initially, whilst gross proximal movements of the shoulder and hip remain unaffected. This too is the pattern of recovery: proximal before distal, gross before fine movements.

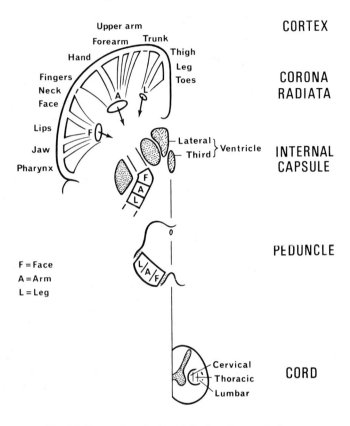

Fig. 1.3 The corticospinal tract. F=face; A=arm; L=leg.

When cortical sensation is deranged there is loss of *two-point discrimination*, the ability to discern that a double touch or pain stimulus is in fact made up of two discrete points. The distance between them which can be detected varies widely on different parts of the body, being most fine on the finger tips, most crude on the back of the trunk; the normal side is the standard for comparison. *Astereognosis* is the inability to appreciate differences in texture of materials and weight, and to recognize an object from feeling its shape or character. Even when astereognosis occurs without any weakness it may seriously limit the use of fingers and hand which will be capable of fine movements only when under direct vision. When *joint position sense* is lost the patient is unaware of the state of the joints or even the location of his or her limb, and this renders a limb almost useless, although muscle strength remains unimpaired. Complex movements depend as much on sensory guidance as on motor control, and loss of either can be crippling. When testing reveals an obviously powerful limb which the patient protests is useless, the patient may be wrongly suspected of exaggerating the disability.

Centrally placed supratentorial masses

Anterior part of third ventricle

In the cavity of the ventricle tumours usually produce only increased pressure, by occluding the foramen of Monro, causing hydrocephalus, (Fig. 2.3). Because the commonest lesion, a colloid cyst, is sometimes mobile in the ventricle, the obstruction may be intermittent with sudden episodes of headache of the utmost severity, and hydrocephalic attacks; drop attacks also occur (p. 9).

Above the ventricle, in the corpus callosum or septum pellucidum, tumours cause the most profound dementia, much more severe than is common either from the increased pressure or from unilateral frontal tumours. Drowsiness and repeated yawning are frequent and the patient may become mentally inaccessible even though there is no increase in intracranial pressure. Hemiplegia is sometimes bilateral, but occasionally affects the two sides alternately, probably due to pressure on the anterior cerebral arteries. Alternating hemiplegia, which is sometimes mistakenly suspected of being hysterical, may also be produced by parasagittal lesions involving the medial surfaces of both hemispheres and by lesions in the brainstem or at the foramen magnum where the pyramidal fibres for the two sides are contiguous.

Lateral to the third ventricle lie the basal ganglia, involvement of which may give symptomatic Parkinsonism characterized by extrapyramidal rigidity of a cog-wheel (as distinct from clasp-knife pyramidal) type, paucity of movement, and occasionally involuntary movements. The internal capsule is very close and there may be hemiplegia which involves all parts of the one side, for the fibres are closely crowded together here; there may be a capsular hemianopia in addition.

Below the ventricle lies the tuber cinereum, disorders of which cause endocrine imbalance with obesity or wasting and occasionally precocious puberty; the wasting state may be mistaken for anorexia nervosa.

Sellar and parasellar masses

Chiasmal compression is a most important condition to recognize because it is frequently possible to save sight by surgical intervention if this is done in time. Careful plotting of the visual fields is essential (p. 15) because certain patterns of field defect are associated with pressure from different directions, although these patterns are seldom pure for long. They take time to develop, and are frequently incomplete at the stage when it is most important to detect a tumour, whilst later the involvement of other parts of the tracts may lead to a mixture of more than one type of field defect. What matters is to realize that the location of the lesion is chiasmal.

Central pressure from below, due to a mass growing out of the sella, causes bitemporal hemianopia which appears first in the upper quadrant (Fig. 1.4). If pressure begins further forwards, one eye alone may become blind from optic nerve pressure; if further back the optic tract may be affected initially, resulting in a homonymous defect. The length of the nerve and tract vary a great deal, prefixed (short nerve) and postfixed chiasms being recognized as anatomical variations, so that conclusions about whether a compressing mass is anterior or posterior cannot be too confident.

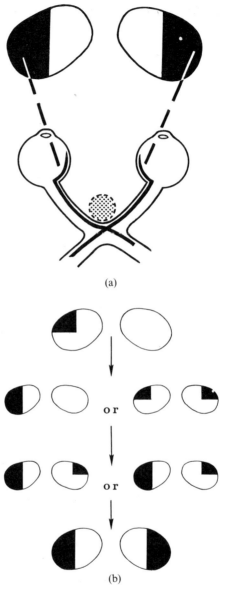

(a)

(b)

Fig. 1.4 Bitemporal hemianopia. (a) Anterior chiasmal lesions affect the nasal fibres from each retina. (b) Pressure from below the chiasm (e.g. pituitary tumour) affects first the upper field; according to the direction of tumour growth, bitemporal hemianopia may evolve in different ways.

Visual acuity is not always tested as part of the examination of the cranial nerves; patients can go blind unnoticed if their remarks about not seeing the print too well go unverified. Standard test types should be used; they allow repeated observations to be made over a period of time, provided that the same glasses are worn (if any are) on each occasion. If distant and near vision are both tested errors of refraction will be detected. Papilloedema and retinal lesions, as well as opacities in the media must be excluded before ascribing failing vision to a lesion of the visual pathways.

Endocrine abnormalities can result from interference with the anterior or posterior pituitary itself, or from involvement of the hypothalamic nuclei, or the portal vessels and nerve fibres in the pituitary stalk. Hypogonadism, hyperprolactinaemia, hypothyroidism and adrénocortical deficiency, diabetes insipidus, obesity and dwarfism may result in varying degrees.

Cavernous sinus syndromes develop from lateral spread involving the third to sixth cranial nerves, which are in the lateral wall of the sinus. Clinically recognizable thrombosis of the sinus with congestion of the conjunctiva seldom occurs, though some degree of proptosis may appear. Fifth nerve dysfunction shows itself as facial pain, usually of the first division (forehead), a local sensation quite clearly distinguishable from headache. Loss of sensation over the trigeminal distribution is less common, but corneal anesthesia, often the first sign, will go undetected unless specifically tested for. Oculomotor palsy is commoner than fourth or sixth nerve weakness, and may begin with squint, a dilated unreactive pupil or ptosis; eventually all three features develop. Diplopia is the earliest sign of imbalance of the external ocular muscles, and before it is sufficiently marked for two images to be appreciated, the complaint is of blurring of vision, which is corrected by closing one eye; this latent diplopia can be mistaken for visual failure. Diplopia will not develop if visual acuity is severely depressed in one eye, as it often is by lesions in this situation; complete ptosis likewise masks it.

Infratentorial masses

It is less easy to be sure that a lesion lies in the posterior fossa than to know that it must be above the tentorium. Manifestations of raised pressure usually dominate the clinical picture from an early stage, and need relief before the appearance of any localizing signs. This is partly due to the smaller size of this compartment of the skull but also to the readiness with which the cerebrospinal fluid (CSF) pathways become blocked by masses in this situation.

Many of these patients are children; two-thirds of intracranial tumours occurring under the age of 15 are in the posterior fossa. In infancy papilloedema may not develop because the skull bones give way, resulting in prominent sutures and a wide tight fontanelle; an unusually large head is always suspicious. Vomiting is a very frequent symptom, and children can become cachexic and acidotic from daily vomiting over a period of time. The prominence of this complaint may be due to the frequency with which these lesions cause raised pressure or sometimes to involvement of the floor of the fourth ventricle. Headache from tumours in the posterior fossa is often confined to the occipital region and radiates down the neck; it may even favour the side of the tumour if this is in the cerebello-pontine angle. Dementia in adults with slowly growing tumours is quite common, and is probably secondary to internal hydrocephalus, though many patients with very high pressure and huge ventricles remain alert. Squint due to non-localizing sixth nerve palsy is very common.

Signs of foraminal impaction or coning are important in pointing to a posterior fossa tumour (p. 38).

Central
Tumours of the vermis and fourth ventricle are apt to be silent in respect of local signs but are very liable to produce severe internal hydrocephalus and raised pressure. Nystagmus and limb ataxia are seldom seen, but truncal ataxia may be disabling: the patient is unable to stand or even to sit up in bed although the limbs can be moved gracefully. Vomiting as a sole sign, before there are signs of pressure, bespeaks involvement of the floor of the fourth ventricle, which may also give nuclear facial palsy and respiratory irregularities.

Lateral
Ataxia of the limbs on one side, usually first noticed in walking, is often the presenting symptom. Even if the classical staggering wide-based gait is not obvious, unsteadiness may be detected by having the patient walk across the room and turn quickly; he or she will usually sway for a moment and need to steady up before beginning to walk again. Hopping on one foot may be more difficult on one side, and intention tremor may be detected when a finger or the big toe is aimed at a small target.

Nystagmus of cerebellar origin is slower and coarser when the eyes are deviated to the side of the lesion; indeed it may only occur in this position. Rotatory or vertical nystagmus usually indicates invasion of the central pathways in the brainstem. Unsustained nystagmus at the extremes of deviation may be found in normal individuals, whilst patients taking high doses of epanutin for epilepsy may have both nystagmus and ataxia. Middle ear disease is probably the commonest cause of nystagmus, but this vestibular type is finer and less obviously lateralized than the cerebellar type and persists when gaze is not fixed; recent head injury is another frequent cause of vestibular nystagmus.

Dysarthria can result from a cerebellar defect, a special form of ataxia, or it may be due to bulbar palsy from a tumour spreading to the medulla or the issuing nerves. In either event this defect of phonation must be distinguished from disorders of language function, and from the slurred and indistinct speech of confused and drowsy patients, and that due to facial paralysis.

Cranial nerve palsies, other than the sixth palsy from pressure, may develop with any lateral cerebellar lesion but are most constant when the tumour is in the cerebellopontine angle. Deafness is often the first sign; tuning-fork tests will help to distinguish nerve and conduction types, but audiometry may be needed to assess mixed types of deafness (p. 127). Vertigo is a frequent complaint, and the function of the vestibular nerve may be tested objectively by the caloric reaction; absence of this reaction indicates that the nerve is dead, provided disease of the inner ear has been excluded (p. 127). Facial palsy may be hard to detect when slight, but diminished blink on one side is an early sign. The bulbar nerves (ix, x, xi, xii) are usually affected as a group as they lie close together on the jugular bulb; dysphagia and dysarthria result. Fifth nerve irritation occasionally gives rise to symptomatic trigeminal neuralgia, but this is much less common than facial anaesthesia which may at first be very limited, often to loss of corneal reflex only.

Transtentorial masses

Lateral tumours either grow through the tentorial hiatus and lie alongside the brainstem both above and below the tent, or arise from the dura of the tent and expand in both directions, indenting the under surface of the occipital lobe and the upper surface of the cerebellar hemisphere. Palsies of the seventh and eighth cranial nerves, combined with lesions of the second and third; hemianopia or dysphasia associated with cerebellar ataxia; these are the kind of surprising combinations to which these tumours may give rise. Intracranial pressure may be very high, either from a block to upward flow through the cisterna ambiens or due to obstruction of the lateral venous sinus retarding venous drainage from the brain and perhaps impeding CSF absorption.

Central tumours exert their effects without encroaching functionally on either of the main compartments of the skull until late in their course. These arise in the region of the pineal gland or the tectal plate but eventually spread more widely, usually above the tent (to cause hemianopia or hemiplegia). Internal hydrocephalus from aqueduct obstruction develops early; and there are signs of dysfunction of the third nerve nucleus – the dilated, sluggishly reacting pupils, with impaired upward movement of the eyes and mild ptosis. This syndrome was for long believed to be pathognomonic of pineal tumours but it may also result from chronic transtentorial herniation of the temporal lobe (p. 38).

Further reading

Asbury A.K., McKhann G.M., McDonald W.I. (eds.) (1992). *Diseases of the Nervous System*, 2nd edn. Philadelphia: W.B. Saunders.

Lindsay K.W., Bone I., Callander R. (1991). *Neurology and Neurosurgery Illustrated*, 2nd edn. Edinburgh: Churchill Livingstone.

Rowland L.P. (ed.) (1989). *Merritt's Textbook of Neurology*, 8th edn. Philadelphia: Lea & Febiger.

Chapter 2

Raised intracranial pressure

Physiopathology

> Blood volume
> CSF volume and circulation
> Brain volume
> The mass itself
> Volume/pressure relationships

Clinical

> Headache
> Papilloedema
> Vomiting

Effects of brain shift

> Transtentorial herniation
> Foraminal impaction

Presenting syndromes

> Increased intracranial pressure with focal features
> Focal features alone
> Raised pressure alone

Physiopathology

Changes in ICP reflect changes in the volume of the intracranial contents, which are made up of brain, CSF and blood (Fig. 2.1). Although each of these can change in volume, brain and CSF do so much less rapidly than intracranial blood volume. Fluctuations in blood volume in patients already suffering from more slowly developing space-taking lesions may aggravate or mitigate the effects on ICP.

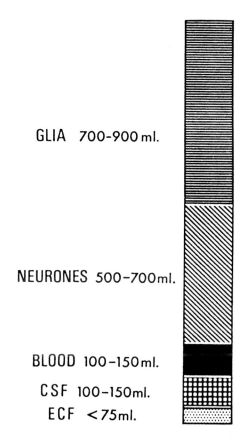

GLIA   700-900 ml.

NEURONES 500-700ml.

BLOOD 100-150 ml.

CSF 100-150ml.

ECF < 75ml.

Fig. 2.1 Intracranial contents, by volume. Only the blood volume can be rapidly altered. Note the small volume of extracellular fluid (ECF).

Blood volume

Changes in blood volume may be physiological (changes in posture, coughing, straining at stool), or pathological (respiratory inadequacy or obstruction). They can also result from clinical interventions, mechanical and pharmacological. Cerebral arterioles are sensitive to changes in $PaCO_2$; when this rises from 40 to 80 mmHg there is a doubling of the cerebral blood flow (CBF), and the increased intracranial blood volume causes the ICP to rise (Fig. 2.2). Changes in blood gases are usually due to respiratory inadequacy, itself the result of hypoventilation or of pulmonary insufficiency. Hypoventilation may be due to respiratory depression from drugs or from some cerebral condition; sometimes it is due to respiratory obstruction from the aspiration of vomit, from swallowing the tongue or from glottic closure during the onset of an epileptic fit. Any element of respiratory obstruction will cause an additional rise in ICP by passive venous engorgement, because the intracranial venous sinuses are in direct contact with the superior vena cava, with no valves intervening; any increase in central venous pressure is therefore immediately

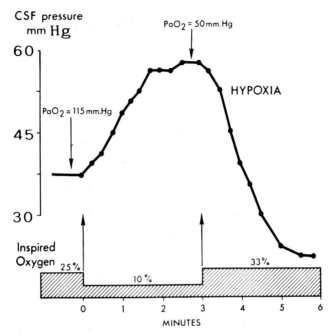

Fig. 2.2 ICP: effect of hypoxia. The response is vasodilation with increased intracranial blood volume; increased inspired carbon dioxide percentage has a similar effect. (Record from an anaesthetized, curarized dog maintained by a mechanical ventilator.)

transmitted to the intracranial cavity. Patients with impaired consciousness are liable to these events, whether their condition is traumatic or not. An epileptic fit may aggravate the situation, as may sedative or analgesic drugs. Alone or in combination, these factors may precipitate a crisis in a patient whose capacity to compensate for temporary rises in intracranial blood volume is already impaired (p. 27).

CSF volume and circulation

CSF is mainly secreted from the choroid plexuses in the lateral ventricles. It then passes by way of the foramen of Monro (interventricular foramen) into the third ventricle, down the aqueduct of Sylvius (iter) to the fourth ventricle. From there it escapes into the cisterna magna through the median foramen of Magendie and the lateral foramina of Luschka (Fig. 2.3). Some fluid then passes into the spinal subarachnoid space but most probably passes up through the cisterna ambiens, a narrow space between the midbrain and the edge of the tentorial hiatus (Fig. 2.4), to gain the subarachnoid space over the surface of the cerebral hemispheres, from which it is absorbed into the sagittal sinus by way of the arachnoid villi. Some CSF is produced and absorbed all along this route, but most originates in the lateral ventricle and most is absorbed by the sagittal sinus. The brain lacks lymphatic drainage channels and the extracellular fluid is in free communication with CSF via the ventricular ependyma. About 15–20% of CSF volume is thus formed this way.

CSF PATHWAYS

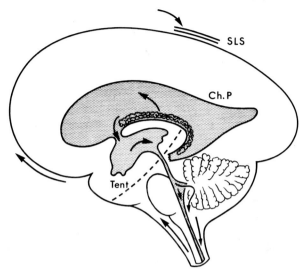

Fig. 2.3 CSF pathways. Most CSF follows the path shown from the lateral ventricle choroid plexus to the fourth ventricle and then via the cisterna ambiens to the supratentorial subarachnoid space. SLS = Superior longitudinal sinus; Ch.P = choroid plexus; Tent = tentorium.

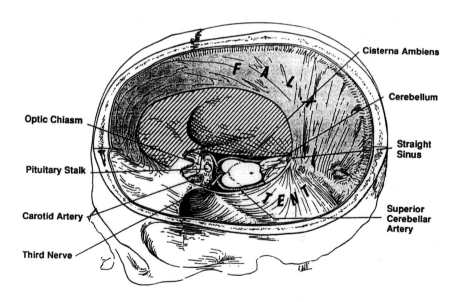

Fig. 2.4 Tentorial hiatus. The midbrain largely fills the hiatus but the cerebellum is visible behind. The third nerve leaves the midbrain, passing between the superior cerebellar artery below and the posterior cerebral artery above (omitted from the diagram). The subarachnoid cisterna ambiens (in black) lies at the side of the midbrain, communicating with the cisterna interpeduncularis in front.

When ventricular pathways are obstructed, CSF may likewise be absorbed via retrograde flow into the extracellular fluid – so-called transependymal absorption. This may be visible on CT scanning as a low-density area around the ventricles. Obstructive hydrocephalus occurs when a mass impairs CSF flow through the ventricular system. In this way a small tumour may have a marked effect on ICP. Blockage leads to dilatation of whatever cavities are above the obstruction, affecting one or both lateral ventricles if the foramen of Monro is blocked. When the aqueduct is involved, the third ventricle also dilates, and so does the fourth ventricle if its outlet is obstructed. Patients with obstructive hydrocephalus can develop very high intracranial pressures which may persist over long periods, although the pressure probably fluctuates; it is such patients who commonly develop secondary changes in the skull related to raised pressure (Fig. 4.1 p. 55).

Brain volume

Brain oedema is a term often loosely used when what is meant is simply swelling of the brain. Its use should be restricted to increase in brain water, which normally comprises 70% of white matter and 80% of the more cellular grey matter.

Two main types can be distinguished, although they may coexist. Vasogenic oedema is characterized by an increase in extracellular fluid, largely due to increased permeability of the endothelium of brain capillaries. This is the type of oedema that is commonly associated with tumour, abscess, contusion or haemorrhage. It is often focal and may therefore contribute to brain shift and herniation. Cytotoxic oedema is associated with swollen cells, glia or neurons, due to the accumulation of intracellular water and sodium. The common cause is hypoxia, particularly due to cardiac arrest; this effect is therefore often widespread throughout the brain. Focal infarcts initially cause cytotoxic oedema but this often progresses to vasogenic oedema.

The mass itself

The accumulation of additional intracranial material, be it tumour, blood or pus, must eventually raise pressure; but first it causes redistribution of intracranial contents, some of which are displaced into the spinal canal. This is a stage of compensation before ICP rises, but eventually this can no longer contain the situation (see below, and Fig. 2.5). The extent of the effects produced will depend mostly on the size of the lesion, but somewhat on the speed of development and on the extent to which the pathological process destroys the brain, rather than expanding it with pathological tissue. Blood flow mapping studies indicate that expanding mass lesions compress surrounding brain and reduce perfusion of tissue around the mass, thus inducing an ischaemic lesion which may worsen brain oedema. These factors, and the amount of cerebral oedema or swelling induced by the lesion, largely account for the wide discrepancy found in the effects produced both clinically and pathologically by what may seem similar masses in terms of size and site.

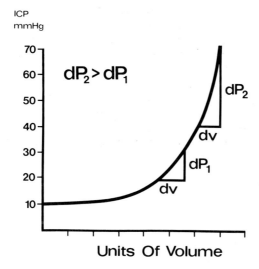

Fig. 2.5 Relationship between ICP and volume of space-occupying lesion. At first compensation is possible, but once these mechanisms are exhausted a small increase in volume causes a large increase in pressure. Compensation takes a finite time, and although the graph is relatively independent of the time scale over days, weeks or months, a sudden increase in volume might produce an immediate rise in pressure, even when the added volume increase is quite small. d = increment of V(olume) or P(ressive).

Volume/pressure relationships

The main factor which influences the effect that alterations in the volume of various intracranial contents have on ICP is the elastance or stiffness of the brain. This depends in part on the extent to which normal compensatory processes have been exhausted. By decreasing the capacitance of intracranial vessels the intracranial blood volume is decreased. Then CSF is displaced from the intracranial cavity into the more distensible spinal canal, and brain then takes up the subarachnoid space vacated by CSF. Brain shifts may also develop, with the formation of internal herniae and the development of the characteristic clinical effects related to these (p. 35). Once these compensatory mechanisms are exhausted, the slightest additional increase in volume, such as due to temporary cerebral vasodilatation, can produce a marked rise in ICP and this may precipitate a clinical crisis. This is because each quantum of additional volume causes a much greater effect on pressure when compensatory reserves are no longer available (Fig. 2.5). Intracranial elastance is not, however, dependent only on the existing volume of intracranial contents and their proportional disposition. Certain other factors, which are to some extent under clinical control, have been found to affect elastance to a greater or lesser degree than they affect ICP directly (Table 2.1).

Table 2.1 Factors affecting brain elastance

Increased elastance	Decreased elastance (more stiffness in brain)
Hypercapnia (any degree)	Hypocapnia (any degree)
Hypoxia (PaO_2 < 50mmHg)	Hyperoxia PaO_2 1000–1500 mmHg)
REM sleep	Hypothermia
Volatile anaesthetic agents	Barbiturates
Nitrous oxide	Neuroleptanalgesia
	Increased intrathoracic pressure

REM = Rapid eye movement.

This quality of the brain is of considerable clinical significance, because on the elastance of the brain at any time will depend the effect of any event which increases intracranial volume, such as oedema, or temporary vasodilatation (due to various causes such as blood gas changes, respiratory obstruction, or epileptic fits, *inter alia*). If elastance is low such an event may more readily precipitate a clinical crisis. When ICP measurements are available the elastance may be tested by observing the volume–pressure response – the change in pressure which immediately follows a 1 ml change in intracranial volume (by intraventricular aspiration or injection): normally the change is less than 3 mmHg.

Measurement of ICP

Increasing use of direct measurement of ICP has revealed what was already suspected – that clinical signs of raised pressure are very unreliable. The measurements have also indicated that the level of pressure is often variable, particularly when it is raised; therefore single observations (e.g. during ventricular tapping or at lumbar puncture) can be misleading. The ICP is normally about 10 mmHg, with pulsations corresponding to the pulse rate, and slower waves reflecting respiration. When pressure is raised abnormal waves may appear; periods of ICP above 50 mmHg lasting at least 5 minutes (more often 10–20 minutes) are termed plateau waves (Fig. 2.6a), whilst briefer (0.5–2 minutes duration) and less high changes are called B waves (Fig. 2.6b).

Although intraventricular catheters provide reliable ICP measurement, they are increasingly being superseded by the use of transducer-tipped measurement systems where a miniaturized electrical or fibreoptic sensor is inserted into the intracranial cavity usually subdurally or a few millimetres into the brain parenchyma itself. Infection risk is reduced with these systems, but drainage of ventricular fluid and volume–pressure response testing are not possible. Where ventricles are large, it is advisable to use a ventricular catheter for ICP measurements; when they are small and slit-like, as usually occurs after severe head injury, transducer-tipped sensors are preferable. Fluid-filled, catheters placed into the subdural space are unreliable, particularly at high ICP because the expanding brain usually occludes the lumen of the catheter. Monitoring ICP aids diagnosis by establishing whether or not pressure is increased; for example in patients with hydrocephalus or suspected benign intracranial hypertension, and in patients with posttraumatic and postoperative deterioration. This makes it possible to monitor treatment, which can be changed if it is not effective in lowering pressure, and it may be of use in prognosis, in that high pressure which fails to respond to treatment indicates an irrecoverable situation.

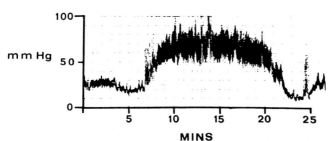

(a) Plateau wave (>50 mmHg for at least 5 min)

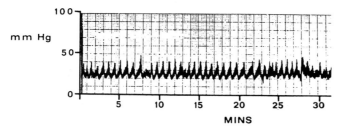

(b) B waves (1–2 per min)

Fig. 2.6 ICP traces (intraventricular catheter).

Effect of raised intracranial pressure on function (Fig. 2.7)

The effect on function of raised ICP alone is difficult to study in clinical practice because almost always the primary pathological process is directly influencing brain function locally, and there are brain shifts affecting areas of brain remote from the primary mass. What is known clinically is that some patients with a high ICP are alert and sometimes quite free of symptoms, as in the condition of benign intracranial hypertension (p. 41). Others are drowsy and disoriented but immediate improvement may follow treatment which deals only with the ICP, such as aspirating CSF from the ventricle. It appears that pressure alone, with no local mass causing brain shifts, produces few symptoms, at least until a certain level of pressure is reached. That critical level is when the perfusion pressure is so reduced that cerebral blood flow falls, so that cerebral oxygenation and other metabolic requirements are no longer adequately met. Mean perfusion pressure is the mean arterial pressure minus the ICP and is normally about 100 mmHg; animal experiments suggest that when this falls below c. 40 mmHg cerebral hypoxia may develop, but no data are available for humans. The importance of considering ICP in conjunction with mean arterial pressure is obvious and is a factor of great importance in considering anaesthesia for neurosurgical patients (p. 77). One effect of a rapidly rising ICP, as occurs for example with extradural haematoma, is to raise the arterial blood pressure and in such circumstances ICP may reach very high levels without any appreciable change in perfusion pressure; it is the brain shift induced by such a lesion which is the vital factor, until the pressure outstrips compensatory mechanisms, when the brain as a whole will suffer. Other interrelationships which affect and are affected by ICP are discussed on page 76.

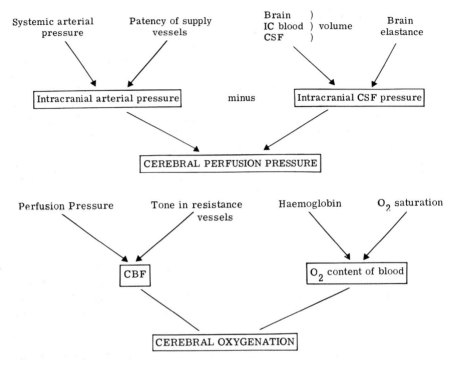

Fig. 2.7 Some inter-relationships affecting cerebral oxygenation. IC, Intracerebral; CSF, cerebrospinal fluid; CBF, cerebral blood flow.

Clinical

Two-thirds of patients diagnosed as having space-occupying lesions are usually said to suffer from the classical triad of headaches, papilloedema and vomiting, with most of the remainder having at least two of these complaints. Many also show some mental disorder, from personality change to profound dementia, from drowsiness to coma (Chapter 3). Fewer patients might be expected to show signs of raised pressure on presentation where there is open access to modern imaging for patients who have common symptoms that occasionally indicate serious intracranial disease; however, there are no systematic data to show this.

None of these features is peculiar to raised pressure; indeed with the exception of papilloedema there are many commoner causes of each of them alone. It is their occurrence together which raises the suspicion of raised ICP. Evidence for a causal relationship between high pressure and the classical symptoms is however, incomplete and there is no consistent correlation between the height of the pressure and the severity of the symptoms. These features are conventionally ascribed to raised ICP, and are commonly referred to as the general symptoms and signs of intracranial tumour, in contrast to localizing features.

Headache

Mechanism of production
Most structures in the head are insensitive to pain. Indeed neurosurgeons used to operate almost exclusively under local anaesthesia, knowing that the bony skull and the brain itself could be handled painlessly. Distension or traction of the arteries of the scalp and at the base of the brain, or the venous sinuses and their main tributaries, gives rise to ill-localized pain. More localized pain results from stretching or distortion of certain areas of the dura mater and of the trunks of the fifth, ninth and tenth cranial nerves. Headache can also originate in spasm of the large muscles at the base of the skull, and this may occur alone or as an added reflex activity when one of the other painful mechanisms is in play. Whatever the origin, the final common path for pain is limited to the trigeminal, glossopharyngeal and vagus nerves, together with the posterior roots of the first three cervical segments.

Characteristics of pressure headache
The patient commonly wakes with a headache which disperse within an hour of so of rising. It may disappear for days or even weeks, and sometimes after months of regular morning headache there may be a complete remission, although the pressure is unrelieved. Pressure headaches are frequently not of very great intensity, being described as throbbing or bursting, aggravated by coughing, sneezing, stooping down or exertion, and may be relieved by simple analgesics or by going to bed for a few days.

The distribution of the headache seldom gives any useful clue to the site of a tumour. Not only is the headache often felt at a situation remote from its production, but the site of production may be remote from the lesion. Most pressure headaches are felt bilaterally in the frontal or occipital regions. However, headache which is initially or exclusively occipital, radiating down the neck, is common with a mass in the posterior fossa: tumours in the cerebello-pontine angle often cause persistent aching in these areas.

Severe obstructive hydrocephalus may produce a syndrome of intense episodic headache associated with acute rises of pressure, which may be precipitated by neck or head movements. These so-called hydrocephalic attacks can be alarming; the patient may cry out with pain, consciousness may be clouded, pulse and respiration become irregular and occasionally death supervenes. These attacks warn of dangerously high pressure requiring prompt intervention.

Some other causes of headache

1. *Hypertension.* Although there may be a specific vascular component to hypertensive headaches, they are largely due to raised ICP and may therefore be indistinguishable from those due to tumour. Occurring in the morning, and sometimes accompanied by vomiting, they are frequently more severe than headaches due to tumour. Episodes of hypertensive encephalopathy can closely resemble hydrocephalic attacks. The relief of hypertensive headaches when the blood pressure is lowered by drugs is not a reliable diagnostic test, for a similar improvement can be expected in patients with tumour due to the lowering of intracranial tension

secondary to a drop in arterial pressure. The remarkable efficacy of splanchnicectomy in relieving hypertensive headache, even when the blood pressure was not greatly altered, has never been satisfactorily explained.

2. *Migraine.* These severe episodic headaches usually begin in the teens, tend to run in families, and are sometimes accompanied by focal neurological disorders such as visual phenomena (fortification spectra, hemianopia or blindness), paraesthesia or weakness on one side of the body, and dysphasia; numbness round the lips on both sides is another common complaint. The headache is often a hemicrania, altering from side to side in different attacks, and lasting for several hours to a day or so. It seldom returns within a fortnight; more commonly attacks recur monthly or even sporadically over the years. Some patients recognize specific precipitating factors such as menstruation, the weekend or emotional stress. Vomiting is common and alarming prostration can occur. Ergot preparations, if given at the outset, may abort an attack.

3. *Anxiety states and neurosis.* Headache is one of the commonest of psychosomatic symptoms, when it tends to have certain characteristics. Unremitting over weeks, months or years, with even an hour's relief denied, it is often said to be worse at times, but never better. The sensation reported is of pressing, burning or 'like a tight band round the head'. It is usually uninfluenced by analgesics.

4. *Ear, nose and throat (ENT), eye and dental disease.* Sinusitis, glaucoma and toothache all give rise to pain in the trigeminal distribution, but there is often radiation or referral to the head. Secondary muscle spasm can cause headache, as frequently occurs with cervical spondylosis.

5. *Meningism.* Irritation of the basal meninges, whether by blood from subarachnoid haemorrhage, or by pus in meningitis, gives rise to severe pain in the head and neck associated often with restlessness and noisiness.

6. *Temporal arteritis.* The elderly patients who suffer this condition complain less of headache than of localized pain or tenderness in the scalp, and the affected artery may be palpated. The pain can be very severe and unremitting until the artery is divided surgically or prednisolone is given. A third develop visual symptoms, sudden blindness or field defects.

7. *Lumbar puncture headache – low-pressure state.* Traction and distortion of structures at the base of the brain, similar to that which occurs with raised pressure, causes the headache which may follow drainage of CSF by lumbar puncture. This often appears to be aggravated by sitting up, and may be relieved by a high fluid intake and recumbency; low CSF pressure may therefore be one factor but headache is very variable after lumbar puncture, some patients denying any discomfort whatever.

Papilloedema

Because the optic nerve is an extension of the brain, complete with meningeal coverings and subarachnoid space, intracranial tension is thereby transmitted to a site where its effects may be directly observed. Two factors that limit the reliability of such observations are the time needed for papilloedema to develop and the possibility that the subarachnoid extension to the optic fundus is blocked pathologically. Although large blot or splash haemorrhages can occur at the time of a severe subarachnoid haemorrhage, it probably takes some days of abnormally high ICP before papilloedema is evident.

Mechanism of production
Papilloedema is probably due to obstruction of axoplasmic flow with resultant swelling of the nerve head. Unilateral disc swelling may result from an orbital lesion affecting the optic nerve, or from generalized pressure when there is anatomical or pathological blockage of the subarachnoid space around the other optic nerve. A tumour may cause optic atrophy on one side from direct pressure and papilloedema on the other from the mass effect (the Foster Kennedy syndrome).

Papilloedema seldom develops in infants, except following sagittal sinus thrombosis, because the skull bones can separate and the sutures spread; the fontanelle tension is the best guide to pressure at this age. The elderly less often have papilloedema as a sign of intracranial tumour because the large subarachnoid spaces and dilated ventricles leave more room for an expanding lesion.

Appearance
The swelling of the nerve head may be measured in dioptres by comparing the lenses required to bring the disc and then the peripheral retina into focus. This manoeuvre requires experience, and even skilled observers often come to conflicting conclusions about the degree of swelling. A qualitative assessment based on a number of factors is more useful.

The earliest change is filling of the depression in the nerve head from which the vessels emerge and where the nerve fibres seen end-on normally form a stippled patch (lamina cribrosa). Then the medial half of the disc becomes pink and its edges indistinct, until no normal disc remains visible and the vessels climb out over the heaped-up pink swelling which has replaced it. The veins appear engorged at an early stage and later flame-shaped haemorrhages may develop, often alongside vessels. In severer degrees small circular 'blob' haemorrhages and exudate appear.

Papilloedema eventually subsides either because of a natural resolution of the process responsible or following surgical relief of pressure. Depending on the severity and duration of the swelling the disc may be restored to normal appearance and the nerve to full function, or consecutive optic atrophy may develop.

Once started, atrophy often progresses, even though the pressure has been relieved. The patient may be left blind, with a pale disc that is permanently blurred at the edges. Fear of this sequel puts urgency into the treatment of patients with severe papilloedema, even when there appears to be no immediate danger from herniation.

Symptoms

Most patients are unaware of papilloedema and are surprised by the seriousness with which their other complaints are taken after their fundi have been examined. A number of brain tumours are first detected by opticians who examine the fundi before prescribing glasses. The visual fields show enlargement of the blind spot and later peripheral constriction of the field. Children under about 9 years of age are curiously reluctant to complain of deteriorating vision, and may present with blindness before other features of raised pressure become obvious.

Intermittent loss of vision is more common than steady deterioration. Episodes termed amblyopic attacks (synonyms: obscurations of vision, amaurosis fugax) consist of brief periods of partial or complete blindness, lasting usually less than a minute, occurring many times a day, often for several months. There may be complete blacking-out of vision, or only blurring, or greying with loss of colour perception. Episodes are sometimes precipitated by sudden rising from the horizontal or sitting position or by stooping. Postural alterations in local blood supply probably account for these symptoms. They occur only with severe papilloedema, usually after some weeks or months of headache. This symptom is often misinterpreted as a form of epilepsy, vertigo, dizziness or fainting. It is important to recognize because it indicates that sight is in peril and relief of pressure is urgently needed.

Differential diagnosis for bilateral fundal changes includes arterial hypertension, pseudopapilloedema and prolonged carbon dioxide retention in advanced emphysema. Unilateral fundal changes are most often due to retrobulbar neuritis, usually due to demyelinating disease. Visual acuity is affected early and severely, due to a paracentral scotoma impairing central vision. The globe is often painful to move and tender on palpation. The marked swelling of the disc may be indistinguishable from papilloedema, but haemorrhages are rare and exudates unknown. Occasionally the second eye is affected. A less common cause is orbital tumour, usually associated with proptosis, failure of vision and sometimes limitation of eye movement.

Thrombosis of the central retinal vein is sudden in onset, with loss of vision, as in retrobulbar neuritis, but the fundal changes are quite different. Haemorrhages spread widely to the peripheral retina, which is oedematous, with severe engorgement of veins. Cavernous sinus thrombosis and carotico-cavernous fistula may give a similar but less acute and dramatic appearance.

Vomiting

This may be a sign of increased pressure but also occurs as a focal manifestation of lesions in the fourth ventricle. Such lesions almost always bring about raised pressure due to obstruction to CSF flow and it may not be easy to determine which mechanism is operative at any one time.

Vomiting due to pressure usually occurs before breakfast, frequently as an accompaniment of morning headache. Although referred to as projectile, this is seldom a striking feature; certainly it can occur without much nausea, and so without warning. Children with tumours more frequently vomit than adults and often without any complaint of headache. This may be related to the frequency in children of posterior fossa tumours which can produce both raised ICP and local pressure on the medulla. Five-sixths of gliomas below the tentorium have vomiting compared with less than half those above the tentorium.

Vomiting due to a local lesion in the fourth ventricle is uncommon and more likely to appear long before headache. It may occur daily for many months before signs of pressure or neurological disorder lead to the correct diagnosis.

The two commonest causes of morning vomiting are pregnancy and migraine, the latter usually recognizable by the episodic nature of the attacks and other features such as hemicrania and visual disorders.

Effects of brain shift

Sooner or later, as pressure rises, the brain itself must move. How it does so depends on the site of the expanding lesion relative to the dural partitions which subdivide the cranial cavity. Part of the brain shifts into the larger subarachnoid spaces, the cisterna ambiens and cisterna magna, displacing CSF; and there is shift from a compartment where pressure is rising to one of lower pressure.

Focal signs related to brain shifts and herniations affecting structures remote from the site of a primary expanding lesion prove false or misleading only if it is assumed that they reflect dysfunction in the immediate neighbourhood of the primary mass lesion. Properly evaluated they can indicate whether the primary mass is more likely to be above or below the tentorium, and they also warn that the brain is dangerously compressed.

The tentorium is the most complete of the dural barriers and divides the posterior fossa from the supratentorial compartment. This division is complete but for the hiatus, which is filled by the midbrain and the narrow cisterna ambiens (Fig. 2.4). Masses above the tentorium push the midbrain and part of the cerebral hemisphere down through the tentorial hiatus, the only exit from this compartment; posterior fossa tumours drive the cerebellar tonsils and medulla through the foramen magnum. These comprise the two most important brain shifts; each puts a vital part of the brain in jeopardy.

Transtentorial herniation
(synonyms: tentorial or temporal cone*)

Pathology
The medial part of the temporal lobe (the uncus and hippocampus) is packed down into the cisterna ambiens forming a hernia (Fig. 2.8). One result is that the midbrain is compressed from side to side, and thrust downwards through the hiatus, suffering strains in its long axis, either longitudinal stretching or buckling. Deterioration in conscious level results from reticular formation involvement. The third nerves and posterior cerebral arteries, being fixed above, are stretched; the ipsilateral nerve may also be compressed against the unyielding petroclinoid ligament as well as being pushed down by the temporal herniation. Posterior cerebral artery occlusion may result in haemorrhagic infarction of the occipital lobe. The pituitary stalk may be stretched across the dorsum sellae, resulting in diabetes insipidus.

* The word 'cone' was first applied to herniation of the cerebellum through the foramen magnum to form a cone-shaped plug of tissue. The verb 'to cone' is in common usage among neurosurgeons and neurologists to describe the development of clinical syndromes associated with transtentorial herniation or foraminal impaction.

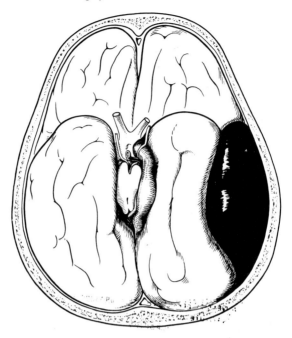

Fig 2.8 Tentorial herniation of the medial part of the temporal lobe, seen from below. This causes dysfunction in the midbrain, the third nerve and the territory of the posterior cerebral artery. A temporal haematoma is shown but a mass in any situation above the tent can produce a hernia.

Not only are the nuclear masses and tracts of the brainstem distorted but so are their intrinsic vessels, frequently resulting in local haemorrhages, most likely due to tearing of stretched arterioles and capillaries. Haemorrhages are most striking after acute compression that does not have time to produce marked tentorial herniation, whilst gross herniation and midbrain distortion can occur without any haemorrhage when compression has developed slowly.

Clinical

Acute tentorial cone
This critical condition is most often encountered by neurologists in patients who have suffered cerebral haemorrhage, a massive infarct followed by oedema, or necrotizing encephalitis; and by neurological surgeons in association with rapidly accumulating traumatic haematoma or rapidly advancing malignant tumours above the tentorium.

Deterioration of conscious level is usually the first evidence of acute coning. At first there may be no more than drowsiness but soon confusion occurs and there is progression down the coma scale (p. 47).

Third nerve palsy on the side of the compression is most readily detected by dilatation of the pupil with loss of both the direct and consensual light reflexes (Fig. 2.9). Other third nerve functions are difficult to test in patients with impaired consciousness, but in the few who will cooperate, some ptosis and loss of eye movement (especially upward) may be discovered. Relief of the

NORMAL LIGHT REFLEX

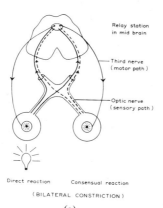

Fig. 2.9 Pupillary light reflex (position of the third nerve is diagrammatic). Both direct and consensual reactions must be tested to localize the lesion. (a) Normal light reflex: whichever eye is illuminated, both pupils react by constriction. (b) Optic nerve lesion: illumination of the affected eye produces no reaction on either side. (c) Third nerve lesion: the affected pupil fails to react whichever eye is illuminated.

compression frequently reverses the oculomotor palsy immediately, but it may recover only gradually over days or weeks. If the condition is not relieved the opposite pupil follows the course of the first one; recovery is rare once the condition has advanced to the stage of bilaterally fixed and dilated pupils.

Other causes may account for unilateral dilated pupil, including atropine drops, posterior communicating artery aneurysm and, after recent head injury, damage to the optic nerve which is the afferent path for the light reflex (Fig. 2.9). In the last case the pupil will constrict normally when light is shone in the opposite eye (consensual reaction). Bilaterally fixed dilated pupils occur during epileptic seizures and this possibility must be considered when pupillary change and coma develop very suddenly: if due to epilepsy the pupils will usually recover within minutes.

Extensor posturing of the limbs (previously often called decerebrate rigidity) results from loss of cortical inhibition. The increased extensor tone in the limbs is often associated with neck retraction. The legs are straight at the knees with strong plantar flexion, the arms hyperpronated with the fists clenched and the elbows extended. This posture is often aggravated during the hyperpnoeic phase of periodic respiration or this abnormal tonus may be assumed only when painful stimuli are applied. Only the stimulated limb may become decerebrate, or the response may be generalized.

Autononic abnormalities include slowing of the pulse and a rising blood pressure. The latter response to rising ICP helps to maintain adequate blood flow to the medulla. If the blood pressure is elevated when a patient first presents, the diagnosis of pre-existing hypertension with a vascular accident must be considered. Respiration may be slow and is sometimes periodic – slow and shallow for a few breaths and then more rapid and deep (sometimes termed Cheyne–Stokes breathing).

Chronic tentorial cone
Any slowly growing supratentorial mass can give rise to this but the most striking examples have been due to chronic bilateral subdural haematoma.

Loss of conjugate upward gaze with bilateral ptosis is probably the result of compression of the dorsal midbrain. Ptosis is easily overlooked when the patient is in bed, but the wrinkled forehead and look of surprise (due to overaction of frontalis), with the eyes only partly open, is characteristic. If cooperation is poor, the eyes may be induced to turn up reflexly by touching the cornea, and a diminution in upward movement detected. Both ptosis and loss of upward movement are sometimes more marked on one side than the other. A tumour in the pineal region may be suspected, but dilated pupils reacting only sluggishly to light, common with a pineal tumour, are rarely a feature of a chronic cone.

A fluctuating conscious level, probably due to impairment of function in the midbrain reticular formation, is a striking feature. A patient who is drowsy and almost inaccessible may appear normally alert only a few hours later, and this cycle may be repeated many times without any obvious precipitating factors.

Ipsilateral hemiplegia, on the same side as a supratentorial mass, is due to pressure of the free edge of the tentorium against the opposite cerebral peduncle, producing the Kernohan–Woltman notch.

Homonymous hemianopia, from posterior cerebral artery compression, is not often detected clinically.

Occasionally a mass in the posterior fossa causes upward displacement of the upper part of the vermis through the tentorial hiatus. This upward trans-tentorial herniation may compress the dorsal midbrain, and is encouraged by lowering the supratentorial pressure, by draining the lateral ventricles, without also lowering the infratentorial pressure by providing a bony decompression of the posterior fossa.

Foraminal impaction
(synonyms: cerebellar or tonsillar cone)

Pathology
When pressure in the posterior fossa reaches critical levels the cerebellar tonsils crowd into the foramen magnum, and the medulla is compressed between them and the anterior bony margin (Fig. 2.10). Normally the tonsils just reach the level of the foramen but with posterior fossa compression they are often found as low as the spine of the axis (second cervical vertebra).

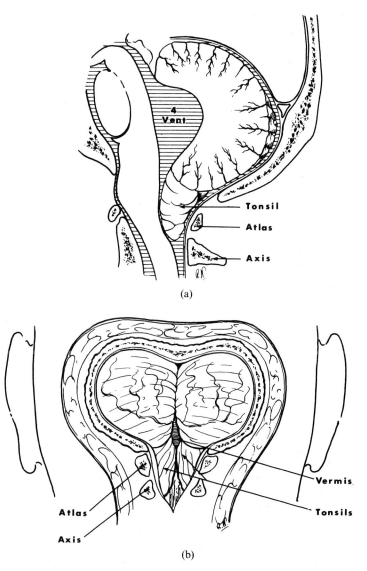

(a)

(b)

Fig. 2.10 Foraminal impaction. (a) Cerebellar tonsils driven between the posterior arch of the atlas and the medulla, which is compressed. (b) Tip of tonsil is normally seen above the arch of the atlas; here it is at the level of the axis.

Clinical

A foraminal cone may lead to apnoea with little or no warning with an acute compression, or it may develop as a late stage of a neglected tentorial cone.

Abnormal neck posture takes several forms. A child may have a head tilt when he or she walks due to vestibular imbalance or due to sixth nerve weakness, the head position being adjusted to avoid diplopia. This head tilt is seldom noticed by the patient or relatives.

Stiff neck, due to irritation of the dura around the foramen magnum by the tightly packed structures, may raise the question of meningitis. Tingling in the arms on extension of the neck is due to pressure on the cervical cord by the prolapsed plug in the foramen magnum, and some patients 'black out' if they extend the neck too far; this movement probably raises pressure by completing the block to CSF circulation in addition to causing pressure directly on the medulla. Opisthotonus can occur (p. 9).

Abnormalities of respiratory rate and rhythm are danger signs in posterior fossa compression. A slow rate, say 9 breaths a minute, may be continued with complete regularity for days but this is uncommon. Periodic breathing is common. In its classical form (Cheyne–Stokes breathing) it consists of a crescendo of breaths of increasing depth and frequency followed by a period of total apnoea of up to a minute or so, probably until the accumulating carbon dioxide reaches a high enough level to stimulate the failing respiratory centre. Any irregularity of respiration should raise suspicion of a foraminal cone, which is probably the final stage of cerebral compression of whatever origin. When the mass is in the posterior fossa, however, apnoea is frequently quite sudden, without impaired consciousness or any other warning signs.

Presenting syndromes

Intracranial space-occuping lesions may present with clinical evidence of increased pressure or with focal neurological disorders, or both. The differential diagnosis varies with the type of presentation, and any evidence of brain shift.

Increased intracranial pressure with focal features

This combination leaves little doubt that the patient is suffering from an intracranial mass. Tumour may be distinguished in most instances from abscess or haematoma by the preceding history. However, neither a sudden onset nor spontaneous remission excludes tumour, and patients with tumour may have raised blood pressure either from pre-existing hypertension or as a reaction to raised ICP.

Focal features alone

This opens a wider field of differential diagnosis. Confusion most often arises with cerebrovascular disease, cerebral atrophy and demyelinating disorders. In making the distinction from brain tumour a careful history is invaluable; the steadily progressive development of dysfunction which is confined to a single, even if extensive, area of the brain is suggestive of tumour. Probably all patients developing focal neurological signs which persist or progress should be investigated as brain tumour suspects, unless there are definite indications of vascular disease or demyelination in the form of previous episodes of transient disturbance of function in parts of the brain remote from that presently affected.

Raised pressure alone

This is a more frequent and a more pressing situation. Likely causes are midline masses blocking CSF flow and causing internal hydrocephalus, silent slowly growing lateral supratentorial masses (usually right frontal or temporal) and chronic bilateral subdural haematoma. Progressive loss of vision from papilloedema can occur with relatively few headaches in patients with a benign meningioma or neurofibroma. Mental disorder can so dominate the scene in some patients with pressure and no signs that they may be referred for psychiatric opinion without any suspicion of underlying organic disease.

A number of patients with raised pressure alone appear after investigation to have no local lesion, and are diagnosed as suffering from the unexplained but not uncommon condition known as pseudotumour cerebri (synonyms: otitic hydrocephalus, serous meningitis, benign intracranial hypertension). It is commonest in young adults, women more than men; it may be associated with pregnancy or obesity, sometimes with infections, especially of the ear. Headaches, seldom of great severity, are followed by diplopia due to sixth nerve weakness from raised ICP. There is severe papilloedema; in some cases obscurations of vision give way to blindness from consecutive atrophy. With all this evidence of severely raised ICP the general well-being of the patient is as surprising as it is characteristic.

The natural history is towards resolution but it may be many months before the papilloedema subsides completely. Treatment is now usually with steroids and diet to reduce weight, if required. Lumbar puncture, previously sometimes done repeatedly as an aid to recovery, shows that the pressure fluctuates widely from day to day; a further curious feature is an abnormally low CSF protein (10–20 mg/100 ml). Some patients require a lumbo-peritoneal shunt, but rarely is a subtemporal decompression required in an attempt to save sight.

The association with otitis media led to the term 'otitic hydrocephalus' and to the theory that it was due to thrombosis spreading from the lateral to the sagittal sinus with impaired absorption of CSF. This explains the symptoms in a proportion of patients, but in most the pathogenesis remains unexplained. The ventricles are never dilated; accurate measurement shows a reduction in ventricular size, giving the impression that they are being squeezed by a swollen brain.

There are other causes of raised pressure than brain tumour; arterial hyptertension, polycythaemia and chronic emphysema are among the more common. Each must be severe before it affects ICP, and is therefore obvious if a general clinical examination is conducted, as it should be in every case of suspected brain tumour.

Further reading

Adams J.H., Graham D.I. (1976). The relationship between ventricular fluid pressure and the neuropathology of raised intracranial pressure. *Neuropathol. Appl. Neurobiol.*; **2**: 323–32.

Hoff J.T., Betz A.L. (eds.) (1989). *Proceedings of International Symposium on Intracranial Pressure VII.* Berlin: Springer Verlag.

Ishi S., Nagai H., Brock M. (eds.) (1983). *Proceedings of International Symposium on Intracranial Pressure V.* Berlin: Springer Verlag.

Jennett W.B., Barker J., Fitch W., *et al.* (1969). Effect of anaesthesia on intracranial pressure in patients with space occupying lesions. *Lancet*; **i:** 61–4.

Johnston I., Paterson A., Besser M. (1981). The treatment of benign intracranial hypertension: a review of 134 cases. *Surg. Neurol.*; **16:** 218–24.

Miller J.D., Dearden N.M. (1992). Measurement, analysis and the management of raised intracranial pressure. In: Teasdale G.M., Miller J.D. (eds.) *Current Neurosurgery*. Edinburgh: Churchill Livingstone.

Miller J.D., Teasdale G.M., Rowan J.O., *et al.* (eds.) (1986). *Proceedings of International Symposium on Intracranial Pressure VI*. Berlin: Springer Verlag.

North B., Reilly P. (1990). *Raised Intracranial Pressure: A Clinical Guide.* London: Heinemann.

Plum F., Posner J.B. (1980). *Diagnosis of Stupor and Coma,* 3rd edn. Philadelphia: Davis.

Reid A., Matheson M., Teasdale G. (1980). Volume of the ventricles in benign intracranial hypertension. *Lancet;* **ii:** 7–8.

Sullivan H.G., Miller J.D., Griffith R.L., *et al.* (1978). CSF pressure–volume dynamics in neurosurgical patients. *Surg. Neurol.;* **9:** 47–54.

Tans T.T.J., Poortvliet D.C.J. (1983). Intracranial volume – pressure relationship in man: clinical significance of pressure – volume index. *J. Neurosurg.;* **59:** 810–16.

Chapter 3

Organic mental dysfunction, coma and brain death

Mental dysfunction in alert patients

Organic dementia
Cerebral irritation or traumatic delirium

Conditions mistakenly interpreted as mental dysfunction

Causes of organic dementia

Syndromes associated with impaired consciousness

Coma and its assessment
Reduced responsiveness with eyes open

Brain death

Acute brain damage (whether due to trauma, haemorrhage or infection) usually causes some degree of impaired alertness. But with slowly developing lesions, such as intracranial tumour, changes are often unobtrusive and noticed only by close relatives or friends. Despite improved understanding and more sympathetic attitudes to mental illness, there is still a stigma which seals the lips of those who suffer and those who witness symptoms which are believed to mean a failing mind. Once intracranial conditions begin to cause raised ICP and brain shift and impaired alertness obscures the earlier features of mental abnormality relatives may admit to having observed such features over a period of weeks or months. It is useful, therefore, to separate the two main types of mental disorder which can be recognized in association with organic brain disease into those occurring in patients whose conscious state is not depressed, but in whom the content of consciousness is abnormal, and those associated with impaired consciousness.

Mental dysfunction in alert patients

Organic dementia

This usually affects three aspects of normal mental function – intellect, memory and personality. However, one may be more severely impaired than the others.

Intellectual function is concerned with problem-solving when dealing with novel situations. Formal tests may indicate marked limitation of ability in this field in patients well able to conduct themselves appropriately both at work and at home provided their lives are largely routine and present few new situations from day to day. With less stereotyped occupations deficiencies at work may be the means whereby illness first comes to light.

Poor memory is a socially acceptable complaint and may be the cliché whereby a patient expresses a wide range of limitations in mental capacity. Testing may reveal the defect to be primarily in intellectual or language function, rather than of memory itself. Impairment of recent memory is, however, a common feature of organic dementia, with distant (childhood) memories remaining intact. When memory is predominantly and severely affected a focal lesion may be suspected.

All available evidence points to the limbic system as vital for active memorizing. A memory record of immediate recent experience is essential for orientation and for the execution of planned, purposeful activity; a crippling dementia results if this record breaks down. Memory involves the perception and temporary storage of experience, followed after some delay by permanent registration; subsequent recall may be deferred indefinitely. Organic lesions usually affect only the permanent registration of new memories, without interfering with the recall of established memories, even those of childhood.

Personality can be regarded as comprising drive, affect and social restraint or social judgement. Lack of drive, or apathy, is the commonest feature and is often first noticed in a falling off in interest in leisure activities. A man may continue to perform quite exacting work under the stimulus of bread-winning and protected by long-established routine, yet come home exhausted, sink in a chair and doze away the evening. This change in personality (if such it is!) may lead to recommendations to take a holiday, to pull himself together or take vitamin pills. Eventually more serious lapses appear, many of which can be traced to failing recent memory: appointments are forgotten, articles mislaid, shopping expeditions left half completed. Carelessness in personal appearance combined with falling standards at work can lead to dismissal, and the patient takes to sitting for long periods looking into space, accessible yet making little spontaneous attempt to keep in contact with surroundings.

Organic dementia seems often to be more marked in older patients and the form it takes may reflect the basic personality of the individual. Insight may be retained, or be lost early on, but in either event memory for distant events, even those of childhood, is well-preserved. When certain aspects of personality are predominantly affected a local lesion in the frontal lobes may be suspected (see below)

Cerebral irritation or traumatic delirium

This state of restless, disorganized behaviour is commonly seen during the recovery of consciousness after head injury, but occasionally after other disorders. It may be looked on as a kind of mental dystonia in which a normal afferent input evokes a disinhibited and uncontrolled response – it could be a state of misdirected rather than impaired alertness. There may be motor restlessness, attempts to get out of bed, and even to attack attendants; a lot of shouting and swearing is common and yet this may be interspersed with periods of apparent lucidity and appropriate response

Conditions mistakenly interpreted as mental dysfunction

Temporal lobe epilepsy can take the form of automatisms during which complicated and purposive, yet entirely inappropriate, activities are carried out for which the patient has no subsequent memory. The clue to the nature of such behaviour is the tendency for it to be stereotyped from one attack to another, and the invariable amnesia for events occurring during the episode. Some temporal lobe seizures consist entirely of subjective mental experiences which, when described, may suggest a functional disorder of the mind.

Disorders of language function are not always recognized immediately for what they are and profound dementia may be suspected when it is only the lines of communication which are affected. Nominal dysphasia, showing itself in the forgetting of names, is often regarded as due to a failing memory, whilst the faltering and inappropriate words slowly forced out by the patient with severe expressive dysphasia are easily taken as evidence of an equally disorganized mind. When the receptive side of language function is also affected, the appearance is even more suggestive of dementia. For here is a person who appears not to be able or willing to cooperate even in simple physical tests – in fact he or she cannot understand what he or she is being told to do, does not know what question is being asked; and the more verbal explanations that are offered, the less likely he or she is to grasp what is wanted. Other evidence of left hemisphere dysfunction, hemiparesis or hemianopia, often accompanies dysphasia.

Topographical disorientation or agnosia is a manifestation of dysfunction of the right parietal lobe (p. 12). There is an inability to recognize even familiar surroundings so that the patient may be unable to pick out his or her own front door on returning from the office, be unable to find the bathroom in his or her own house. The nature of this disorder may be suspected from its association with other signs of right hemisphere dysfunction such as hemianopia. Tests involving the drawing of maps and plans or the copying of designs may bring out the defect quite clearly. If these additional signs are not elicited, primary dementia may be suspected, and a psychiatrist may be called before a surgeon.

Causes of organic dementia

Head injury and slowly developing *space-occupying lesions* are the commonest causes of organic dementia in surgical practice. Other causes are:

Cerebral atrophy in its pure form consists of progressive dementia occurring usually in men in their fifties and associated with marked shrinkage of brain substance and dilation of the ventricles. There are no signs of pressure because the hydrocephalus is secondary to atrophy of the brain; CT scan shows the enlarged ventricles and subarachnoid spaces with the shrunken gyri.

Presenile dementia, associated with the names of Pick and Alzheimer, is rapidly progressive. There are many organic signs, such as dysphasia and hemiplegia, but not signs of raised pressure.

Cerebral arteriosclerosis betrays itself by small vascular accidents and by the appearance of sclerotic vessels in the retina. There may be characteristic neurological syndromes such as Parkinsonism or pseudobulbar palsy, and epilepsy is common. Generalized arteriosclerosis is usually evident.

Psychosis. A tumour rarely produces symptoms which closely resemble primary psychiatric disorders, although if insight is retained for long with organic dementia, the awareness of failing mental powers may give rise to secondary depression. But mania, endogenous melancholia, schizophrenic withdrawal, violent behaviour, persecution, obsessions and hallucinations are rarely encountered. Nevertheless, some neurosurgeons know patients who have had courses of electroconvulsive therapy in an attempt to disperse symptoms which were due to brain tumour or chronic subdural haematoma.

It is not possible from the nature of the mental symptoms to reliably distinguish these organic conditions from dementia due to a space-occupying lesion; absence of pressure is not a reliable criterion because tumours may grow for long periods without evidence of raised ICP. For this reason patients developing dementia which is thought to be organic are usually investigated to exclude a mass – a very important step to take before accepting the uniformly gloomy prognosis associated with other conditions.

Syndromes associated with impaired consciousness

Impaired responsiveness is an expression of dysfunction of the brain as a whole – it could be said that coma indicates brain failure, as uraemia bespeaks renal failure. The agents responsible may be reversible, such as depressant drugs, metabolic disorder and acute but transitory lesions like mild concussion or meningitis.

The mechanism underlying impaired consciousness is not understood but is presumed to be reduced activity of a significant amount of the cerebral cortex. This may be the result of direct pathological involvement of the cortex, or of impaired function in the subcortical white matter connecting the cortex to the reticular formation of the brainstem. Lesions in the brainstem itself have to be very extensive before the patient becomes unconscious due to failure of the upward-projecting reticular activating system.

Coma and its assessment

The first sign of reduced responsiveness is a tendency to fall asleep in spite of surrounding stimuli that would normally keep a person awake. The patient may be described as drowsy but can be roused to speak and to obey commands, and at first may be oriented when attention is focused in this way. The next stage is of confusion – about time and place, later even of personal identity. The term 'stupor' is sometimes applied to states of drowsiness or reduced responsiveness in which the patient can be roused to speak, but it seems better simply to describe what the patient is like, and what he or she will and will not do, rather than using terms that are not widely used or understood.

The term coma is now usually reserved for patients who do not obey commands, do not utter any comprehensible words and who do not open their eyes, even in response to pain. This definition makes use of the Glasgow Coma Scale (Fig. 3.1a), which has been adopted in many countries as a practical means of recording the depth and duration of coma. Although originally introduced for the monitoring of recently head-injured patients, many of whom are cared for by non-specialist hospitals and units, it is also applicable to non-traumatic coma. It can be incorporated in a general observation chart for nurses (Fig. 3.1b).

Observer-error trials have shown it to be reliable in the hands of non-specialist medical and nursing staff, including those for whom English is not their first language. The scale is a simple descriptive one, which avoids complex definitions, and it acknowledges that different types of response may vary independently. It avoids making an arbitrary division between consciousness and unconsciousness, because altered consciousness is a continuum. The three behavioural responses recorded relate to motor activity, verbal performance and eye opening.

If commands cannot be obeyed, motor activity is reported as the response to a standard painful stimulus – pressure on the supraorbital nerve or to the nailbed with a pencil. The response is recorded as localizing if the hand comes above the chin on the side of the stimulus; as flexor if the elbow flexes, as extensor if it extends. This avoids the use of the terms decerebrate and decorticate, with the anatomical implications which these carry. The response of the upper limbs is usually the most reliable but the lower limbs should also be tested. It is the response of the best limb which is indicative of the conscious level; if one limb (or side) is clearly worse than the other, this is evidence of focal damage in the nervous system.

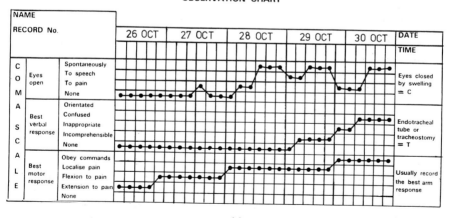

(a)

Fig. 3.1 Glasgow Coma Scale. (a) Coma chart.

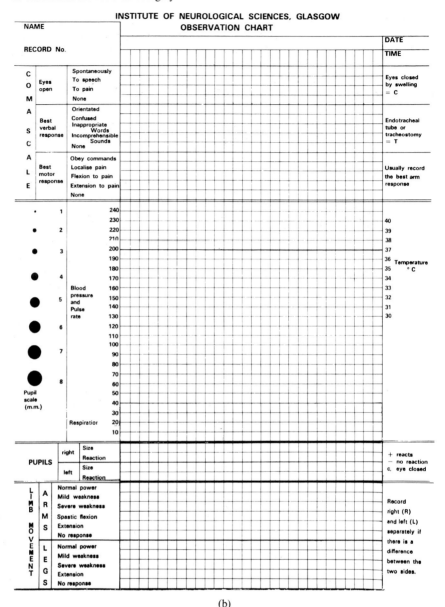

(b)

Fig. 3.1 *(cont)* (b) General observation chart.

In the verbal sphere orientation implies awareness of self and environment – the patient knows where he or she is, why he or she is there, and also the year, the season and the month. *Confused conversation* covers varying degrees of disorientation and confusion in a patient able to respond to questions in a conversational manner. *Inappropriate speech* indicates intelligible articulation limited to exclamatory or random words, usually shouting and swearing, with no sustained conversational exchange. *Incomprehensible sounds* refers to moaning and groaning without recognizable words. In previous assessments of conscious level too much emphasis has probably been placed on the failure to speak – there are several reasons why patients may not speak, including dysphasia, tracheostomy and inability to converse in a particular language.

Eye opening indicates that the arousal mechanisms in the brainstem are active. Eye opening to speech is a response to any verbal approach, spoken or shouted, and not necessarily the command to open eyes; eye opening to pain should depend on a stimulus in the limbs, because facial stimulation may cause reflex eye closure as part of a grimace. Eye opening without awareness is a feature of the persistent vegetative state (see below).

An advantage of this scale is that a measure of conscious state may be obtained even when one of the elements of the scale cannot be tested (e.g. a tracheostomy or when eyes too swollen to open after local injury). In gauging deterioration or improvement during the acute stage of many conditions the degree and duration of coma or altered consciousness usually overshadow all other clinical features in importance, and are the main determinants of prognosis. The depth of coma can be expressed in terms of the Glasgow Coma Score (Table 3.1) by adding the individual scores; the sum ranges from 15 (fully awake, oriented and obeying) to 3 (eyes closed, no sounds, flaccid).

Table 3.1 Coma scales for adults and children

Adult scale

Eyes open	Score	Best motor response	Score	Best verbal reseponse	Score
Spontaneously	4	Obeys commands	5	Oriented	5
To speech	3	Localizes pain	4	Confused	4
To pain	2	Flexion to pain	3	Inappropriate words	3
None	1	Extension to pain	2	Incomprehensible sounds	2
		None	1	None	1

Paediatric scale

Normal score at age	Eyes	Motor	Score	Verbal	Score	Total
0–6 months	4	Flexion	3	Cries	2	9
6–12 months	4	Localizes	4	Vocalizes	3	11
1–2 years	4	Localizes	4	Words	4	12
2–5 years	4	Obeys	5	Words	4	13
>5 years	4	Obeys	5	Oriented	5	14

Adult (Glasgow) scale has aggregate score of 14 in this version; in specialized units abnormal and normal flexion are scored as 3 and 4, localizing and obeying as 5 and 6, and the maximum score is 15. Paediatric (Adelaide) scale takes account of expected verbal behaviour at different ages, so that normal aggregates vary with age, as shown.

Reduced responsiveness with eyes open

Although sometimes described as states of prolonged coma, this term is inappropriate because these patients are in an aroused state. Three quite different conditions should be clearly distinguished.

Vegetative state

The cerebral cortex is functionless, either because of extensive traumatic damage to its ascending and descending fibres, or of anoxic neocortical necrosis. The brainstem and deep subcortical structures are spared, so that breathing and arousal are normal and a range of reflex responses are possible. The eyes are open for long periods, alternating with hours of 'sleep'. When awake, the patient may briefly follow a moving object or 'look' to a bright light or loud sound. Relatives may regard these responses, together with withdrawal of the spastic limbs from pain and a grasp reflex when the fingers are stroked, as signs of returning consciousness. However, careful observation reveals no psychologically meaningful responses, and although grimacing and groaning sounds may occur, no recognizable words are ever uttered. After an anoxic episode (e.g. cardiac arrest) this state may be suspected after a day or so, but after head injury it is usually suspected only 10 days or more before the eyes open (as the concussive effect of injury on the brainstem wears off). It is the failure of any other evidence of neurological improvement once the eyes are open that makes vegetative survival likely, but it requires observation over some weeks before a persistent vegetative state can be confidently diagnosed.

Locked-in syndrome

Selective brainstem damage that spares the arousal mechanisms but destroys the motor system leaves the patient fully conscious but unable to communicate by word or gesture. Blinking and vertical eye movement are usually preserved and patients may be taught to use these movements to communicate by code. Most cases are due to brainstem ischaemic strokes, but trauma can occasionally result in this tragic state.

Brain death

Brain death is a product of our time, a result of efficient and widely available resuscitation procedures which result in many patients with respiratory arrest being intubated and ventilated as a routine resuscitative measure. When the cause of respiratory failure is remediable the patient may recover, for example if brainstem compression is relieved or the effects of depressant drugs are reversed. But if there is irrecoverable brainstem damage, continued mechanical ventilation serves only to prolong the process of dying, as other organs cease to function. The heart is among the last to fail in many cases, and may beat for 10–14 days after brainstem death. It is now widely agreed that when the brainstem is dead the brain is dead; and when the brain is dead the person is dead. The time of death is therefore when brain death is diagnosed – not some time later when the heart stops. To continue ventilation after brain death has occurred is undignified, and is needlessly distressing to relatives; it also involves inappropriate use of intensive care facilities.

Criteria for the diagnosis of brain death, published by the UK Royal Colleges in 1976, indicate beyond doubt that the brainstem has irretrievably ceased to function. A set of preconditions have to be satisfied before proceeding with the tests of brainstem function. The preconditions stipulate that the patient is in apnoeic coma due to irremediable brain damage, and that reversible causes of brainstem depression have been excluded (depressant drugs, including alcohol; neuromuscular blocking agents; hypothermia; gross metabolic imbalance). The diagnosis of the cause of brain damage is seldom in doubt;

half of all the cases of brain death in the UK each year are due to head injury, and almost a third are the result of spontaneous intracranial haemorrhage. Sufficient time must pass to determine that the damage is irremediable – time to restore normotension and normoxia, and to attempt reduction of raised ICP. This usually needs at least 6 hours, but if drugs are suspected, or the brain damage is due to an anoxic episode, then the time must be longer – at least 24 hours.

The *brainstem tests*, performed only when the preconditions have been met, are to confirm that all brainstem activity is absent (Fig. 3.2). The final and most crucial test is to confirm that there has been no return of spontaneous respiratory activity. The $PaCO_2$ is allowed to rise to 50 mmHg by disconnection from the ventilator for 5–10 minutes, whilst preventing hypoxaemia by diffusion oxygenation (6 litres per minute of oxygen by tracheal catheter). If $PaCO_2$ is below normal the patient should be ventilated with 5% carbon dioxide in oxygen for 5 minutes before disconnection. No respiratory activity is observed if the patient is brain-dead. The brainstem tests should be repeated after an interval of 30 minutes, and two doctors of adequate seniority and experience should be involved. It is wise to record the examination of the patient in a standardized fashion in the patient's case notes (Fig. 3.2).

NAME ....   UNIT NO

PRECONDITIONS
What condition has led to irremediable brain damage?   Time of onset of coma:

Dr A. ....

Dr B. ....
Are you satisfied that potentially reversible causes for the patient's condition have been adequately excluded, in particular:

	Dr A	*Dr B*
Depressant drugs	. . . .	. . . .
Neuromuscular blocking (relaxant) drugs	. . . .	. . . .
Hypothermia	. . . .	. . . .
Metabolic or endocrine disturbances	. . . .	. . . .

TESTS FOR ABSENCE OF BRAINSTEM FUNCTION

	Dr A	Dr B
Do the pupils react to light?	. . . .	. . . .
Are there corneal reflexes?	. . . .	. . . .
Is there eye movement on caloric testing?	. . . .	. . . .
Are there motor responses in the cranial nerve distribution, in response to stimulation of face, limbs or trunk?	. . . .	. . . .
Is there a gag/cough reflex?	. . . .	. . . .
Were any respiratory movements seen following disconnection from the ventilator ($PaCO_2$ to reach 50 mmHg)	. . . .	. . . .
Have the recommendations* for apnoea testing been followed?	. . . .	. . . .

Date and time of first testing	. . . .	. . . .
Date and time of second testing?	. . . .	. . . .
Dr Signature	. . . .	. . . .
Status	. . . .	. . . .

*UK Medical Royal Colleges, 1976: reproduced in *Cadaveric Organs for Transplantation: A Code of Practice including the Diagnosis of Brain Death*. London: HMSO, 1983.

Fig. 3.2 Model checklist for diagnosis of brain death.

Further reading

Conference of Medical Royal Colleges and their Faculties in the UK (1976). Diagnosis of brain death. *Br. Med. J.*; **2:** 1187–8.

Conference of Medical Royal Colleges and their Faculties in the UK (1979). Diagnosis of death. *Br. Med. J.*; **1:** 322.

Gentleman D., Easton J., Jennett B. (1990). Brain death and organ donation in a neurosurgical unit; an audit of recent practice. *Br. Med. J.*; **301:** 1203–6.

Jennett B. (1981). Brain death. *Br. J. Anaesth.*; **53:** 1111–19.

Jennett B. (1991). Vegetative state: causes, management, ethical dilemmas. *Curr. Anaesth.*; **2:** 57–61.

Jennett B., Plum F. (1972). Persistent vegetative state after brain damage. *Lancet*; **1:** 734–7.

Plum F., Posner J. B. (1980). *Diagnosis of Stupor and Coma*, 3rd edn. Philadelphia: F. Davis.

Reilly P. L., Simpson D. A., Sprod R. *et al.* (1988). Assessing the conscious level in infants and young children: a paediatric version of the Glasgow Coma scale. *Child's Nerv. Syst.*; **4:** 30–3.

Teasdale G, Jennett B. (1974). Assessment of coma and impaired consciousness: a practical scale. *Lancet*; **ii:** 8–4.

Williams S. E., Bell D. S., Gye R. S. (1974). Neurosurgical disease encountered in a psychiatric service. *J. Neurol. Neurosurg. Psychiatry*; **37:** 112–16.

Chapter 4

Investigations

Several procedures can be employed to supplement the clinical assessment of patients suspected of harbouring an intracranial lesion, some of them available in general hospitals or on an outpatient basis. These may dispense with the need to investigate the patient more elaborately, for example, if underlying disease is revealed which will account for the disorder in the nervous system. On the other hand the initial suspicion may be strengthened, and there may be clear indications as how best to plan neuroradiological investigation.

Search for extracranial disease

The range of conditions which may develop central nervous system (CNS) complications is enormous. The commoner ones should be considered, whenever intracranial disease is suspected, especially if the problem is one of focal signs without pressure. Evidence of *arterial disease* and hypertension is important, and *a source of cerebral emboli* such as atrial fibrillation or subacute bacterial endocarditis will suggest an alternative explanation for symptoms. *Infective foci* in the ears, sinuses or lungs, hydatid disease of the liver, cysticerci in the muscles – all will raise the possibility of CNS symptoms related to the spread of infected material or parasites to the brain.

Metastatic intracranial tumours are so common that a diligent search for a *primary extracranial tumour and other secondary tumour* is essential. All patients suspected of having a brain tumour require pelvic and abdominal examination, palpation of the breasts and lymph nodes and a chest X-ray.

Plain (straight) skull X-rays

Skull X-rays remain a useful preliminary investigation, particularly after trauma, where they guide further management. In patients presenting without physical signs (e.g. presenting with headache, dementia or epilepsy) a single lateral film is adequate for screening purposes; this will show the pituitary fossa, dorsum sellae, state of the sutures, size of posterior fossa, angle of the clivus and the presence of calcification either above or below the tentorium. Other views, which may be indicated because of abnormalities seen in this lateral film, or because of certain physical signs are:

1 Posteroanterior (PA) to show the frontal region, sphenoidal wings and orbits.
2. Towne's view to show the occipital region, foramen magnum, posterior clinoid processes and petrous bones.
3. Basal (occipitomental) to show the petrous and sphenoid bones, foramen magnum and other basal foramina.
4. Special views are required for detailed examination of the internal auditory meati and the optic foramina.

While normal skull films do not necessarily preclude the need for further imaging, plain X-rays can be useful as a triage tool; the degree of clinical suspicion of an intracranial lesion will determine whether to investigate further.

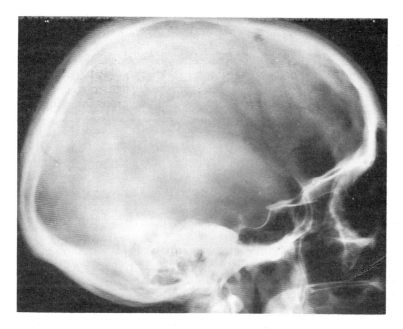

(a) Posterior clinoid processes (dorsum sellae) eroded.

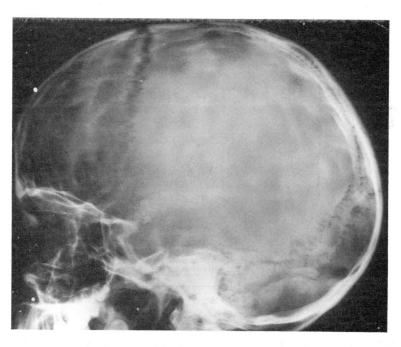

(b) In a child: widened coronal sutures, eroded dorsum sellae and digital impressions on the vault. (Note the enlarged pituitary fossa and suprasellar calcification – craniopharyngioma.)

Fig. 4.1 Radiological signs of raised pressure.

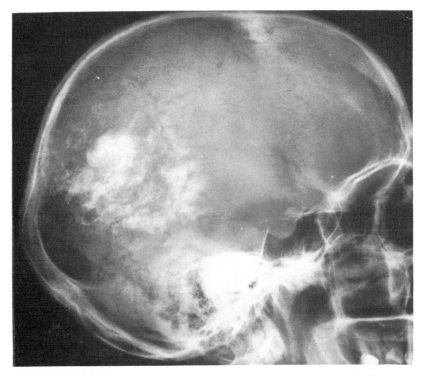

Fig. 4.2 Calcification in an intracranial tumour – parietal oligodendroglioma.

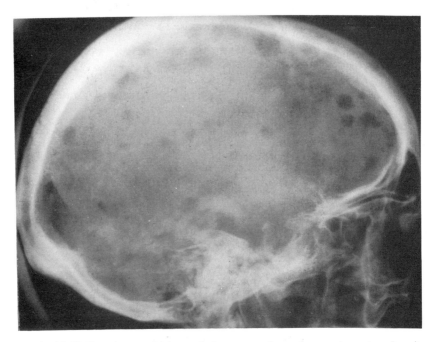

Fig. 4.3 Skull erosion – multiple punched-out areas of secondary carcinomatous deposits.

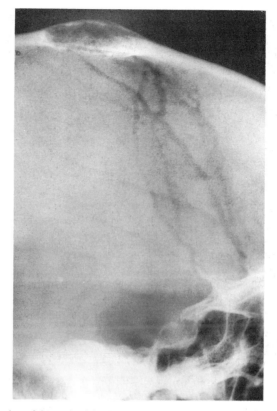

(a) Expansion of the vault with sclerosis and dilated vascular channels.

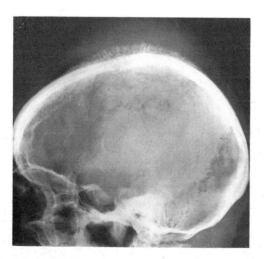

(b) Sun-ray appearance associated with a palpable lump.

Fig. 4.4 Meningioma on plain films.

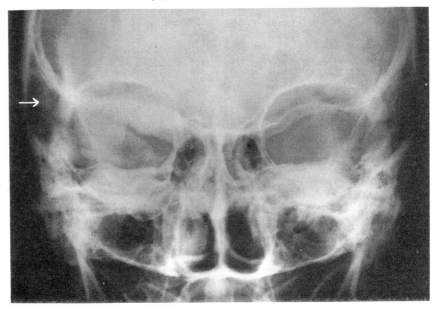

Fig. 4.4 (*cont*) (c) Thickening and sclerosis of sphenoid wing.

Information from plain skull films

Plain films can yield many different kinds of information. Thinning of the dorsum sellae and erosion of the posterior clinoids indicate long-standing raised ICP (Fig. 4.1a), which in young children can produce widening of the sutures (Fig. 4.1b). Calcification may develop in certain tumours (oligodendroglioma, craniopharyngioma, chordoma and meningioma; Fig. 4.2) but may also occur within the walls of aneurysms and atherosclerotic vessels and in other non-tumorous conditions including cysticercosis, toxoplasmosis, and the Sturge–Weber syndrome. Tumours can also erode bone (Fig. 4.3), dilate cavities (e.g. pituitary fossa) and enlarge foramina. Meningiomas, fibrous dysplasia and Paget's disease may produce thickening and increased density (Fig. 4.4).

CT scanning

This method of obtaining a density picture of a series of horizontal slices of the intracranial cavity revolutionized investigation of the brain in the mid 1970s. Multiple 'pencil' beams of X-ray are directed through the head from a succession of positions on an arc. Their attenuation is measured by an array of fixed detectors arranged around the head. A computer solves the equations necessary to calculate the attenuation values of multiple cubes of tissue (voxels) from the slice of brain under examination. The attenuation values of the voxels are converted to a grey scale and displayed as 'pixels' on a two-dimensional image. With modern scanners the matrix size is 250×250 or more. The attenuation is different for brain, CSF, haematoma, infarcted brain, oedema and tumour. Abnormal appearances may be enhanced by intravenous injection of iodinated contrast media (Figs 4.5 and 6.2, p. 102); increased density reflects breakdown of the blood – brain barrier, leading to leakage of

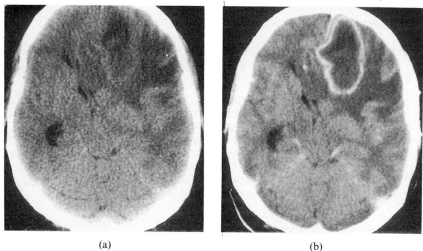

(a)   (b)

Fig. 4.5 CT scan with and without contrast enhancement. (a) Plain scan: frontal low-density lesion with mass effect. (b) After intravenous iodinated contrast medium: ring enhancement delineates the capsule of a cerebral abscess.

contrast, or excessive vascularity. Scans are usually taken in the transaxial plane, normally at 5 or 8 mm intervals. High-definition slices (i.e. 1 or 2 mm) can be reconstructed in the coronal or sagittal plane. Angling the X-ray gantry and extending the patient's neck permit direct-coronal scanning and this technique is often employed for sellar and parasellar lesions.

CT scanning clearly delineates bone, brain tissue and the ventricular system. Not only is the displacement of structures seen, but the pathological nature of the lesion can frequently be recognized. Fresh blood appears as a high-density lesion, gradually becoming less dense over a 10–20-day period, and hypodense beyond that. Enlargement of the cortical sulci and sylvian fissures suggests cerebral atrophy. Tumours, abscess and infarction all have characteristic appearances, with which we will deal in a later chapter.

The safety of scanning makes it appropriate for use in circumstances that would not have justified the use of previously available neuroradiological techniques, because of the risks that these carry. This means that demand for the use of scanning can soon outstrip availability, and some kind of triage is required, depending on local circumstances. One limitation is that it does not show the vascular tree, although large vessels and even aneurysms can often be recognized on high-quality scans. Another is the need for the head to remain stationary for the duration of the scan, so that general anaesthesia may be needed for young children or for patients who are confused or restless.

Unless there is close cooperation between surgeon and radiologist, inappropriate or unnecessary investigations may be carried out, adding only information which is unhelpful and at the price to the patient of added discomfort and possibly of increased risk. The problem of the particular patient should be kept in mind during the performance of each test because with critically ill patients a decision may have to be made whether to persist with or abandon an examination at a certain stage; the right course can be followed only if the radiologist has a clear idea of what information is required, and what can be dispensed with if circumstances are difficult.

Magnetic resonance imaging (MRI)

The novelty of this method is that it does not use ionizing radiation. Instead it depends on the tendency of the protons of atoms to align in the direction of a powerful magnetic field. As the protons of each element spin at a specific frequency, each can be recognized. MRI was originally developed for chemical analysis and its clinical use depends on displaying the distribution of hydrogen protons, and therefore of water, in the parts of the body examined. Further developments now make it possible to image other elements (e.g. sodium and phosphorus), and this enables various chemical processes to be detected by spectroscopy.

How protons react in the latticework of surrounding molecules can be deduced from the rate of return of protons to equilibrium when they have been displaced by a radiofrequency pulse (T1 component of the signal or spin-lattice relaxation time (Fig. 4.6a, b). This relates to thermodynamic equilibrium and is the main contributor to the anatomical image produced. The T2 component (spin-spin relaxation time) depends on the electromagnetic characteristics of surrounding protons (Fig. 4.6c), and this helps to distinguish different pathological processes (haemorrhage, oedema, tumour etc.; Table 4.1). Prolonged T1 relaxation produces a less intense signal, prolonged T2 a more intense signal. The intravenous injection of gadopentetate produces paramagnetic enhancement in lesions associated with impaired blood – brain barrier, given a hyperintense signal due to shortening of the T1 component. Bone produces an image void, although marrow gives an anatomical outline, and CT or plain X-rays are the method of choice to show lesions in the skull bones. The void resulting from rapidly moving protons enables intracranial vessels to be recognized by these flow voids, and this may eventually replace angiography.

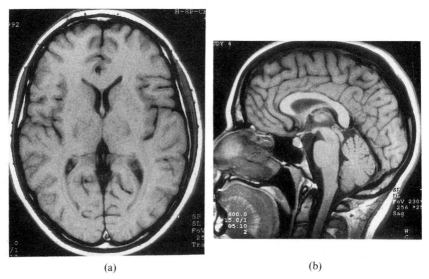

(a)   (b)

Fig. 4.6 Normal magnetic resonance scan (T1/T2 weighting in relation to normal grey/white matter). (a) T1-weighted axial view; (b) T1-weighted sagittal view.

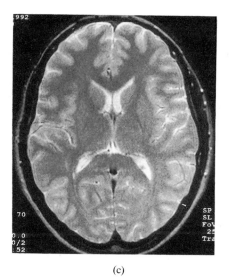

(c)

Fig. 4.6 (*cont*) (c) T2-weighted axial view.

Table 4.1 Signal changes caused by various lesions on T_1 and T_2 weighted magnetic resonance scans relative to normal grey and white matter

Tissue/lesion	T_1	T_2
CSF, Cystic fluid, Cerebromalacia	↓↓ Intensity	↑ Intensity
Oedema, ischaemia Demyelination Malignant tumours	↓ Intensity	↑ Intensity
Extravasated blood subacute/chronic	↑ Intensity	slight ↑ Intensity
Fat dermoid lipoma atheroma	↑ Intensity	↑ Intensity
Extravasated blood acute	Isointense	↓ Intensity
Meningioma	Isointense	Isointense

CT or MRI?

Modern-generation MRI scanners give greater definition than modern CT scanners and are more likely to detect small lesions. But MRI scanners are more expensive and at present are less widely available. CT scanning is adequate for many neurosurgical conditions and is the method of choice in neural trauma and when imaging bony detail. A few patients experience claustrophobia due to the enclosed nature of the field coils and require general anaesthesia. Patients with pacemakers or ferromagnetic implants are restricted to other forms of imaging.

MRI is of greatest advantage in:

1. Lesions around the cervicomedullary junction.
2. Midline lesions of the pineal, third ventricle and pituitary regions (Fig. 6.9).
3. Intramedullary spinal cord lesions (Fig. 12.9).
4. Multiple sclerosis.

Angiography

Angiography is now so ordinary a procedure that it is becoming available outside special centres. But the interpretation of films is not always straight-forward or easy and patients may not always benefit from the availability of angiography in isolation from the other techniques of neuroradiology, and without surgical facilities at hand. Moreover the risk of complications is substantially greater with occasional operators (see below).

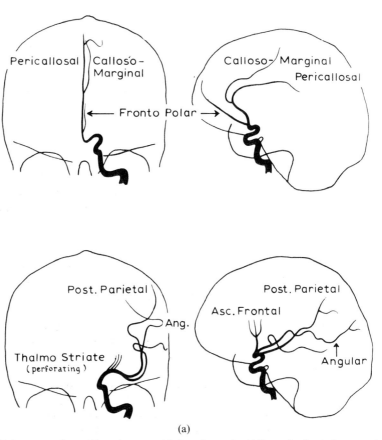

(a)

Fig. 4.7 Anatomy of carotid angiograms. (a) Anterior and middle cerebral arteries separately displayed with the internal carotid. The anterior cerebral artery becomes the pericallosal artery after the anterior communicating branch.

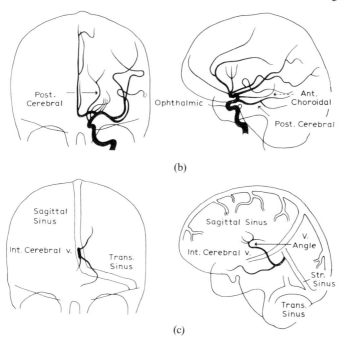

(b)

(c)

Fig. 4.7 (*cont*) (b) Complete arterial tree – anterior and middle cerebral branches and vessels arising directly from the carotid (ophthalmic and anterior choroidal). The posterior cerebral artery fills in about one-third of carotid angiograms via the posterior communicating artery. (c) Venogram.

Technique

Angiography is now performed by the retrograde femoral catheterization technique, with selective injection of the carotid and vertebral arteries. This makes it possible to investigate the whole intracranial arterial tree without the confusing pictures produced by simultaneous four-vessel angiography by a single aortic injection. Carotid injection displays the vessels in the territory of the anterior and middle cerebral arteries and sometimes of the posterior cerebral also (Fig. 4.7). Vertebral injection displays the basilar and posterior cerebral arteries and their territories. Subtraction of a preinjection skull X-ray removes unwanted bony detail and may aid identification of small lesions. Anteroposterior and lateral views are standard and are often supplemented by oblique and Towne's views when investigating subarachnoid haemorrhage. Rarely catheterization fails and the older technique of direct carotid or vertebral puncture becomes necessary. In view of lesser risk, retrograde injection after percutaneous puncture of the brachial or subclavian artery may be preferred to direct vertebral puncture.

Angiography is frequently performed under local anaesthesia with suitable premedication, although the inevitable sudden hot flush in the head and neck when the contrast is injected is vividly described and remembered by most patients. In addition the elaborate apparatus, lead screens and masked figures, the click and thud of exposure and cassette changer all makes for a somewhat alarming experience. Some centres use general anaesthesia as a routine, others confine its use to children and difficult patients.

Digital subtraction angiography (DSA)

Digital computing allows subtraction of an image obtained before contrast injection from that after injection, while further data manipulation permits magnification or enhancement of the resultant angiographic image as required. This technique requires less contrast and an intravenous injection of contrast is sufficient to display the extracranial vessels. Unfortunately, due to limited spatial resolution, an intra-arterial injection is required to display the intracranial vessels. The resolution even then does not match standard angiography, but it is sufficient for most needs and is preferred for interventional techniques (see below) which involve multiple injections of contrast.

Complications

Development or aggravation of CNS signs is reported with varying frequency, reflecting variations in the skill of the operator, in the concentration and volume of the contrast injected and in the care with which temporary signs are sought. Hemiparesis and/or dysphasia are usually transient but occasionally permanent. They may result from manipulation of the catheter tip, or dislodging fragments of atheromatous plaques into the distal circulation. Systemic arterial hypotension, induced by anaesthesia or by the injection of contrast, may aggravate the situation. If there is already occlusion of the opposite carotid artery, or of either of the vertebral arteries, any of these accidents may result in ischaemia, and most complications arise in patients with arterial degeneration. With modern techniques the risk of a permanent deficit is very small and lies in the region of 1 in 5000 in skilled hands with large-volume throughput. However, angiography is so much less often used since the appearance of CT and MRI that there is some risk from occasional operators.

Sensitivity to iodine is rarely seen with Urografin or Hypaque, but if there is an allergic or asthmatic history it is wise to do a preliminary skin test. Reactions include allergic rash, bronchospasm and cardiorespiratory failure.

Renal damage may delay the excretion of the contrast medium, which can further add to the damage, and the method is contraindicated in patients with advanced renal disease.

Increased ICP is sometimes suspected after angiography, usually in patients already critically compressed. Oedema may increase around a malignant tumour, perhaps due to excess contrast medium (or large quantities of saline injected between films) acting on abnormal vessels with an altered blood-brain barrier.

Haematoma in the neck may complicate direct carotid puncture, but is seldom alarming if a finger is kept firmly on the puncture point for a minutes after withdrawing the needle. But it is important to ascertain before the procedure that patients are not receiving long-term anticoagulants. Tracheal deviation and respiratory embarrassment occasionally develop.

An *epileptic fit* occasionally occurs as soon as contrast is injected. *Nausea* is often complained of immediately after the first injection, but rarely after subsequent ones. With direct puncture *syncope* can occur from the needle being in the carotid sinus, and calls for replacement of the needle. *Carotid aneurysms* and *caroticojugular (arteriovenous) fistulae* are rare late developments of direct puncture.

Complications are uncommon in experienced hands, but may occur in up to 10% of cases. The risk of their developing, the quality of films produced, and the amount of discomfort suffered by the patient under local anaesthesia depend very largely on the skill of the operator and team – skill which takes time to acquire and continued practice to maintain. There is little place for the occasional operator.

Information

Identification of the source of subarachnoid haemorrhage or intracranial haematoma is the commonest indication for angiography (provided CT or MRI is available for the investigation of suspected mass lesions). Four-vessel angiography may reveal an aneurysm or an arteriovenous malformation.

Cerebrovascular disease
Angiography may identify extracranial vascular disease in patients with transient ischaemic attacks or in patients who have recovered from a small stroke and are potential candidates for vascular surgery. In some patients angiography is necessary to diagnose intracranial vessel disease.

Cerebral tumours
Angiography shows the vascularity of a tumour and should indicate whether it encompasses or displaces main blood vessels. For certain tumours this is an essential prerequisite to operation.

Embolization

With advancing interventional techniques, neuroradiologists may now play an important therapeutic role. In some conditions (e.g. meningioma, glomus jugulare tumours and arteriovenous malformations), preoperative embolization of feeding vessels can minimize blood loss during operation. In other conditions (e.g. carotid-cavernous fistula, dural arteriovenous malformations and some giant aneurysms), embolization may provide definitive treatment, avoiding the need for surgery.

High-flow systems involving large vessels require occlusion with detachable balloons, while particles of Ivalon sponge or dura are sufficient to occlude low-flow systems. In some centres, radiologists inject acrylic 'glue' into arteriovenous malformations or insert fine platinum coils into aneurysms.

These techniques are not without risk as particles or balloon fragments may pass beyond their intended site, causing an embolic stroke. Patients must be fully informed that they are not simply undergoing a test but an extensive procedure with inherent risks, which can be compared with those of surgery or of no treatment.

Radioisotope tests

The distribution of *gamma-emitting isotopes* within the brain can be detected through the intact skull, using scintillation counters. These isotopes permit several different types of investigation. Display of the gamma emission on a two-dimensional map localizes intracranial lesions (conventional gamma-camera scanning). Although this technique carries negligible risk and serves as a useful screening procedure, it has no place when CT scanning is available. Radioisotopes also provide a method for measuring CBF (xenon clearance) and for mapping the distribution of blood flow throughout the brain (single photon emission tomography). Positron-emitting isotopes, when bound to specific compounds, give a quantitative measure of CBF, oxygen extraction and utilization and drug and neurotransmitter receptor sites (positron emission tomography, PET). Techniques permitting measurement of CBF, although occasionally of direct clinical value, tend to be restricted to research use.

Conventional gamma scanning

Technetium (Tc^{99m}), with a half-life of 6 hours, is the most commonly used isotope. Scanning begins about an hour after intravenous injection. Most machines produce a lateral and an axial view of the intracranial cavity; a rotating gamma-camera or multiple detectors ranged in a halo around the head give three-dimensional localization of areas of increased uptake. The gamma-camera can give rapid serial views of the uptake and distribution of isotope, thus adding the fourth dimension – time.

The physicochemical abnormalities which determine the accumulation or exclusion of isotope from pathological areas are not yet understood, but seem likely to be related to alterations in the blood – brain barrier. To a large extent therefore the method remains empirical, and its discriminative value has still to be assessed. It is of most use in detecting supratentorial lesions, but with optimal collimation lesions can be shown in the posterior fossa. Meningiomas have the densest uptake, but this does not seem to relate to vascularity; metastases usually show clearly, and the demonstration of more than one area of increased uptake may be of considerable help in management; gliomas can usually be recognized, although they do not as a rule show up as strikingly as meningiomas or metastases unless they are rapidly growing. Abscesses, infarcts and haematomas may show up satisfactorily. Gamma-camera scanning carries negligible risk and serves as a useful screening procedure; it has no place when CT scanning is available.

Xenon clearance and cerebral blood flow

The brain is more critically dependent on the integrity of the circulation than any other organ in the body. Neurons are uniquely vulnerable to ischaemia; cerebral ischaemia is the penultimate common path by which most types of brain damage are caused, whether due to head injury, space-occupying lesion, blockage of a main arterial trunk or sudden loss of perfusion pressure due to a fall in cardiac output. There is therefore concern about the cerebral circulation in many conditions other than those due to occlusive vascular lesions.

The outstanding characteristic of the microcirculation in the brain is the efficiency of its autoregulation, which ensures a constancy of flow under widely varying conditions. Regulation depends chiefly on alteration of arteriolar diameter, and flow is critically dependent on the arterial tension of carbon dioxide and of oxygen ($PaCO_2$ and PaO_2), less so on arterial blood pressure. When measuring CBF and when comparing values in one patient on two or more occasions, it is important to show that these other factors are constant, especially the $PaCO_2$. Accurate estimates of the regional cerebral blood flow (rCBF) can now be made using gamma-emitting isotopes. With inert and freely diffusible isotopes the rate of disappearance of the radioactivity from the brain will depend only on the blood flow, and by using gases which are excreted into the air by the lungs during one circulation, the reintroduction of radioactivity into the brain by recirculation is avoided. The blood flow in milliliters per 100 grams per minute can be calculated from the exponential curve of clearance from the brain. Multiple detectors allow comparison of different parts of the brain, but the geometry of collimators and the high energy of the isotope result in some overlap between adjacent detectors and limit the degree of resolution.

This technique originally involved injection of isotope into the carotid artery in the course of angiography or of carotid surgery. An intravenous method is now available in addition to the inhalation method. These techniques can be used in outpatients and repeated as required to demonstrate pathological progression or recovery, or the effect of drugs.

Single photon emission computed tomography (SPECT)

This technique uses gamma-emitting radiopharmaceuticals to measure CBF. The Tc 99m-labelled derivative of propylamine oxime (HMPAO) when injected intravenously diffuses across the blood – brain barrier and becomes trapped within the cells. Gamma activity is detected with either a rotating gamma-camera or, preferably, a bank of fixed detectors arranged around the head. Similar computing techniques to CT scanning produce a two-dimensional image composed of pixels of radioactivity for a selected plane. The amount of radioactivity indicates the distribution of CBF at the time of the HMPAO injection, but does not permit quantitative estimation. SPECT scanning provides early evidence of ischaemic changes in cerebrovascular disease. Although awaiting full evaluation, SPECT appears to be extremely useful in the preoperative evaluation of patients with intractable epilepsy by detecting the dramatic increase in blood flow which occurs around the epileptic focus during a seizure.

Positron emission tomography

PET scanning uses compounds labelled with a positron-emitting isotope (ligands). The selected ligand and the route of administration depend on the required measurement (e.g. intravenous deoxyglucose is labelled with fluorine 18 to study cerebral glucose metabolism). Each decaying positron interacts with an electron to release two gamma photons in diametrically opposite directions. These coincidentally activate one pair of an array of fixed detectors around the head. CT analysis produces an accurate measurement of the radioactivity emitted from each pixel. This is displayed as a two-dimensional colour-coded image. In addition to cerebral glucose metabolism, use of the appropriate ligand gives a quantitative measurement of cerebral blood volume, CBF, cerebral oxygen utilization and extraction and drug and transmitter-binding sites.

Since positron-emitting isotopes depend on a cyclotron for their production, PET scanning is extremely costly and only available in a few centres. Limited access inevitably restricts its clinical use, but PET scanning has considerably improved our understanding of the mechanisms of ischaemic damage in cerebrovascular disease and dementia, of brain tumours and of epilepsy. Identification of drug and transmitter receptor sites has helped elucidate the biochemical basis of psychiatric disease and movement disorders and should guide future treatment.

Ultrasound

B-mode

Sound waves of high frequency (5-100 MHz) emitted from a probe applied to the skin surface are reflected from the interface of structures of varying acoustic impedance and are detected by the same probe. These waves are reconverted into electrical energy and displayed on a two-dimensional image (B-mode). Skull thickness limits the value of this technique in intracranial imaging, but in infants application of the probe over the anterior fontanelle clearly images the ventricular system and may detect intracerebral and subdural haematoma.

Doppler

When ultrasound waves are directed towards moving structures, e.g. red blood cells within a blood vessel lumen, frequency shift occurs proportional to the velocity of the blood flow. Pulsed waves allow identification of frequency shift at a specific depth and when combined with B-mode scanning give an image of the vessel from which the velocity is being measured (Duplex scanning). With modern refinements and using low frequency (2 MHz), some skull penetration is possible, permitting assessment of intracranial as well as extracranial vessels (see p. 151).

Electroencephalography and evoked potentials

The development of new imaging techniques has diminished the need for the EEG as a screening test, but it still has a role in the management of epilepsy and in the investigation of encephalitis and certain encephalopathies.

Electrodes are applied to the scalp with collodion. Most centres use the internationally agreed 10/20 system, which is based on a percentage of the nasion – inion distance and the sagittal skull base distance.

The normal frequency is 8 – 11 Hz*, known as the alpha rhythm; this is most consistently found in the occipital region when the eyes are closed and the mind is relaxing; it appears to be an 'idling' rhythm, normally replaced by

*Hz = Hertz = cycles per second.

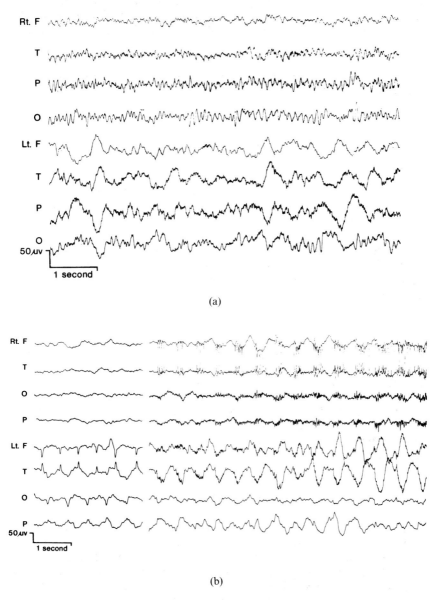

(a) Left hemisphere lesion: the right side shows normal alpha rhythm (8 Hz), most marked posteriorly; the left side is slow with delta activity (4 Hz), but some alpha remains in the occipital lead. (b) Focal spikes: these are most marked in left frontal and temporal leads in an unconscious patient: 1 minute later, right-sided facial twitching produces bursts of muscle spikes in right frontotemporal leads, associated with high voltage activity in left frontotemporal leads. Note the phase reversal between left frontal and temporal channels, denoting origin of abnormal activity near the electrode common to these two leads.

Fig. 4.8 EEG abnormalities (only eight channels are displayed).

desynchronized or random activity when the eyes are open or the subject engages in active thinking, such as doing mental arithmetic.

Focal abnormalities cause local slow waves, either theta (4 – 7 Hz) or delta (less than 4 Hz; Fig. 4.8a), but slow waves also occur normally in children and young adults, predominantly in the frontal and temporal regions. More accurate localization is possible if phase reversals are seen, with waves in opposite directions occuring simultaneously in two channels which share a common electrode, under which the maximum abnormality is assumed to be located. Intracranial infections often produce a very dramatic abnormality and emergency EEG can be of value in such instances. Herpes simplex encephalitis produces generalized slowing with periodic high-voltage wave complexes over the affected temporal lobe, whilst coma produces generalized slowing.

In epilepsy the EEG is only of benefit if an attack occurs during the recording period (Fig. 4.8b); even so, there are occasional seizures which are electrically silent. When it is essential to establish the diagnosis of epilepsy or to determine the exact site of seizure origin (e.g. prior to surgical intervention – see p. 303) then telemetry is used to record EEG activity over a 24-hour period; this is often combined with video-monitoring. Implantation of additional electrodes, into the cheek (sphenoidal) or through the foramen ovale, provides more accurate sampling of electrical activity in the important medial temporal structures.

The limitations of the EEG must be fully appreciated if it is not to be misleading; a high degree of skill both in recording and interpretation are essential and the investigation is better not done if these are not available.

Evoked potentials

Averaging electrical activity recorded in response to a specific sensory stimulus produces a characteristic wave pattern which gives information about the pathway under study. Visual evoked potentials are recorded over the occiput in response to a flash stimulus or to an alternating checkerboard pattern. Brainstem auditory evoked potentials are recorded over the vertex in response to a 'click' stimulus, applied through headphones. Somatosensory evoked potentials are recorded over the parietal region while stimulating a peripheral nerve.

Evoked potentials aid the diagnosis of certain conditions (e.g. multiple sclerosis, acoustic schwannoma) and provide a prognostic guide after brain injury. They also provide a way of monitoring sensory pathways during operative procedures (e.g. removal of acoustic schwannomas or complex spinal procedures).

Development of the magnetic stimulator which induces an electrical current within small regions of the motor cortex has produced a more acceptable method of examining motor pathways, rather than using direct electrical stimulation. The value of this technique in clinical practice awaits further assessment.

Lumbar puncture

Where imaging is readily available, lumbar puncture will seldom be justified except in specific conditions. When infection is suspected or scanning has failed to confirm subarchnoid haemorrhage, then CSF examination is essential.

Raised pressure may be detected on lumbar puncture, but it should not be. If there is papilloedema a lumbar puncture should not be done. One can only rely on the pressure measurement when this is measured with the patient horizontal, fully relaxed and the legs extended so that the thighs are not pressing on the abdomen.

Lumbar puncture is dangerous in patients with raised ICP in whom herniations and brain shifts are already established. The removal of CSF from below allows the brainstem to move caudally through the tentorial hiatus and the foramen magnum. The patient may die suddenly while the needle is still in place, but more often coning is delayed for several hours, even until the next day. Continual leakage of CSF through the puncture hole in the lumbar dura decompresses the system long after the needle has been withdrawn. This leakage can occur with or without raised ICP, and explains the severe headache which sometimes follows lumbar puncture and which is associated with a low CSF pressure. The possibility of its occurrence means that even 'careful' lumbar puncture, using a fine needle and letting off only a small amount of fluid, is not without risk; once the theca has been punctured, the situation is out of control.

Raised protein occurs in patients with tumour or infection, or following a haemorrhage when the red cells break down. Those patients with tumours abutting the ventricles or subarachnoid spaces give the highest levels – neurinomas, in particular, where levels may reach 400 mg per 100 ml. Any meningitic infection increases the CSF protein, but in tuberculous meningitis levels are particularly high, often rising to 100–400 mg per 100 ml.

Xanthochromia occurs when red blood cells break down in the CSF. It confirms the presence of subarachnoid blood existing prior to the lumbar puncture, rather than resulting from a 'traumatic tap'.

Pleocytosis usually means infection, but not always. In bacterial meningitis the CSF white cell count rises to over 500 cells/mm^3 and often reaches several thousand. Viral and tuberculous meningitis increase the CSF lymphocyte count to several hundred cells/mm^3; when tuberculosis develops acutely, as many as 1000 polymorphs/mm^3 may be found. Brain abscess causes only a mild reaction, 100 cells or so, unless complicated by frank meningitis.

Tumours give rise to cells in the CSF in about 10% of patients; about half of those that do are gliomas. Although less than 50 cells is the rule, up to 1000 cells, either polymorphs or lymphocytes, can occur, probably due to necrosis in a malignant glioma close to the ventricles or subarachnoid pathways. Centrifuging the CSF and staining the deposit after fixation in formalin may aid recognition of tumour cells, which in routine counts are usually reported as large mononuclear or bizarre white cells. Medulloblastoma, malignant glioma or metastasis (especially meningitis carcinomatosa) are the most likely to shed cells into the CSF but it is unusual to be able to identify the primary cell type in the fluid.

Ventriculography, air encephalography and basal cisternography

These techniques have become redundant in many places with the increasing availability of modern CT scanners. In the absence of CT scanning, angiography may suffice, although in some patients outlining the ventricular system, basal cisterns or cortical subarachnoid space gives further necessary information.

Ventriculography

In patients with suspected raised ICP, water-soluble contrast is introduced through a ventricular catheter into the lateral ventricle. Varying the patient's position allows the contrast medium to enter and outline various parts of the ventricular system. Ventriculography may demonstrate shift due to a supra- or infratentorial mass without identifying the exact lesion site, but if the lesion encroaches on the ventricular system, the resultant filling defect provides accurate localization.

Ventriculography is most useful in the investigation of patients with hydrocephalus or suspected intracranial mass lesions. The risks of haemorrhage, infection and seizures are small. Alteration of intracranial dynamics may occasionally induce a tentorial cone.

Air encephalography

This technique is used in patients with unlocalized symptoms such as epilepsy or dementia, without signs of raised ICP. Air is introduced into the lumbar theca and allowed to run up to the ventricular system, basal cisterns and the subarachnoid space over the cerebral hemispheres. Information from ventricular displacement matches that from ventriculography, but additional information is gained from abnormalities of the subarachnoid cisterns. The technique is less valuable in demonstrating blockage of CSF flow.

Air encephalography tends to produce troublesome headache and vomiting. Although it can reveal the displacement effect of tumours, it should never be used when clinical signs or symptoms suggest a mass lesion in view of the risk of precipitating tentorial herniation.

Basal cisternography

Water-soluble contrast media, injected either through the lumbar theca or into the cisterna magna, will clearly outline the basal cisterns, demonstrating filling defects caused by tumours of the cerebellopontine angle or parasellar region. As with air encephalography, this technique is restricted to patients without clinical features of raised ICP.

Further reading

Ashid R., Markwalder T.M., Nornes H. (1982). Non-invasive transcranial ultrasound recording of flow velocity in basal cerebral arteries. *J. Neurosurg.*; **57**: 569 – 774.

Baker H.L., Houser O.W., Campbell J.K. (1980). National Cancer Institute Study: evaluation of computed tomography in the diagnosis of intracranial neoplasms. *Radiology*; **136**: 91 – 6.

Duncan R., Patterson J., Hadley D.M. *et al.* (1990). CT, MR and SPECT imaging in temporal lobe epilepsy. *J. Neurol. Neurosurg. Psychiatry*; **53:** 11 – 15.

Greenberg R.P., Newlon P.G., Hyatt M.S., *et al.* (1981). Prognostic implications of multimodality evoked potentials in severely head injured patients. A prospective study. *J. Neurosurg.*; **55:** 227 – 36.

Hadley D.M. (1992). Magnetic resonance imaging – how has it helped the neurosurgeon? In: Teasdale G.M., Miller J.D. (eds) *Current Neurosurgery.* Edinburgh; Churchill Livingstone.

Hadley D.M., Teasdale G.M. (1988). Magnetic resonance imaging of the brain and spine. *J. Neurol.*; **235:** 193–206.

Naylor A.R. (1992). Transcranial Doppler sonography. In: Teasdale G.M., Miller J.D. (eds) *Current Neurosurgery.* Edinburgh: Churchill Livingstone.

Stevens J.M., Valentine A. R., Kendall B.E. (1988). *Computed Cranial and Spinal Imaging.* London: Heinemann.

Chapter 5

Principles of treatment

Non-operative relief of raised intracranial pressure

Brain – lung interactions

Brain-protective agents

Anaesthesia for intracranial operations

Intracranial pressure
Cerebral oxygenation
Recovery phase
Neuroleptanalgesia
Position on table

Operative approaches

Burr holes
Supratentorial exploration
Posterior fossa exploration

Surgical means of reducing intracranial pressure

Intracranial clot

Pyrexia and infection

The wound
Meningitis
Abscess
Osteomyelitis
Extracranial infection

Epilepsy

Care of the eyes

Once a space-occupying lesion has been localized, it remains to determine its pathological identity, and to manage the particular lesion appropriately. In many instances the history and investigation may leave little doubt as to the nature of the lesion, say temporal lobe abscess in a patient with chronic otitis, or meningioma when there are classical bone changes and angiographic appearances. Sometimes, however, the matter is nothing like so obvious and the final steps towards diagnosis are taken in the operating theatre, and the further management depends on the findings. Later chapters will deal in detail with the management of intracranial tumours, infections and haemorrhage, but general principles are outlined here and certain measures described which may apply to any space-occupying lesion. They are concerned with the relief of ICP and the problems of access to the lesion such that at least a diagnosis is established; in favourable circumstances this will lead to effective treatment.

Non-operative relief of raised intracranial pressure

A number of manoeuvres can reduce pressure and these may be employed not only by the anaesthetist in the operating theatre but also in the ward before or after operation.

Hypertonic solutions, given intravenously, depend for their effect on osmotic dehydration of the brain; as a result blood volume is increased and a diuresis induced. Reduction of ICP is evident within about 15 minutes of rapid infusion and lasts for about 4–6 hours. A saturated solution of mannitol (20%) is most commonly used, but this must be kept in a warm cupboard to prevent crystallization. The full dose is 200 ml given over 20 minutes, but smaller amounts may be effective; it is preferable to urea (1.5 g/kg body weight) which is locally irritant and which also requires some preparation immediately before injection. Frusemide may itself be effective, and if given 30 minutes before mannitol will largely prevent the rise in blood pressure which is normally observed as the result of an increase in blood volume. In the theatre mannitol may be given as a routine after induction of anaesthesia, so that its maximal effects are established by the time the bone flap is turned. However, in most situations a properly conducted anaesthetic with good positioning on the table and controlled respiration will give a sufficiently slack brain, but disadvantages may result, in that brain shrinkage may tear bridging veins or avulse olfactory nerves, causing permanent anosmia.

Corticosteroids are less rapid in action but their effects can be none the less dramatic in patients with intracranial tumours. Although side-effects tend to develop with prolonged use, patients with inoperable tumours may tolerate a low maintenance dose of 2 mg/day of dexamethasone and maintain a sustained improvement over many months, only to develop symptoms again as soon as this drug is withdrawn. In acute situations a dose of 4 mg 4 times a day is reduced to 2 mg 3 times a day after 3 days and eventually to 2 mg/ day. Although sometimes employed as a routine postoperative measure to prevent oedema and brain swelling, steroids are probably not useful in the treatment of spontaneous or aneurysmal intracerebral haematoma. They have no place in the treatment of head injury (p. 204).

Hyperventilation, by inducing cerebral vasoconstriction secondary to hypocapnia, reduces ICP within minutes. Anaesthetists frequently employ this as a routine measure but if unusually high levels of ventilation are maintained, the reduction in CBF can result in a degree of cerebral hypoxia.

Brain – lung interactions

Since Cheyne described periodic respiration, it has been increasingly recognized that brain damage may affect not only the rate and rhythm of breathing but also the efficiency of pulmonary gas exchange. The latter may be affected by central respiratory depression, by respiratory complications of the unconscious state and also, according to some reports, by ventilation – perfusion abnormalities in the lungs produced by neural influences, acting either directly or through the cardiovascular system. Whatever the reasons for respiratory dysfunction, alterations in blood gas levels affect the brain and are particularly adverse if the brain is recently damaged, or if there is reduced intracranial compliance. Both hypercapnia and hypoxia cause cerebral vasodilatation, which will raise ICP; they occur together if ventilation is inadequate. But, more often in brain-damaged patients, hypoxia is associated with hypocapnia. The threat to the brain is then related to the reduction in arterial oxygen content and to the net effect on cerebral blood flow of hypocapnia, which causes both vasoconstriction and reduction of ICP. Hypocapnia may occasionally be due to a brainstem lesion causing central neurogenic hyperventilation. This is now believed to be a rare condition, and hyperventilation is more likely to be due to other abnormal drives to breathing, arising from cerebral acidity, interstitial lung oedema and hypoxia.

Awareness of the deleterious effect of respiratory insufficiency on the brain has led to great care being taken in the course of neurosurgical operations to avoid conditions which are not only bad for the brain but which also, by producing a 'tight brain', make the surgeon's task more difficult. It has also led to increased attention to the respiratory care not only of postoperative patients but of all unconscious patients. Enthusiasm has sometimes overtaken understanding in this complex field and there are still divided opinions about the place and value of controlled ventilation for unconscious brain-damaged patients, particularly those who have recently sustained a head injury. No one disputes the importance of maintaining a clear airway at all times (p. 201). If, once this is established, there is hypoventilation, with raised PCO_2, the need for increasing the ventilation by controlled or assisted ventilation is clear. If PCO_2 is normal or low, but if the PaO_2 is less than 9 kPa despite efficient delivery of a raised inspired percentage of oxygen, there is need to consider controlled (assisted) ventilation to correct hypoxia. Another reason advanced for controlled ventilation is in order to eliminate the work of breathing in the patient who is hyperventilating. In these instances controlled ventilation may be recommended to reduce rather than to increase ventilation, in order to benefit the brain by reducing the vasoconstriction of hypocapnia. It may, however, be unwise to reduce the ventilation, even if there are other good reasons for taking it over mechanically, since the hypocapnia may be an important compensation for cerebral tissue acidity. Indeed, the reason most often advanced in support of controlled ventilation is that hyperventilation can be used to reduce ICP. The question is whether the patient does in fact have significantly raised pressure; and if he or she has, whether there may not be a possible threat to cerebral oxygenation in seeking to reduce ICP by producing reduce CBF. The more frequent use of jugular bulb oxygen saturation monitoring in intensive care units may serve as a guide. A low jugular venous oxygen saturation indicates a high cerebral oxygen consumption;

in these patients, an increase in ventilation and a further reduction in P_{CO_2} risks cerebral anoxia from vasoconstriction.

There are other possible disadvantages to controlled ventilation, carried out over a period of several days; one is the effects on the lungs, including the possibility of infection, particularly if tracheostomy becomes necessary. Another is that the clinician is deprived of most clinical indications of the state of the brain function, and so cannot judge whether the patient is improving or, more significantly, is showing evidence of developing intracranial complications. Whatever the theoretical case for its value, it must be appreciated that in large series of similarly severely brain-damaged patients there is no good evidence that outcome is better when controlled ventilation is used routinely than when it is reserved only for those circumstances which clearly require it. That will usually be in patients with associated chest injuries or specific pulmonary complications. If controlled ventilation is used for these purposes, then the Pa_{CO_2} should not normally be lower than 4 kPa, in order to avoid undue cerebral vasoconstriction.

Brain-protective agents

Ventilated patients often receive some form of sedation, either with *benzodiazepines*, e.g. midazolam, or with *anaesthetic agents*, e.g. propofol or barbiturates, and these may help control ICP. In addition to their sedative effects, these drugs also reduce cerebral metabolism. The reduction is metabolic demand may provide a degree of cerebral protection, but benefits remain uncertain.

Much attention is now focused on drugs which can provide protection against cerebral ischaemic damage. The *calcium antagonist* Nimodipine reduces ischaemic complications following subarachnoid haemorrhage, by either improving collateral circulation or by preventing a harmful influx of calcium into ischaemic brain cells. The use of such drugs in head-injured patients requires further study. Experimental studies have confirmed the benefits of *NMDA (glutamate) antagonists* in preventing the toxic effects of glutamate accumulation in ischaemic regions; some success has also been obtained with *free radical scavengers*. Many such neuronal-protective drugs, potentially suitable for clinical use, await full evaluation.

Anaesthesia for intracranial operations

The neurosurgeon demands three conditions from an anaesthetic technique: that it should not increase ICP; that it should not impair cerebral oxygenation; and that its effects should not persist after leaving theatre. These conditions are reliably met only by local anaesthesia, and this was indeed the method of choice for many years.

Intracranial pressure

Any degree of ventilatory insufficiency or obstruction will result in raised ICP, due to the vasodilatory effect of hypercapnia and hypoxia and to the transmission of raised central venous pressure to the intracranial venous sinuses.

These factors are most reliably avoided if controlled respiration is employed so that the patient never strains; supplements of relaxant drugs must be given regularly because as soon as the patient does begin to 'fight the pump', the brain will become tense, and will bulge if the skull is open.

Even if ventilation is adequate and unimpeded the ICP may rise due to the direct effect of volatile anaesthetic agents on CBF. In the presence of an intracranial mass, even a small rise in pressure may precipitate brain shift and cause brain damage. All volatile anaesthetic agents have this potentially harmful effect, but normally this is well-controlled with hyperventilation.

Cerebral oxygenation

This depends on CBF, oxygen saturation and the haemoglobin level; all three factors may be impaired during operation under anaesthesia. Normally CBF remains constant over a wide range of systemic blood pressure, but under anaesthesia autoregulation may be imperfect; moreover, if ICP is raised the effect of a fall in blood pressure on perfusion pressure becomes more pronounced (see p. 30). Factors which may lower the blood pressure are the induction dose of thiopentone and the initial or supplementary doses of d-tubocurarine. Both halothane and methoxyflurane induce hypotension (and, as they also raise ICP, perfusion pressure may be markedly affected); if the patient is placed in the sitting position the blood pressure often falls abruptly and sometimes fails to return to normal levels; blood loss may contribute to hypotension at a later stage in any procedure. Patients already on treatment with hypotensive drugs have a labile blood pressure and are much more liable to develop falls in pressure in these various circumstances.

Induced arterial hypotension was once frequently used, particularly for surgery on intracranial aneurysms. With hypotension, manipulation of the aneurysm sac becomes easier and blood loss from premature rupture is more readily controlled. Various agents can be used, such as halothane or nitroprusside; whatever the method, the degree and duration require careful control, with arterial pressure being continuously monitored via an arterial line. Concern that this technique might increase cerebral ischaemic complications has considerably reduced its usage.

Hypothermia was formerly employed in an attempt to protect the brain from hypoxia associated with induced or accidental hypotension, or when major vessels were to be temporarily occluded. It is now seldom used.

Recovery phase

Intracranial operations may be followed by intracranial haematomas, similar to those which develop after accidental trauma to the head. The same rules apply in each situation, in that a deteriorating conscious level or developing signs signal cerebral compression and the need for urgent repeat investigation. But after an operation such signs may be the direct result of the intracranial surgery, hence the need for early evaluation of whether or not the patient can speak, can move all four limbs and has reacting pupils. Otherwise it may be impossible to judge whether signs, if first observed a few hours later, represent a newly developing complication. For this reason the anaesthetic technique should allow rapid recovery of consciousness.

Neuroleptanalgesia

This term is applied to combinations of a neuroleptanalgesic drug (droperidol) with a narcotic analgesic (fentanyl or phenoperidine). These produce a quiet inactive patient who will, however, respond rationally when spoken to; the respiratory-depressant effect of these drugs is definite but with appropriate dosage is not serious. They may be of value for procedures such as angiography, stereotaxic surgery and burr holes in patients unlikely to tolerate only local anaesthesia. Because these drugs do not increase ICP, even in patients with space-occupying lesions, they may be more appropriate as supplements to nitrous oxide oxygen anaesthesia than the volatile agents in these patients.

Position on table

This can be crucial in achieving good operating conditions by ensuring there is no venous congestion. Care must be taken to ensure that excessive neck rotation does not obstruct venous drainage from the head; a lateral approach demands the full lateral position with kidney and chest rests to stabilize the patient. Occipital approaches require either the lateral, three-quarters-prone or fully prone position, and the hips and shoulders must then be built up with bridges or sandbags to keep the chest and abdomen free from pressure. Venous pressure can be further lowered by raising the head-end of the table and dropping the feet. If three-pinhead fixation is used, it is essential to ensure that the patient is well-secured to prevent movement and traction on the neck.

The logical extension of this principle is to have the patient sitting up and many prefer this for posterior fossa explorations (as well as for cervical laminectomies). *Air embolism* is a danger, however, due to air sucking into large muscle, diploic or emissary veins, or into an inadvertently opened dural venous sinus. Because the venous pressure is so low that no blood escapes, the surgeon may be unaware that he or she has opened venous channels. Continuous monitoring for flow turbulence with praecordial Doppler and of end-tidal carbon dioxide provides early detection and minimizes risk. If an air embolus is suspected, the surgeon floods the operative field with saline while the anaesthetist compresses the jugular veins. Air bubbling from open veins identifies the source and permits coagulation. Since nitrous oxide diffuses into air cavities and expands, this anaesthetic agent should be avoided in the sitting position. Pressure stockings help to maintain venous pressure; a pressurized space suit, if available, is ideal. When these measures are taken, a catastrophic fall in blood pressure or cardiac arrest is rare. If this does occur, the patient must be laid down on the left side to keep air away from the opening of the pulmonary artery in the right ventricle. It may be possible to aspirate air from the heart through a central line; apart from this, the management is that of cardiac arrest. Probably most cases which develop cardiac arrest could have been suspected by a vigilant anaesthetist of having an embolus at an earlier and more readily reversible stage.

Operative approaches

Burr holes

These are commonly made for tumour biopsy, for aspiration of a chronic subdural haematoma or abscess, or for the insertion of a ventricular drainage catheter or ICP monitor. The burr hole must be so placed that a needle can be passed to the lesion without traversing vital areas of brain; and it must take account of what kind of skin flap and bone removal might be required if an open exploration should subsequently be required. The initial burr hole may form part of the flap and the direction of the skin incision is then vital (Fig. 11.2, p. 216); or the burr hole may be placed so that it will lie in the middle of a flap and the skin incision should then lie approximately at right angles to the base of the flap.

Supratentorial exploration

Before a surgeon can plan an approach to a lesion in this compartment of the skull, he or she must have fairly precise information about its situation, and should understand the relationships between the skull and the underlying structures (Fig. 5.1). The shape of the skin incision is also dictated by the need to preserve an adequate blood supply to the scalp flap, and by cosmetic considerations. When possible the incision is kept within the hair-line but if it must come down on the forehead it is usually least conspicuous if it remains strictly in the midline (Fig. 5.2). For these reasons the scalp flap may be made larger than the bone flap, the size of which depends only on the region to be explored; the bone is cut between burr holes and turned down on a pedicle of periosteum (and of muscle in the temporal region), or removed as a free flap.

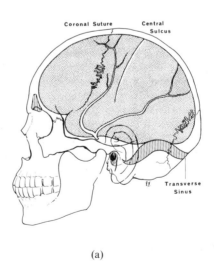

(a)

Fig. 5.1 Skull anatomy related to deep structures. (a) The upper part of the central sulcus (Rolandic fissure) lies just over 1 cm posterior to the midpoint of the arc between nasion and inion. The floor of the middle fossa is at the level of the zygoma. The frontal lobe is anterior to the central sulcus: frontal bone is anterior to the coronal suture. The middle meningeal artery soon divides into anterior and posterior branches.

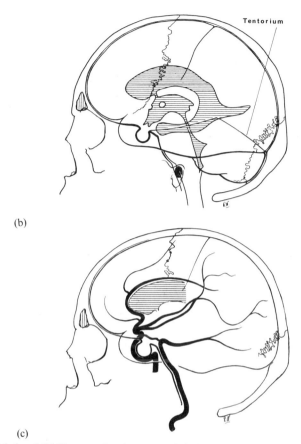

(b)

(c)

Fig. 5.1 (*cont*) (b) The tentorium is not a straight line from torcula to posterior clinoid, but is in fact a tent rising medially to a ridge; one result is that the occipital lobe overlies the cerebellum laterally. (c) The callosomarginal artery is closely applied to the roof of the lateral ventricle. The posterior communicating artery connects the carotid and basilar systems.

The most commonly used flap is the frontal, which allows access to all of the brain in front of the central sulcus, enables a frontal lobectomy to be done as an internal decompression and is also used for approaching the optic chiasm and suprasellar tumours. A satisfactory exposure of these basal structures is usually obtained by turning a large bifrontal skin flap, taken well down across the supraorbital margin where medially it may open into the frontal sinus. Unless the sinus is infected no special precautions need be taken if it is opened, but some surgeons attempt to seal off the lower opening with a graft of temporal fascia.

Posterior fossa exploration (Fig. 5.3)

Although the whole of this compartment can be explored through a midline incision, if the lesion is situated laterally, for example in the cerebellopontine angle, a lateral vertical incision allows a more direct approach. No skin or bone flap is used; instead sufficient of the occipital squama is nibbled away to form a craniectomy. A combined approach from above and below the tentorium (Fig. 5.3b) allows removal of tumours such as a tentorial meningioma lying in both supra-and infratentorial compartments.

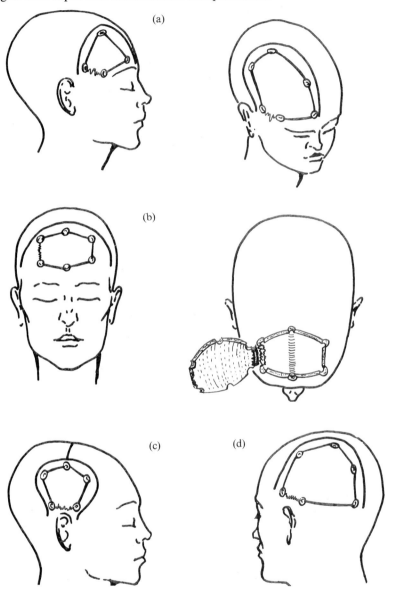

(a) Frontal (unilateral); (b) coronal (frontal bilateral); (c) lateral – split-ring incision allows access beyond the flap if necessary; (d) occipital. Many variations are possible, limited only by cosmetic considerations and the need for a sufficiently wide base to assure viability. Flaps may be rectangular rather than rounded and extra exposure can then be gained by extending one limb rather than by a split-skin incision.

Fig. 5.2 Supratentorial operative approaches.

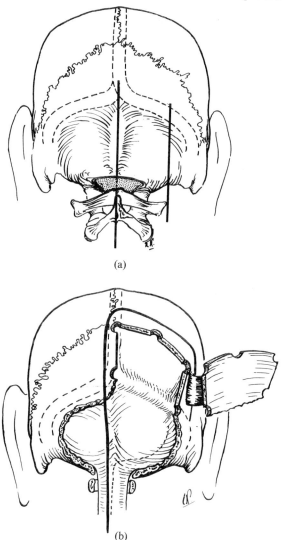

(a) Midline or paramedian incision allows sufficient access for most procedures; the incision may curve laterally at its upper end for further exposure (hockey-stick incision). (b) An additional bone flap allows division of the lateral sinus and tentorium to improve access to difficult tumours.

Fig. 5.3 Posterior fossa approaches.

Surgical means of reducing intracranial pressure

Removing the intracranial lesion is the most satisfactory method of reducing raised ICP. But with some lesions, for example infiltrative tumours, complete removal is not always possible. In these patients an *internal decompression* can be produced by removing part of the lesion or, in some instances, by performing frontal, temporal or occipital lobectomy (frontal lobectomy entails removing only the anterior half of the frontal lobe in front of the Sylvian fissure). These two methods may be combined, when a lobectomy is carried out across an infiltrative tumour, part of which is taken with the lobe, but leaving as much of it as invades areas of the brain which could not be removed without causing serious disability. If the tumour is slowly growing, an internal decompression can give a patient several years of useful life before symptoms recur.

In the posterior fossa a large portion of one cerebellar hemisphere can be removed along with the lesion without causing any serious disability. Some surgeons routinely remove part of the cerebellar hemisphere to gain access to certain lesions in the cerebellopontine angle. When there is a possibility of postoperative cerebellar swelling it is wise to carry out a wide suboccipital decompression, removing the occipital squama, the posterior rim of the foramen magnum and usually the arch of the atlas; this ensures relief of pressure on the medulla by prolapsing cerebellar tonsils. So thick is the muscle and scalp in this region that it may be almost impossible after some years to feel the bone defect at all.

An acute obstructive hydrocephalus, from a lesion around the foramen of Monro, in the pineal region or in the posterior fossa, requires urgent *ventricular drainage*. A ventricular catheter inserted through a burr hole temporarily relieves pressure. CSF drains to a sterile transfusion bottle, the height of the loop of tubing being fixed at about 150 mm above the head. A patient who is very ill with high pressure may be in better condition for operation after 24–72 hours of continuous drainage, but the risk of infection increases with a more prolonged period; another danger is upward herniation of the cerebellum through the tentorial hiatus (p. 35). Unless the causative lesion is removed and the CSF obstruction cleared, permanent CSF drainage will be required as described in Chapter 14 (p. 284). In communicating hydrocephalus, CSF drainage through the lumbar puncture route can serve as a temporary measure, perhaps avoiding the need for an internal shunt if the absorption block spontaneously clears.

CSF drainage through an intrathecal spinal catheter is often used to aid brain retraction when access to deeper structures is required.

Intracranial clot

Every neurosurgeon fears this complication, which may spoil the best operation. It may deprive the patient of some function which was carefully preserved at operation a few hours before or it may prove fatal. The cavity left when a benign tumour (e.g. meningioma) has been removed can readily bleed, as may the overlying dura which strips away from the bone to sag into the cavity. Before closing the skull the surgeon must meticulously stop all bleeding, having ensured that the blood pressure has regained its normal level if it has been low. Observation of the patient over the next 2 days is directed primarily at detecting clot formation; to establish a baseline as soon as possible, the anaesthetist is encouraged to have the patient answering simple questions and moving limbs to command before leaving the operating theatre. Any subsequent change in conscious level, power of the limbs or size of the pupils must then be explained in terms of secondary changes – haemorrhage, infarction or oedema. A clot may form within hours of leaving the theatre, and the patient who is allowed to 'sleep off' the operation, with either long-acting anaesthetic agents or postoperative sedation, may never wake up. Discomfort after craniotomy is seldom great and can be alleviated without masking changes in the conscious level by codeine, aspirin or other simple analgesics.

The signs looked for after a supratentorial operation are those sought after head injury (p. 200) – deteriorating conscious level, larger ipsilateral pupil, hemiplegia, rising blood pressure and falling pulse rate with stertorous periodic respiration. Observations of pulse, blood pressure, pupil reaction and conscious level should be recorded at least hourly for 24 hours, and for longer if there is any doubt about progress, however unkind it may appear to the patient or relatives. Sometimes a relapse is delayed till the second or third day; oedema rather than clot may be suspected. Postoperative monitoring of ICP may help to distinguish between deterioration from a haematoma or that due to infarction; pressure does not rise for 24 hours or so after infarction, if at all. CT scanning may be useful, but can be difficult to interpret in the early postoperative period; if any doubt remains the flap must be reopened.

Clot may be extradural or intradural, or both, and a single sizeable bleeding point is less often found than a general ooze. The brain is frequently oedematous after this second handling; if the bone flap is difficult to replace comfortably it is best left out and stored in deep freeze for replacement after a few weeks or months. Suturing galea a second time at this early stage is difficult; it is best to insert only a few stitches and rely on more deeply placed skin sutures than usual, and these should lie between the original skin suture marks. Infection is a risk after reopening; prophylactic antibiotics are probably a wise precaution, given in two or three large doses over 24 hours.

Posterior fossa haematomas are more treacherous because they may produce few signs before causing terminal apnoea. Continual complaint of headache, especially if accompanied by vomiting, should raise suspicion, but the respiratory rate is the most critical index; a persisting fall below 16 breaths per minute calls for careful review of all aspects of the case and inspection of the wound to see if it is tight and bulging. Even more than with supratentorial haematomas, the slightest suspicion of a clot calls for investigation, and for operation if doubt remains.

Pyrexia and infection

Early pyrexia is unlikely to be due to infection; up to 38°C in the first 48 hours may reasonably be ascribed to *reaction to blood* at the operation site or in the subarachnoid space. Hyperpyrexia may occur following operations in the region of the upper brainstem and hypothalamus; this calls for vigorous treatment (p. 207).

Delayed pyrexia, after the third day, must be presumed to indicate infection and the most likely sites must be systematically searched.

The wound

Some surgeons inspect operation wounds routinely on the first or second day; blood-soaked dressings, which are an excellent culture medium for bacteria, are removed. Subgaleal suction drains, left for 24–48 hours, avoid distension of the wound by blood or CSF. Aspiration using a sharp needle inserted into the centre of the flap or with a blunt cannula inserted through the suture line is rarely required.

The occurrence of pyrexia calls for inspection of the wound, whether this is routine or not. Stitch abscesses, once commonly seen when silk sutures were routinely used for deep and subgaleal layers, rarely occur with absorbable materials. Skin sutures or clips removed on the third day seldom provide an infective source; posterior fossa sutures are left 7–10 days and do have time to become infected. The affected stitch should be removed to allow the pus to come out and a culture taken to identify the organisms and test their sensitivity to antibiotics. Occasionally cellulitis of the wound develops, calling for systemic antibiotics. The dura is an effective barrier to infection and provided it is intact, meningitis and brain abscess rarely develop from superficial infections.

Prophylactic antibiotics probably do reduce wound infection, but since the rate is low (about 3–5%), no controlled trial has as yet produced conclusive evidence of benefit. Generally one large dose of a broad-spectrum antibiotic is given before making the incision, followed by one or two further does in the subsequent 12–24 hours. Prophylaxis is most important in circumstances known to carry a risk of infection. These include all operations in which frontal sinuses have been opened, those which were prolonged (contamination rises abruptly after about 4 hours), and wounds which were reopened for any reason.

CSF leak carries the threat of meningitis; rhinorrhoea may follow the removal of a basal anterior fossa tumour, whilst CSF may leak directly from a posterior fossa wound when the dura has been left open. Every effort must be made to stop the leak by keeping the pressure low with repeated lumbar punctures and elevation of the head of the bed; an additional skin stitch may be needed where the leak is occurring, followed by a plastic sealing. Pressurized antibiotic sprays should not be used too close to a leaking wound; a jet may distend it and carry in contaminants.

Meningitis

Blood in the CSF may produce meningism and pyrexia at an early stage, but if these develop later, meningitis must be suspected and a lumbar puncture promptly done. Even though the fluid is blood-stained the pathologist must be urged to count the cells because meningitis may be diagnosed if there is a marked excess of white cells for the amount of blood contamination (one white cell per thousand red cells). About 100–200 excess leukocytes can be accepted as a reaction to blood spilt at operation, but more than this is best regarded as evidence of infection. The fluid should be cultured, as should every aspirate in the early postoperative days, even when no infection is suspected; treatment with antibiotics should not be delayed until bacteriological confirmation (p. 180).

Abscess

The operative cavity is occasionally the site of a late intracranial abscess, weeks or months after recovery. Although this may be due to a foreign body, such as a stitch or fragment of cotton wool, it may develop with no such provocation. There may be repeated mild attacks of meningitis due to leakage of infected material, or the patient may present with raised pressure and signs of a local mass. This may suggest tumour recurrence but occurs too soon after operation for this possibility to be seriously considered. Treatment is by burr hole aspiration or by reopening the craniotomy and excision (p. 176).

Osteomyelitis

Infection of the bone flap is suspected when a sinus forms with intermittent discharge of pus, often weeks or months after operation. The chronicity is typical, whereas a brief episode of local infection, due to a loose deep suture, rapidly resolves once the offending stitch comes out.

Bone changes are difficult to detect radiologically but a frank sequestrum can be recognized as a relatively dense white shadow, and such a fragment must be removed before healing can be expected. If a sinus persists or recurs after local excision and removal of the granulation tissue, osteomyelitis must be presumed and the whole flap reopened. The inner surface of the bone is usually found to be 'worm-eaten' for several centimetres from the region of the sinus, with granulation tissue, filling the interstices of eroded bone and extending into the scalp (Fig. 5.4). Nothing short of removal of the whole bone flap will ensure immediate and permanent wound healing unless the area of bone involvement is very local indeed and can be removed by nibbling. The diseased bone flap may be replaced several months later after boiling or sterilization by gamma rays from a cobalt source, but if the bone is extensively destroyed some form of cranioplasty will be needed (p. 231).

Extracranial infection

The chest and the bladder are frequent sites of infection in a patient who is unconscious for any period, and with the inevitable absence of specific complaints, requires an active effort to exclude these sources if pyrexia develops. The management of chest complications is dealt with in relation to head injury (p. 205)

Epilepsy

Every supratentorial operation, even a burr hole, carries some risk of epilepsy, even if the underlying condition does not predispose to fits. The risk depends on the underlying pathological lesion and on the amount of cortical damage caused by the surgery. Explorations in the frontotemporal region carry a higher risk than in the occipital. Fits are more likely if epilepsy has occurred before operation, and such patients must accept that surgery does not guarantee relief from this symptom. If there is a fit in the first week after operation there is a greater risk that epilepsy will develop as a late complication. The immediate significance of an early postoperative fit is that it may herald (or precipitate) postoperative complications; but a fit in itself is not a reason for suspecting an intracranial clot.

The implications of epilepsy as a later complication are similar to those associated with traumatic epilepsy, as are prophylaxis and treatment (p. 227). Many surgeons now recommend anticonvulsants for a year after a craniotomy even when there is no definite predisposing factor, because the social consequences of a fit are so serious. Patients who are vocational drivers may have to postpone their return to work, according to local regulations.

Care of the eyes

Swelling of the eyelids develops in varying degrees after frontal craniotomy. The extent of the swelling appears to reflect individual susceptibility and anatomy rather than the nature of the operative procedure. Swelling is often very marked when a postoperative clot is developing and this can make it difficult to observe the pupil. The swelling may be mainly haematoma or oedema and usually develops several hours after operation, sometimes not until the following day, when it may blow up in a matter of minutes.

It is kind ot warn patients that one or both eyes may close temporarily after operation. Some surgeons attempt to minimize this annoying sequel by applying a pressure sponge to the eye at the conclusion of the operation, and incorporating it in the crêpe bandage securing the dressing. If this is done, great care must be taken to ensure that the eye is closed tightly so that the cornea is not abraded. Ice compresses help to reduce swelling, especially if the patient is sufficiently alert to apply them frequently for him- or herself.

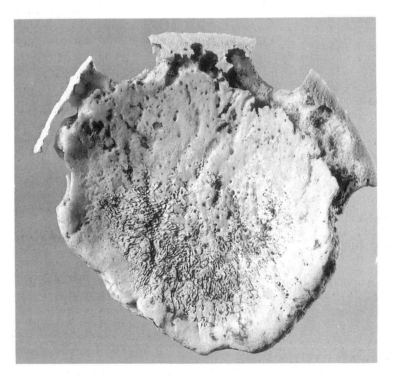

Fig. 5.4 Osteomyelitis affecting an operative bone flap. On either side of the two burr holes (on the upper circumference) the bone edge is eroded; the lower half of this bone flap is quite healthy.

Neuroparalytic keratitis is liable to develop whenever the cornea is rendered anaesthetic, either by surgical interference with the first division of the trigeminal nerve or when this is affected by tumour. The anaesthetic cornea is insensitive to small foreign bodies which, because they are ignored, abrade the cornea. Keratitis rapidly progresses to corneal ulceration, and because the condition is quite painless there is no compulsion on the patient's part to seek urgent aid. This complication can develop years after the cornea is denervated, but most instances are in the first few weeks, after which some resistance may develop.

Prevention should begin as soon as the patient returns from the theatre if it is known that the nerve may have been damaged (or has been deliberately cut). The cornea must be shielded from dust either by closing the lids with adhesive, or by wearing protective goggles. Whatever method is used, the eye must be inspected 4-hourly, when saline irrigations are carried out and hypromellose drops instilled.

If the cornea is still anaesthetic when the patient goes home, he or she must be fitted with protective spectacles to wear out of doors. A clear plastic side-piece (Everest frame) is attached to the patient's own spectacles or to a pair with plain glass lenses. He or she should be instructed to inspect the eye in the mirror, night and morning, and to report immediately if there is any redness, regardless of the presence of pain or discomfort.

When *facial palsy* accompanies trigeminal anaesthesia the risks of keratitis are very high because the eyelid cannot close efficiently. In these circumstances a prophylactic tarsorrhaphy is required: stitching the lids together in the lateral third of the palpebral fissure is sufficient protection as a rule. No anaesthetic is needed for this simple operation as the area is already insensitive. The lid margin is made raw by slicing off a thin margin of the edge and a single mattress suture of nylon is tied over thin rubber tubing. This should be left in for 14–18 days, after which the closure is normally secure but if it comes apart the stitch is simply replaced after freshening the lid margin again.

Once keratitis develops, treatment must be instituted without delay, and patients should be told where they can receive this in an emergency. When there is no ulceration the frequent instillation of Chloromycetin drops or ointment, and atropine if the patient is not elderly, with gentle closure of the middle of the lids with strapping, should be tried for 24–48 hours. If there is not rapid improvement, or ulceration develops, tarsorrhaphy must be performed immediately, and usually a more extensive one than is done prophylactically. Once the acute inflammation settles it is easy to snip it partly open with sharp scissors (without an anaesthetic).

Further reading

Campkin T.V., Perks J.S. (1973). Venous air embolism. *Lancet;* **i: 235–7.**

Cottrell J.E., Turndof H. (eds.) (1986). *Anaesthesia and Neurosurgery,* 2nd edn. St Louis: Mosby.

Dempsey R., Rapp R.P., Young B. *et al.* (1988). Prophylactic antibiotics in clean neurosurgical procedures: a review. *J. Neurosurg.;* **69:** 52 – 57.

Foy P.M., Copeland G.P., Shaw M.D.M. (1981). The incidence of postoperative seizures. *Acta Neurochir.;* **55:** 253 – 64.

Grenvik A, Safar P. (eds.) (1981). *Brain Failure and Resuscitation.* New York: Churchill Livingstone.

Jennett B. (1983). Anticonvulsant drugs and advice about driving after head injury and intracranial surgery. *Br. Med. J.*; **286:** 627 – 8.

Jennett S. (1983). Respiratory aspects of head injury. In: Fitch W., Barker J. (eds.) *Anaesthesia and Head Injuries.* Amsterdam: Excerpta Medica.

Jennett B. (1987). Epilepsy after head injury and intracranial surgery. In: Hopkins A. (ed.) *Epilepsy.* London; Chapman Hall.

Jennett W.B., Barker J., Fitch W. *et al.* (1969). Effect of anaesthesia on intracranial pressure in patients with space-occupying lesions. *Lancet*; **i: 61 – 4.**

Miller J.D., Dearden N.M. (1992). Measurement, analysis and management of raised intracranial pressure. In: Teasdale G.M., Miller J.D. (eds.) *Current Neurosurgery.* Edinburgh: Churchill Livingstone.

North J.B. (1989). Anticonvulsant prophylaxis in neurosurgery. *Br. J. Neurosurg.*; **3:** 425 – 8.

Price D.J.E., Sleigh J.D. (1970). Control of infection due to *Klebsiella aerogenes* in a neurosurgical unit by the withdrawal of all antibiotics. *Lancet*; **ii:** 1213–15.

Wirth F.P., Ratchison A.R. (eds.) (1987). *Neurosurgical Critical Care.* Baltimore; Williams & Wilkins.

Part II:

Particular Intracranial Lesions

Chapter 6

Intracranial tumours

General management

    Surgical principles
    Radiotherapy
    Chemotherapy

Classification of tumours

Glioma

    Astrocytoma
    Ependymoma
    Oligodendroglioma
    Cerebellar astrocytoma and ependymoma
    Astrocytomas in other sites

Medulloblastoma

Meningioma

Pituitary region tumours

    Hypersecreting tumours
    Hyposecreting tumours
    Clinical syndromes
    Treatment

Neuroma (schwannoma)

Acoustic neuroma

Metastatic tumours

Vascular tumours

Congenital tumours

Orbital tumours

Endocrine exophthalmos

Suspected tumour recurrence

General management

Only when an anatomical diagnosis has been made, from clinical and radiological evidence, are the pathological possibilities considered and arranged in order of likelihood. This order will depend chiefly on a knowledge of the tendency of different tumours to favour certain sites, to occur at various ages and to evolve symptomatically according to characteristic patterns.

Benign and malignant primary tumours are less clearly contrasted in the cranium than elsewhere in the body because brain tumours rarely metastasize outside the nervous system. The concept of malignancy depends therefore on other aspects of tumour behaviour such as *rate of growth* and the tendency to *infiltrate diffusely*, as contrasted with a tendency to remain circumscribed.

Whatever its nature, the *location* of an intracranial tumour is critical for many reasons: involvement of vital centres may threaten life directly or limit surgical accessibility; hydrocephalus may result from a small tumour blocking CSF flow; brain shifts and herniations, which vary with the site of the mass, may dominate the clinical picture and constitute the chief immediate danger to the patient. The paradox can arise of a small, discrete and slowly growing mass having a relentless course because it lies in a vital site such as the hypothalamus or medulla, whilst a large and histologically malignant tumour (e.g. some pineal tumours) may be compatible with long survival, if producing only symptoms due to obstructive hydrocephalus, which can be relieved by short-circuiting procedures. It is impossible to separate the nature from the location of a tumour when discussing its clinical significance and prognosis.

A surgeon's natural reaction to a tumour is to remove the whole of it. Such a straightforward solution is not always possible in the brain, where loss of function may be too high a price to pay for radical surgery.

Judging the benefits of treatment for brain tumours is difficult because crude survival rates are unsatisfactory, and the quality as well as the length of survival needs to be examined critically. Most neurosurgeons have had the experience of a patient living for years, mentally or physically crippled, after surgical endeavours which in retrospect were over-ambitious. Yet if no risks are taken a patient may be denied the only chance of cure, and surgery that is too timorous can carry as high an ultimate mortality and morbidity as that which is too bold.

Radiation treatment and, more recently, chemotherapy are also available for dealing with intracranial tumours; however, the susceptibility of the still-functioning brain, which surrounds and often traverses the tumour, places limitations on their use, as it does on the application of conventional surgical methods.

Improvements are slowly occurring with all three methods – surgery, radiation and chemotherapy; there are now clinical trials to find out what combinations of these are most effective. It is hoped that by using combined-modality therapy it may be possible to achieve additive or synergistic effects without increasing the side-effects. For example, even incomplete surgical removal almost always reduces tumour bulk by a greater proportion than either radiation or chemotherapy ever can; it is therefore logical to use these as means of dealing with residual tumour, in the hope of achieving long-term survival. Their use for palliation of inoperable tumours aims at a different objective, and it is in this context that the quality of survival has to be balanced with the mere increase in survival time.

Before dealing with the characteristics and management of specific tumours, the general principles governing the use of these three methods will be outlined.

Surgical principles

The technical feasibility of completely removing a tumour depends on many factors. The tumour may be inaccessible except by causing irreparable local damage; it may share a blood supply with more distant vital structures; regardless of situation, it may be prohibitively vascular, as are large angiomatous malformations; it may be infiltrative, like gliomas where no clear plane of cleavage from surrounding brain can be found.

Although imaging may reveal the size, blood supply and relation to vital structures of a particular tumour and strongly suggest its pathological nature, this can never be diagnosed with absolute certainty; histological confirmation is usually obtained before declaring a tumour irremovable. Even if a tumour is removable, a particular patient's interest may not always be best served by total resection, having regard to its rate of growth and the patient's natural expectation of life. A satisfactory alleviation can often be gained by partial removal with much less risk than a radical operation, and some tumours show little tendency to recur. Patients with a brain tumour are *managed* rather than *cured*; the success of treatment depends on always balancing the probable neurological morbidity of the measures employed with that expected from the natural course of the disease.

Palliative procedures
The wide range of useful procedures available for certain tumours which are irremovable contrasts with the rather bleak outlook for such growths elsewhere in the body. Properly planned palliative surgery can give the patient with a brain tumour many years of useful life even though complete removal is never attempted. Two main groups of symptoms call for palliation.

1. *Symptoms of raised ICP* always demand treatment unless the tumour is so malignant histologically or is so advanced in causing unrecoverable defects as to be quite hopeless. Raised pressure constitutes a threat to life, and often to vision (from consecutive optic atrophy). The methods available for relieving it are described in Chapter 5.
2. *Symptoms of local brain dysfunction* respond less reliably to incomplete surgical measures, even to complete tumour removal. Recovery depends on how long-standing the defect in function is, and how much extra damage either to brain itself or to its blood supply is inflicted during operation. *Vision* recovers well when chiasmal compression is relieved unless marked optic atrophy is already established. *Hemiplegia* due to hemisphere involvement is usually at least partially improved when a tumorous cyst is evacuated; but the manipulation of a vascular infiltrative tumour often aggravates the paralysis, although this effect may be only temporary. *Epilepsy* may undergo a temporary or permanent remission following surgery, or the pattern of the seizures may be altered; but it is unwise ever to promise that the attacks will cease. *Cerebellar symptoms*, ataxia and vertigo, are often satisfactorily relieved by subtotal removal of a laterally placed tumour, even when a considerable part of the cerebellar

hemisphere is sacrificed, provided that the dentate nucleus and vermis are left intact.

Radiotherapy

Although susceptibility of the normal brain to irradiation produces some limitations, radiotherapy remains a useful adjunct in the treatment of many cerebral tumours. The dose can be restricted to the region of the tumour (partial brain irradiation) or focused on a 3 cm target (stereotactic radiosurgery), but this is not always appropriate. Some tumours, such as medulloblastoma which can disseminate along CSF pathways, require whole neural axis treatment, irradiating both brain and spinal cord. Even a glioma, appearing well-circumscribed on imaging, may infiltrate widely throughout surrounding brain. For these reasons irradiation should extend at least 3–4 cm beyond the margin of those parts of the lesion which enhance with contrast on CT scan. Many patients require whole-brain therapy.

Measures designed to radiosensitize the tumour are currently under study. The hypoxic cell sensitizer (misonidazole) has produced no obvious benefit but second-generation analogues (etanidazole) may prove more promising. Another biochemical approach involves halogenated pyrimidines which are incorporated into DNA of rapidly proliferating tumour cells; preliminary results look hopeful.

The stereotactic implantation of radioactive seeds (brachytherapy) achieves a very high local radiation dose without significant risk to surrounding tissues. Encouraging results in non-randomized studies treating recurrent glioblastoma have led some centres to use brachytherapy within the initial treatment plan.

Complications

Radiotherapy does not usually cause any immediate upset and constitutional disturbances such as normally accompany irradiation of the thorax or abdomen. Some temporary *epilation* may occur, depending on dose, and occasionally this is permanent. Sometimes a rapidly growing tumour appears to swell during the early stages of a course of radiation, and it is wise to provide a decompression of some kind for such tumours before radiation is begun; such protection may be conferred by a course of steroids (p. 75).

The susceptibility of normal brain tissue to radiation is the factor limiting dosage, even when treating a sensitive tumour in a circumscribed situation, e.g. a pituitary adenoma. Because the harmful effects from excessive radiation (radionecrosis) to an area of brain may take from 6 months to 10 years (usually 2 years) to appear, the importance of this risk was only gradually appreciated. Many patients died of recurrent tumour without living long enough to develop radionecrosis, whilst those who did succumb to an overdose of X-rays were often assumed to have died of recurrence. The affected tissue becomes ischaemic due to a fibrinoid necrosis in small vessels; the mechanism of the necrosis and the reason for the long latent period are unexplained. The hypothalamus is particularly vulnerable to X-rays, and is liable to be in the target area when the pituitary is irradiated; delayed radiation effects here are usually fatal. Elsewhere, however, there may be no more than the rather sudden reappearance of symptoms similar to those originally caused by the tumour; these may as rapidly subside without treatment.

Now that the dangers of radionecrosis are appreciated and more refined methods of irradiation are available, there should be little risk of producing any additional brain damage.

Chemotherapy

Most known cytotoxic drugs have been tried for malignant glioma. Administration has been by oral or intravenous route as well as by local intralesional and intracarotid injection. The nitrosourea group (BCNU, CCNU, Methyl CCNU) are cell-cycle non-specific agents which are fat-soluble and enter the brain well. These agents have shown promise in prospective clinical trials, with significant responses in up to 40% of patients with malignant glioma of the brain. The most striking results have been obtained using adjunctive chemotherapy in combined-modality treatment in an attempt to achieve additive or synergistic effects without increasing toxicity. Further improvement in results may come from the use of different combinations of drugs for chemotherapy. Considerable interest has developed in attempting to improve methods of drug delivery to the tumour bed. Direct intracarotid injection, however, whether or not combined with disruption of the blood – brain barrier, has produced no obvious benefit.

Monoclonal antibodies can serve as carriers of cytotoxic drugs but transfer through the blood – brain barrier and lack of specificity have presented problems. Intrathecal or intraventricular use in patients with carcinomatous meningitis however appears to prolong survival. The use of liposomes, bound to the cytotoxic agent alone or in combination with monoclonal antibodies, may improve access to the tumour bed, but these techniques await evaluation. Systemic toxic effects of cytotoxic agents in the doses required for brain tumours are seldom marked, but marrow depression can occur. Toxic peripheral neuropathy occurs with some drugs, and brain necrosis sometimes develops after combined chemotherapy and radiotherapy.

Corticosteroids are widely used, often with dramatic effect, to control symptoms associated with brain tumour (p. 75). Steroids act by reducing oedema in surrounding brain rather than by producing any significant oncolytic effect.

Classification of tumours

The natural history and gross anatomy of tumours claim most attention in the account which follows, and microscopic characteristics are dealt with only briefly. The cellular origin of many brain tumours remains controversial and there is no close correlation between minor histological differences and the clinical behaviour of tumours.

Even when *histological criteria* are considered alone there are difficulties in attaching useful or practically significant labels to many tumours. Well-differentiated tumours may recur relentlessly because their diffuseness defies total surgical resection. Any one tumour may not be homogeneous; histological sections from one part may appear more benign than from another. Diagnosis based on a relatively small biopsy is therefore less reliable than an autopsy study of the whole tumour. Furthermore tumours may change their character over a period of time, with increasing anaplasia, and difficulties are then encountered when a single name is sought for a tumour which has been observed in a patient over many years.

The published accounts of the frequency of different tumour types depend on the source of the series which is analysed: surgical series commonly contain more benign, and necropsy figures more malignant, tumours.

The approximate distribution of 950 intracranial tumours encountered over 5 years in the Institute of Neurological Sciences, Glasgow was:

Neuroectodermal		53%
astrocytoma		
(all grades, including glioblastoma)	48%	
ependymoma	1.3%	
oligodendroglioma	1%	
medulloblastoma	2.4%	
Metastatic		15%
Meningioma		15%
Pituitary		3.3%
Acoustic neuroma		5.3%

Neuroectodermal tumours arise from cells derived from the primitive neuroectoderm which is represented in the mature nervous system by the neuroglia, viz. astrocytes, oligodendrocytes and ependymal cells, and by nerve cells. The great majority of cerebral tumours arise from the neuroglial cells and are known collectively as the gliomas.

Glioma

The neuroglia is structurally the connective tissue of the nervous system and is found throughout the brain and spinal cord; gliomas, likewise, may be widely distributed. These tumours are most difficult to put in clear-cut categories which reflect a consistent natural history; even their accurate pathological classification is difficult because of the great histological variations that may occur within an individual tumour.

Pathology

For many years after publication in 1926, the authoritative scheme of Bailey and Cushing was accepted. They held that the tumours fell into 14 discrete groups, each derived from a different embryonic cell type. Most subsequent classifications have been based on this scheme, although many attempts have been made to simplify it. Kernohan and Adson in 1949 reduced the field to five main groups, in four of which they believed that they could recognize four grades of malignancy – viz. astrocytoma grades 1–4, ependymoma grades 1–4, oligodendroglioma grades 1–4, neuroastrocytoma grades 1–4 (rarely encountered) and medulloblastoma (homogeneous group). The propriety of classifying the last two groups as gliomas may, however, be questioned as the most prominent cell types belong to the neuronal series of cells and not to the glial series. Recently the World Health Organization proposed a more workable system, classifying astrocytoma into three grades: astrocytoma, anaplastic astrocytoma and glioblastoma multiforme, the last being separated from its predecessor by the presence of necrosis. Criticism of any system is that if the grading of the tumour is based on a burr hole biopsy, it implies a much greater degree of accuracy than can legitimately be claimed, particularly if any prognostic significance is placed on a biopsy showing the features of a well-differentiated (grade 1) tumour.

Astrocytoma

This is by far the commonest of the gliomas and includes a wide range of tumours from those composed of well-differentiated cells where the predominant cell type is very similar to particular types of astrocyte, e.g. fibrillary, protoplasmic, gemistocytic, to highly anaplastic tumours. All grades of anaplasia may be encountered in different parts of the same tumour, and initially mature astrocytomas above the tentorium display a strong tendency to become anaplastic with the passage of time.

Diffuseness is often the chief characteristic of a *well-differentiated astrocytoma* and it is often impossible to define any edge to the tumour: the affected area of the brain is simply expanded, firm and often rather pale. Even on microscopic examination there is a very gradual transition from obvious tumour to normal brain. In this transitional zone the appearances may be very difficult to distinguish from reactive gliosis. In extreme examples of diffuse astrocytoma there may be no real tumour mass. More often, however, there is a fleshy or friable tumour of low cellularity within which there may be small cysts. Large cysts filled with clear yellow fluid, which clots when exposed to air, are of frequent occurrence in well-differentiated astrocytomas of the cerebellum, where tumour cells may be confined to a circumscribed mural nodule. Similar cysts are less frequently encountered in astrocytomas in the cerebral hemispheres.

Anaplastic astrocytomas are characterized by the presence of poorly differentiated anaplastic and pleomorphic cells of astrocytic type. In most anaplastic tumours, there are sheets of closely packed tumour cells, the majority of which are usually small, although there may also be numerous multinucleate giant cells in some tumours; mitotic figures are frequent and endothelial hyperplasia is often intense. These tumours may appear to have a more clearly defined edge than low-grade astrocytomas, though this is not necessarily borne out by microscopic examination.

Glioblastoma multiforme, the most malignant type, is characterized by the additional presence of necrosis. The lack of differentiation may mask the astrocytic cell origin. Growth is rapid and areas of haemorrhage often occur within the tumour. Cysts, when present, usually contain fluid which is turbid or even creamy and pus-like – the result of necrosis.

Anaplasia is a very frequent occurrence in astrocytoma and may develop at any stage in its life history. The more carefully it is sought, the more likely it is to be found and this is the principal reason why some pathologists are reluctant to apply a particular grade to an astrocytoma on the basis of a small biopsy. Because of the great variation that may be present in any one tumour, a biopsy from one area may have the typical appearance of a well-differentiated tumour while a biopsy taken from a different area may show a highly anaplastic tumour.

The growing edge of a tumour may appear to be confined within a gyrus but sometimes the pia arachnoid is invaded and a carpet of tumour spreads over the surface of the brain. More rarely the dura is involved, but only by malignant tumours. The ependyma may also be breached so that tumour occupies the ventricular cavity; seeding can occur in the subarachnoid or ventricular spaces (but is much less common than from an ependymoma or medulloblastoma) and may give rise to tumour cells in CSF and secondary blocks to CSF flow. Subarachnoid haemorrhage, rare with any tumour, is most frequently found to come from an astrocytoma which abuts on CSF pathways.

Astrocytomas may occur in any age group but some types of mature fibrillary astrocytoma are particularly common in childhood. In the cerebellum and optic nerve these tumours are more benign than any other type of glioma. Even after incomplete removal they may stop growing, or even regress, leading to the suggestion that growth is arrested when the child reaches maturity, as with hamartomas.

Anaplastic change in an astrocytoma may also occur at any age but is more common in adults. Primary glioblastoma multiforme is, however, distinctly rare under the age of 30. These rapidly growing tumours occur mainly in the cerebral hemispheres, particularly in the temporal lobe, and are rare in the cerebellum and brainstem. In the latter site, astrocytomas are usually of the diffuse infiltrating type and are usually well-differentiated and slow-growing.

Ependymoma

Over 50% are in children, mostly aged 8–15 years. Some 60% occur below the tent although ependymomas make up only 10% of posterior fossa tumours under the age of 12. The tumour normally grows from the floor of the fourth ventricle, making total removal impossible, but occasionally the tumour arises in the cerebellopontine angle and spares the fourth ventricle; only 10% are cystic.

Supratentorial ependymomas are usually related to some part of the lateral ventricle but they may also occur in the third ventricle. The lobulated tumour may develop a large cyst anteriorly which may block the foramen of Monro. Supratentorial tumours calcify more frequently than those in the fourth ventricle.

This red nodular tumour, tufty like a cauliflower, and firm because of the dense network of branching vessels, tends to conform to the shape of its surroundings. Histologically there are rosettes and solid clusters of cells. Metastasis by CSF pathways occasionally occurs from paraventricular growths and sometimes it appears to have been precipitated by operation. As with astrocytomas, ependymomas may become anaplastic, as shown by the increased cellularity, necrosis and haemorrhage.

Oligodendroglioma

This occurs superficially in the cerebral hemisphere, and may mushroom through the surface and become adherent to the dura and be mistaken for a meningioma. Mucoid cysts and necrosis occur, and there is a special liability to spontaneous haemorrhage which may lead to sudden clinical deterioration. Calcification, related to vessel walls, is visible on X-ray as irregular strands over a wide area (Fig. 4.2); over half of these tumours calcify. Widespread meningeal and ventricular metastases may develop, possibly precipitated by surgery; this event bears no relation to histological malignancy but depends more on the proximity of the tumour to CSF pathways. Microscopically there are uniform sheets of small polyhedral spaces (clear cytoplasm) containing round nuclei. In keeping with other gliomas this tumour may become anaplastic. Most cases are in adults.

Clinical

Diffuse astrocytoma of cerebral hemisphere

The greater part of one hemisphere is swollen and firmer than normal. The white matter is expanded and rubbery in consistency, and the affected brain retains its shape when cut into, staying stiffly open instead of falling together as normal brain does. A cannula passed through the affected area at operation is 'gripped' by the tumour tissue.

The clinical history is often already long by the time the patient comes for investigation, perhaps several years after the onset of epilepsy. Gradually slight weakness of a limb appears, and there may be mild mental changes; eventually more definite hemiplegia develops, perhaps with signs of raised pressure. CT scanning shows a low-density region, seldom enhancing with contrast and usually without mass effect.

Surgery cannot help the patient with this tumour, except for a decompression when there is raised pressure. Radiotherapy has less effect on slowly growing tumours and it is not known whether or not it influences the course of these tumours. When a patient presents with a history of epilepsy and has no physical disability, the question of management is difficult. Untreated the tumour may grow only slowly and the patient may continue to live usefully for years, whereas operation may add to the disability without improving the prospects. In these patients histological verification may be deferred, provided the clinical history and radiological investigation leave no serious doubt about the diffuse and consequently irremovable nature of the tumour. Moreover the recognition of this tumour histologically is not always easy, especially when

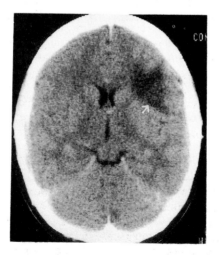

Fig. 6.1 CT of a low-grade astrocytoma showing a diffuse low-density region, unchanged after contrast enhancement, without significant mass effect.

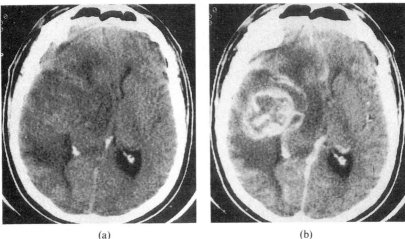

(a)   (b)

(a) Plain scan showing a marked low-density area with ventricular compression and displacement. (b) With contrast enhancement, showing irregular tumour enhancement with surrounding oedema.

Fig. 6.2 CT of glioblastoma multiforme.

only a fragment of tissue is recovered from a burr hole biopsy. In reaching a decision the particular needs of individual patients have to be sympathetically appraised. A semiliterate artisan, a practising barrister, a harassed young mother and a lonely old widow: each has very different requirements – reasons perhaps for wanting to postpone for a year or so any measure which might result in additional disabilities, or reasons for wanting to have the diagnosis confirmed beyond doubt and without delay. Such matters must be given due weight in reaching a decision both in regard to how far to investigate, and how vigorously to treat a patient suspected of having this type of tumour.

Localized astrocytoma of cerebral hemisphere

Any region can be involved but the occipital pole is rarely affected; frontal tumours tend to cross the midline in the region of the corpus callosum, forming a 'butterfly' tumour constricted in the middle. Only part of the tumour is in fact circumscribed, and elsewhere it blends with tough, expanded white matter like a diffuse tumour; the circumscribed area may be cystic. Localized astrocytomas in the cerebral hemispheres show a marked tendency to anaplastic change (p. 100); one series of astrocytomas, reported on surgical biopsy as benign, showed anaplasia in over 90% at subsequent autopsy, mostly years later.

According to the rate of growth, the history of epilepsy, hemiplegia and raised pressure may spread over many years or be telescoped into months or even weeks. Worsening is sometimes associated with a cyst, and simple aspiration may reverse the clinical course for a time. Terminal deterioration is more often due to brain shifts developing than to any new event in the tumour itself.

CT scanning is the investigation of choice in these patients. Not only will it reveal the site of the tumour but it will also show the extent of its mass effect. A low-density lesion extending through white matter with little mass effect suggests a diffuse low-grade astrocytoma (Fig. 6.1). Anaplastic astrocytomas or glioblastoma tend to enhance irregularly after contrast and cause considerable ventricular compression and midline shift. Cystic or necrotic low-density regions may be evident within the tumour mass. Surrounding low density represents oedema but the exact tumour margin is never clear (Fig. 6.2). Calcified regions within the tumour substance suggest oligodendroglioma.

MRI provides limited additional information. The anatomical effects are more clearly delineated and gadolinium may help distinguish the true tumour – oedema interface.

Angiography is now seldom performed if CT or MRI is available. Astrocytomas of intermediate degrees of anaplasia usually show only local displacement, whilst highly anaplastic tumours, including glioblastoma, often have an obvious tumour circulation with abnormal vessels and small arteriovenous fistulae.

If CT scanning is unavailable, isotope scanning will provide a high detection rate but fails to demonstrate whether the lesion is tumour, abscess or stroke.

Treatment of cerebral gliomas

Anaplastic astrocytoma and glioblastoma multiforme are the commonest types of brain tumour and unfortunately the least satisfactory to treat. Even those gliomas which at first appear circumscribed are generally discovered to merge indistinguishably with the brain at some point; many spread across the midline as well as extensively in the hemisphere in which they arise. Radical surgery is therefore misdirected zeal, for even hemispherectomy may not ensure complete eradication. As many of these tumours are slowly growing, however, limited surgical removal offers a fair prospect of palliation.

For a relatively circumscribed glioma in the frontal or occipital pole, or the right temporal lobe, a lobectomy will provide an internal decompression, and most of the tumour may be removed. The hope that a really small tumour in this situation may be found and totally removed is seldom realized because diagnosis in these clinically silent sites is not usually made until the tumour is large. If the tumour is near the central sulcus, in the posterior frontal or the parietal region, an extensive resection risks hemiplegia if this has not already developed. When a tumour in this situation is causing raised pressure without severe hemiplegia a limited intracapsular removal is sometimes attempted. By keeping within the tumour substance the surgeon hopes to remove the centre of the tumour and reduce its bulk without endangering the surrounding and still functioning brain. But such a technique cannot be relied on to preserve function; during the operation embarrassing bleeding may develop, which can be controlled only by removing more tumour than was intended, and the operation then becomes much more extensive than was originally planned. The coagulation of a large vessel in the neighbourhood can be enough to precipitate hemiplegia or dysphasia.

When a glioma has already caused profound hemiplegia or dysphasia there is little hope of restoring function by operation unless there is a large cyst to be drained. Few people wish to see the lives of such seriously disabled patients prolonged by the simple relief of pressure; but before accepting such a case as hopeless it is often necessary to confirm the diagnosis; should this reveal a meningioma or granuloma, the outlook is quite different.

Burr hope biopsy will usually provide enough tissue for a firm diagnosis, and also enables a cyst to be drained, whilst avoiding a major operation and external decompression. A blunt brain cannula is advanced into the brain, guided by an ultrasonic probe if available. The surgeon may detect a change in consistency when the cannula tip penetrates tumour. Suction with a well-fitting 5 ml syringe will usually leave a small plug of tissue in the end of the needle. By smear or frozen section it should be possible to recognize a malignant tumour; the distinction between a metastasis and glioblastoma may not always be possible, nor is it very important at this stage. Very necrotic tissue, almost like pus, may be aspirated from a metastasis, less often from a glioblastoma; such material is often too degenerate for any cells to be recognized. Clear yellow fluid indicates a gliomatous cyst, even though no tissue can be aspirated from the wall. Sometimes biopsy is unsuccessful, either because the tumour is missed by the needle or because a firm tumour is encountered from which no material can be aspirated; in these circumstances there is no option but to turn a bone flap and confirm the diagnosis directly. Small and deeply situated midline lesions require a stereotactic biopsy. This technique is described in detail in Chapter 16. It allows accurate placement of the fine biopsy cannula tip to within 1 mm of the chosen site; the surgeon can select one or more regions from which to obtain tissue. The specimen size is however small and histological recognition at times proves difficult. Biopsy through a burr hole may provoke bleeding in a vascular tumour and the patient's condition may deteriorate rapidly afterwards. This danger is inherent in the method, which must therefore be employed only in circumstances that make it proper to accept such a risk. Because of this it is essential to have a pathologist available to give an immediate report, so that if the patient deteriorates a few hours later the surgeon is in a position to decide what action to take.

Prognosis of cerebral gliomas

In cerebral gliomas of the astrocytoma series the outlook depends on grade site and age. In one series covering all sites in the brain, 66% of patients with low-grade gliomas were alive at 3 years compared with less than 4% of patients with glioblastoma. For patients with malignant tumours of the cerebral hemispheres, most of which are glioblastomas, the median survival is 4–6 months after diagnostic biopsy alone with no further treatment. In one study radical surgery with radiotherapy and BCNU resulted in a median survival of 40 weeks, which contrasted with 17 weeks for those treated with surgery alone. At 18 months, nearly all patients who received only one or two modalities of treatment were dead, whereas 25% of those receiving surgery supplemented by radiotherapy and chemotherapy were alive.

Although of uncertain benefit in glioblastoma, BCNU and PCV (procarbazine, CCNU and vincristine) do appear to extend survival in anaplastic astrocytomas – one series reported a doubling of survival from 82 to 157 weeks when treatment with PCV followed surgery and radiotherapy. Similarly, patients with oligodendroglioma do appear to show some response to chemotherapy. Some non-randomized studies suggest that brachytherapy, first used for the treatment of recurrent glioblastoma, may improve survival when incorporated into the initial treatment plan.

Every surgeon has a few patients who survive 5 years or more, and some with diffuse astrocytomas whose total history spans 10 or 20 years before treatment. The duration of survival after operation may give a false notion of the natural history of a tumour, because surgery is somewhat arbitrarily timed in the course of the disease. Those tumours which will have a long survival cannot yet be recognized in advance, nor does their favourable course reflect particularly effective treatment – they are as likely to have had a burr hole biopsy and radiation as an extensive resection. Indeed, of 13 patients in whom frontal lobectomies were believed to have totally extirpated a glioma, 11 were dead with recurrence within 3 years. Ependymomas behave like relatively favourable astrocytomas, oligodendrogliomas in much the same way.

Cerebellar astrocytoma and ependymoma

These are tumours of childhood. The astrocytoma is usually a well-differentiated fibrillary tumour, forming a cyst with a mural nodule; the rest of the cyst wall is made up of condensed non-tumorous tissue. Probably most originate near the midline, but spread into the hemisphere. A few astrocytomas and most ependymomas grow into the cavity of the fourth ventricle; they are mainly solid and may undergo anaplasia. Adults occasionally develop cerebellar astrocytomas, which then have the unfavourable characteristics of cerebral growths.

These children, commonly aged 6–12 years, present with signs of obstructive hydrocephalus – morning headache and vomiting. It is often possible to elicit an account of long-standing unsteadiness of gait, occasional vomiting without headache, and a head tilt. Chronic papilloedema, a biggish head, nystagmus and limb ataxia have usually developed by the time the surgeon sees the patient. CT scanning or MRI confirms the diagnosis (Fig. 6.3a).

Cystic astrocytoma calls for removal of the mural nodule only; the rest of the wall of the cyst is non-tumorous. More solid tumours may have to be incompletely removed because of invasion of the floor of the fourth ventricle,

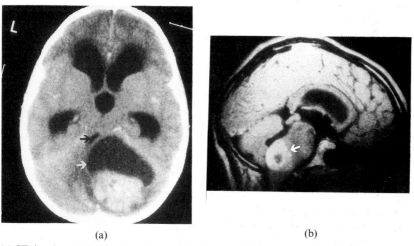

(a) (b)

(a) CT showing cerebellar astrocytoma with a large cystic component (white arrow), compressing the fourth ventricle (black arrow) and causing obstructive hydrocephalus. (b) T1-weighted MRI scan with gadopentetate contrast, showing astrocytoma within the brainstem.

Fig. 6.3 Astrocytoma in the posterior fossa.

although the outlook may still be good even without radiation. Recurrences after 30 years have been recorded, sometimes with the histological appearance of the tumour indistinguishable from that removed years previously.

Ependymoma is rather less benign, because involvement of the floor of the fourth ventricle often limits tumour removal. It is relatively radiosensitive, however, and long survivals are possible if radiation is given to the site of any remnants of tumour; recurrences after many years can still occur, however.

Astrocytomas in other sites

In the *third ventricle* astrocytoma takes the form of a piloid growth in childhood. This dense white mass remains well-demarcated above, but below invades the hypothalamus, producing endocrine disturbance – obesity, diabetes insipidus, and either infantilism or sexual precocity. The optic chiasma may be involved with subsequent visual failure, and eventually hydrocephalus supervenes from blockage of the foramen of Monro. Although this tumour remains histologically benign, involvement of vital structures prevents complete removal and death usually follows within a year; pressure may be temporarily relieved by a ventriculoperitoneal shunt or ventriculocisternostomy.

In the *basal ganglia* in adults local astrocytoma has the same tendency to anaplasia as in the hemisphere. Dense hemiplegia from involvement of the internal capsule may be associated with hydrocephalus from blockage of the foramen of Monro. Palliation may be achieved by CSF drainage followed by radiotherapy.

In the *brainstem* an astrocytoma usually grows diffusely, expanding the pons, which retains its shape. This condition has been known in the past as diffuse hypertrophy of the pons. Although most common in children aged 3–8 years, and fibrillary in type, it also occurs in adults and may undergo malignant change. Multiple cranial nerve palsies predominate over pyramidal signs, and evidence of raised pressure may never develop. In children personality and behavioural changes may be early signs. A sagittal MRI gives most information and usually defines the tumour margins (Fig. 6.3b). A CT scan may show diffuse low-density change within a thickened pons. Biopsy is seldom feasible. Radiotherapy, although often given, is unlikely to prolong survival and most patients die within a year.

In the *optic nerve* astrocytoma is also piloid and occurs in children, who often show stigmata of neurofibromatosis. It presents as a suprasellar mass with visual deterioration. Extension into the orbit causes proptosis (p. 136).

Medulloblastoma

Tumours of the neuron series are much less common than gliomas, and those containing identifiable ganglion cells are extremely rare. Medulloblastoma is the only frequently encountered tumour in this group.

Pathology
This highly malignant tumour forms a soft purplish mass which grows in the vermis of the cerebellum, invading the cavity of the fourth ventricle from the roof and obstructing the flow of CSF. It may spread up the cavity of the

aqueduct to the third ventricle and *seed* through the subarachnoid space. This takes the form of grey sheets, tough with connective tissue, in the spinal arachnoid and over the convexity of the cerebral hemisphere. Distant *metastases* occasionally occur, when growth has breached the dura after operation; bones, lymph nodes and connective tissue of the trunk have been involved in reported cases. Microscopically the closely packed uniform round cells with frequent mitoses and occasional rosettes resemble no normal adult cells.

Clinical

This tumour of childhood is twice as frequent in boys as girls and is commonest between the ages of 6 and 10 years.

The clinical syndrome is remarkably similar from patient to patient. Morning vomiting, sometimes accompanied by headache, is followed after a few weeks by staggering gait. Lateralized cerebellar signs and nystagmus are unusual, but trunkal ataxia may be so severe that the child cannot sit up in bed and is quite unable to stand. Neck stiffness is common. Distant CNS signs suggest spread, directly or by seeding, to other parts of the nervous system.

This tumour does occasionally occur in young adults, affecting the cerebellar hemisphere. It behaves like a local cerebral astrocytoma without a tendency to seeding and with a better prognosis than the vermis tumour in children.

Treatment

Medulloblastoma is a consistently malignant tumour and about 5% of children die within a month of operation; the average survival without radiation is about 6 months. As much tumour as possible is removed at operation as is compatible with avoiding serious postoperative deficit. Exploration is also essential to confirm the diagnosis because clinically and radiologically this tumour may be indistinguishable from astrocytoma and ependymoma. Radiation is the sheet anchor of treatment, and should be given as soon as the diagnosis is confirmed. Because of the tendency of this tumour to spread through the CSF pathways the whole neuraxis is treated, making a spade-like field of brain and spinal cord; for the same reason a CSF shunt should be avoided if possible. Of those who live long enough to have this radical radiation, 60% are alive 5 years later. Adjunctive chemotherapy is often given, but its benefits have not been established in randomized studies.

Meningioma

The surgeon's interest in meningiomas springs from the prospect of total removal and cure in a number of cases. This accounts for a greater concern than may seem to be deserved by a tumour which makes up only a fifth of the intracranial growths seen.

Pathology

Causative factors

Preceding *trauma* is associated with several of these tumours, especially those arising from the meninges of the vault. A relationship between trauma and neoplasia is always difficult to confirm, but cases are recorded of blows on the head followed years later by a meningioma, the stalk of which lies exactly underneath the scalp scar. The association seems more frequent than chance would explain, and no such coincidence has been noticed with other and more common brain tumours.

An aggravating, rather than precipitating, factor is *pregnancy*. Patients with slowly growing and inaccessible tumours have suffered worsening of neurological signs in successive pregnancies, and sometimes also at the menses, with complete remission between these episodes.

Gross appearance

Regardless of histology, meningiomas conform to two growth patterns. *Global* tumours are approximately spherical except where local rigid anatomy distorts this outline; they often arise from a small area of dura, although more extensive secondary dural attachment may develop. *En plaque* growth implies a flat pancake of tumour, usually under an area of thickened and involved bone; this type is mainly confined to the pterion and bregma and tends to invade pia arachnoid and blend intimately with the brain. Both types of tumour are firm, pink masses with a lobulated or finely nodular surface on which supplying vessels ramify. Most tumours are clearly demarcated from the brain, but limited invasion may occur without other evidence of malignancy or any great tendency to recur, provided a complete removal is effected. Some of the firmer tumours are gritty with flecks of calcification, a few are rock hard and may contain formed bone. Cysts are highly unusual, but when they occur are usually at one pole of the tumour between it and the brain. Multiple meningiomas, apparently unrelated, occur in 5–15% of patients with meningiomas examined at autopsy.

Bone changes

The great majority of meningiomas are related to the skull, of which the dura is the inner periosteum. Bone reacts to neighbouring tumour growth in different ways. Most often a conical overgrowth of bone butts into the base of the tumour; this *endostosis* is a non-specific reaction to periosteal stripping and increased vascularity and may contain no tumour. Bone reaction involving the outer table gives rise to a palpable lump on the skull – an *exostosis*. Even without obvious erosion, tumour may invade the Haversian canals of the thickened, vascular bone and recurrence can stem from this source. Bone changes indicate both the site and the nature of the tumour in over a third of meningiomas. Skull X-ray may also show increased diploic venous channels and meningeal arterial grooves; only a few meningiomas undergo sufficiently dense calcification to cast a shadow on X-ray (Fig. 4.4).

Spread

Tumour may erode either hyperostotic or otherwise normal bone to form a mushroom of tumour under the scalp, but the galea prevents its further outward spread. Once bone is breached meningioma may spread to temporal muscle or invade the surrounding cavities of the orbit, air sinuses or the middle ear. Rarely an undifferentiated meningioma metastasizes to viscera, but this is a pathological oddity not usually considered in managing patients with these essentially benign tumours.

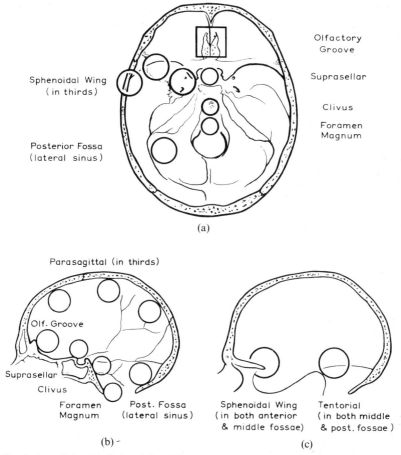

(a) Basal – lateral sites labelled on left; midline on right; (b) parasagittal section; (c) more lateral parasagittal section.

Fig. 6.4 Meningioma: sites of predilection (excluding convexity tumours).

Microscopic appearance

Arachnoid villi buried in dura give rise to these largely fibrous tumours, but whether they are essentially endothelial or mesothelial is an open question. Cushing's term 'meningioma' was purposely chosen to avoid implicating any one theory of origin.

Many subgroups have been labelled by various authorities, but most show a preponderance either of whorls of spindle cells around central hyaline material which eventually calcifies, forming psammoma bodies, or of interlacing bundles of elongated fibroblasts with narrow nuclei. Some are angioblastic and may be indistinguishable histologically from a cerebellar haemangioblastoma.

A sarcomatous variety occurs, particularly in children; it favours the posterior third of the parasagittal region in both children and adults.

Histological appearance has little to do with biological behaviour except for the sarcomatous type which is apt both to infiltrate and to recur. Tumours growing *en plaque* tend to invade pia arachnoid, yet histologically they conform to no single pattern. The recurrence of a fifth of meningiomas, even after apparently adequate surgical removal, appears to result from a failure to perform a sufficiently radical operation rather than to a more malignant type of tumour.

Clinical

The site of the tumour determines not only the clinical features but also the surgical accessibility. Over 90% are supratentorial and over two-thirds of these are in the anterior half of the skull (Fig. 6.4). Meningiomas are most common in adults, especially in middle-aged women, but occasionally occur in children. The frequency of tumours in the more commonly affected sites is approximately as follows:

Parasagittal   25%
Convexity   20%

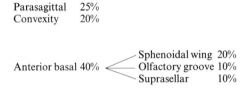

Anterior basal 40% Sphenoidal wing 20%
Olfactory groove 10%
Suprasellar   10%

Parasagittal

These arise in relation to the sagittal (superior longitudinal) sinus, most often in its *middle third* where they frequently cause focal epilepsy and later paralysis, both of which affect mainly the foot. This may lead to detection whilst the tumour is still quite small. *Anterior third* meningiomas tend to be bilateral and to cause only mental symptoms, so that the presence of a tumour is sometimes not suspected until it is so large that the patient is blind from papilloedema.

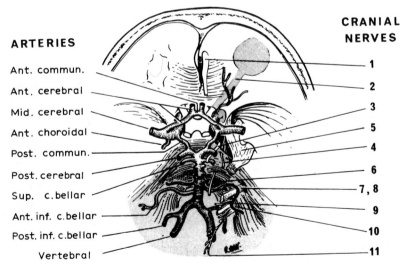

ARTERIES

Ant. commun.
Ant. cerebral
Mid. cerebral
Ant. choroidal
Post. commun.
Post. cerebral
Sup. c.bellar
Ant. inf. c.bellar
Post. inf. c.bellar
Vertebral

CRANIAL NERVES

1
2
3
5
4
6
7, 8
9
10
11

Fig. 6.5 Anatomy of the skull base showing structures which may be involved by basal meningiomas.

Tumours arising primarily *from the falx* also favour the anterior third and tend to be bilateral, producing a similar syndrome. At the *bregma* a parasagittal meningioma often gives rise to marked exostosis, and a lump may have been noticed on the head since childhood. The intradural component of this hyperostotic tumour is usually *en plaque*, frequently bilateral and sometimes consists of only a carpet of tumour down both sides of the falx; no marked indentation of the brain occurs and there may be neither neurological disorder nor any evidence of raised ICP, unless this develops due to sinus obstruction by tumour. The few parasagittal meningiomas which develop in the *posterior third* of the sinus tend to grow large before papilloedema or hemianopia leads to their being detected; they tend to be sarcomatous.

Convexity
These are initially free of any sinus attachment, and more than 70% are frontal, anterior to the central sulcus; more than half arise from the region of the coronal suture. Like parasagittal tumours they may, if growing well in front of the central sulcus, remain silent until they become large. Further back they soon cause faciobrachial hemiplegia and focal epilepsy.

Anterior basal
Half of these arise from the sphenoidal wing and grow into both the anterior and middle fossae of the skull (Figs 6.4 and 6.5). At the *inner* end of the wing the cavernous sinus is involved with the nerves (3, 4, 5, 6) in its wall, as well as the optic nerve and carotid artery; proptosis often develops. At the *outer* end meningioma may take the form of a global tumour growing into the Sylvian fissure, causing temporal epilepsy, facial weakness and, on the left, dysphasia; or it may grow *en plaque* with little encroachment on the brain but forming a hyperostosis which causes proptosis and an obvious swelling in the temporal region.

Olfactory groove meningiomas usually grow bilaterally, the falx indenting the mass from above. With an anteriorly placed tumour there are usually no complaints until raised pressure asserts itself. Anosmia, the only localizing

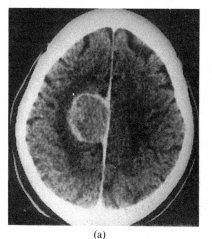

(a)

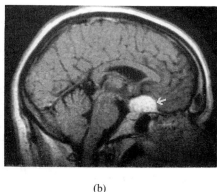

(b)

(a) CT scan with contrast showing parasagittal meningioma; (b) T1-weighted MRI with gadopentetate showing suprasellar meningioma.

Fig. 6.6 Meningiomas.

sign, is rarely complained of, and will be detected only if the sense of smell is tested. More posteriorly placed tumours encroach on the optic nerve if unilateral, and this may result in a Foster Kennedy syndrome (atrophy in one fundus, papilloedema in the other). Mental symptoms are seldom striking until a late stage and epilepsy is not very common.

Suprasellar meningiomas arise from the tuberculum sellae and compress the optic chiasm, leading to early diagnosis whilst the tumour is still quite small. Bitemporal hemianopia with optic atrophy may simulate a pituitary tumour, but endocrine symptoms are less constant and the sella is not ballooned, though minor bone changes can usually be detected.

Posterior fossa

Midline growths arise from the *basilar groove*, high ones on the clivus, low ones at the foramen magnum. Predictably these tend to give rise at an early stage to multiple cranial nerve palsies and long tract signs. Laterally, the commonest site is the *cerebellopontine angle*, the tumour arising from the back of the petrous in relation to the sigmoid sinus.

Tentorial meningiomas appear in most series as posterior fossa tumours, but at least half grow upwards as well as downwards. A variety of symptoms results; raised pressure, cranial nerve palsies and ataxia suggest a posterior fossa tumour, but hemianopia and epilepsy may also develop.

Tumour remote from dura

Intraventricular meningiomas grow into the lateral ventricle, usually on the left side. Raised pressure may be accompanied by hemianopia and slight hemiplegia.

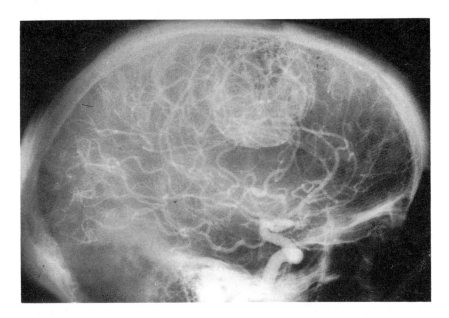

Fig. 6.7 Meningioma. Angiogram – late arterial phase showing dense network of tumour vessels.

Deep Sylvian tumours are presumed to arise from arachnoid condensations deep in the fissure, perhaps from the carotid sheath.

Diagnosis

Plain X-rays are often of value in detecting meningiomas. Sphenoidal wing growths constantly produce changes, either erosion or dense hyperostosis, and a number of vault tumours do also. Large meningeal arteries running to a convexity tumour may make an obvious channel in the bone (Fig. 4.4).

CT scanning is more useful than MRI in the detection of intracranial meningioma and in demonstrating its mass effect. The tumour is well-circumscribed, usually of higher density than brain, sometimes containing calcification and enhancing homogeneously with contrast; surrounding low density represents oedema (Fig. 6.6a). The improved detail provided with MRI may more clearly demonstrate the anatomical relationships of some basal meningiomas. (Fig. 6.6b).

Angiography can be most informative in supratentorial meningiomas, which show a tumour circulation more often than do glioblastomas; not only may the nature of the tumour be recognized but its vascularity can be assessed. A ring of feeding vessels or of veins may outline the tumour; vessels entering the tumour are regular and often take on a sun-ray pattern. A blush in the capillary phase may give a striking picture of the entire tumour which persists after all the normal veins have emptied (Fig. 6.7). Much of the blood supply of these tumours is derived from the external carotid circulation which is normally slower than the internal carotid circulation and readily amenable to preoperative embolization.

Treatment

Meningiomas are generally thought of as benign because most are non-invasive and amitotic. Yet they may occur in situations, such as the cavernous sinus and the clivus, where total extirpation is impossible, and even accessible tumours sometimes present formidable technical problems by reason of their rich vascular attachments.

Convexity and parasagittal

The control of blood loss is an important consideration during the removal of these tumours. Enlarged external carotid branches can give an unduly vascular scalp flap and hyperostotic bone bleeds freely when saw cuts are made; preoperative embolization makes this stage considerably less hazardous. The dura over the tumour may still bleed heavily when separated from bone, and there is still the inevitable bleeding from vessels in and around the tumour during removal.

Unless the growth has eroded completely through the skull the bone flap can be turned down off the underlying tumour; but if there is an endostosis or exostosis with obvious tumour invasion this part of the bone must be nibbled away before closure. When the area involved is large the whole bone flap may be removed and boiled before replacement, or the bone flap may be discarded and the defect made good by cranioplasty at a later date (p. 231).

There is no need to dissect dura off the base of the tumour, because this area of dura must be excised, and is best removed in one piece with the tumour. The dural incision encircles the base of the tumour which will then extrude whilst the remaining dura protects surrounding brain. If falx is involved a generous segment should be resected and the opposite side inspected.

There is no absolute need for the dural defect to be repaired, but a dural substitute is desirable to prevent the underlying brain becoming adherent to scalp or bone, which would make dissection tedious at any subsequent operation and may also predispose to epilepsy. Fascia lata from the thigh, or a synthetic dural substitute, can be used.

Involvement of the sagittal sinus presents a problem because division of the *patent* sinus in its posterior two-thirds is liable to be followed by congestion and haemorrhagic infarction in part of the hemisphere. Care must be taken to shave tumour off the sinus as closely as possible if it is patent; but, if it is already blocked by tumour, it can safely be excised because collateral drainage channels will already have opened up. Sinus patency may be determined preoperatively by sinograms (late phase of carotid arteriograms), MRI, or at operation by needling or catheterizing the sinus. If a patent sinus is inadvertently opened it must be closed with stitches.

Anterior basal tumours
To prevent undue retraction in the confined spaces in which these tumours grow no attempt should be made to deliver them whole. The interior of the tumour is excavated, using suction, ultrasonic aspiration, laser or the diathermy cutting loop, depending on tumour consistency, and the remaining capsule then dissected free of surrounding structures. Radical excision of dura is not always feasible, but the area of tumour origin is burnt black in the hope of destroying all tumour remnants in it. If dura is sacrificed from the floor of the anterior fossa over the ethmoidal sinuses, it must be repaired to prevent CSF rhinorrhoea and the risk of meningitis.

Olfactory groove tumours should be totally removed; the greatest hazard is damage to the anterior cerebral arteries which are closely applied to the posterior pole of the tumour and must be preserved at all costs.

Suprasellar tumours can be completely removed, but the larger they are, the harder this becomes. Considerable care is required to protect the adjacent carotid and anterior cerebral arteries and the optic nerves and chiasma. Larger tumour carry a risk of hypothalamic damage and incomplete removal may be wise in certain cases, leaving small fragments firmly adherent to critical structures.

Inner sphenoidal wing tumours must often be incompletely removed because of their close relation to the carotid artery and cavernous sinus. Global pterional growths demand total removal, but the *en plaque* type are best left alone, once an angiogram has confirmed that there is no large intradural component. These are indolent tumours which may not shorten life, but bone involvement is so widespread and diffuse that complete extirpation is impossible, whilst partial removal seldom improves the proptosis or local swelling.

Prognosis
This is good if the tumour is totally removed, though epilepsy often persists. However, a fifth of tumours regarded by surgeons as having been completely resected have been found to recur, usually within 5 years. Recurrence is probably more often due to inadequate removal rather than to a malignant tumour type, except for the small number of sarcomatous growths. The

commonest sources of recurrence are an invaded venous sinus; parasagittal tumours are therefore the most likely to recur. Less often invaded bone is the site of recurrence, or dura in the region of the tumour base where a subdural carpet of tumour cells may spread beyond the naked-eye limits of invasion. Occasionally a small nodule becomes detached and is overlooked, or there may be multiple tumours from the start.

Recurrence may re-enact the clinical evolution of the primary tumour. If suspected, CT scanning is the most reliable investigation. 'False recurrence' occurs from time to time, especially in ageing patients who have had convexity tumours removed years before; the reappearance of hemiplegia is probably due to vascular insufficiency as arterial disease progresses and affects first an area already short of vessels.

The outlook for tumours not completely removed, because of their critical situation, may be quite good. Very long survivals are common, and little or no progress in the size of the tumour may be apparent over 10 years or more. Some meningiomas never declare themselves in life, and a third of one series of 300 intracranial tumours found incidently at post-mortem were meningiomas, mostly parasagittal. This must be remembered when assessing claims for radiotherapy restricting the growth of these tumours; an incompletely removed sarcomatous growth is, however, certainly worth treating by radiation.

Pituitary region tumours

Tumours in and around the pituitary fossa may cause endocrine effects, compression of the chiasm and sometimes of other cranial nerves, or obstruction of the foramen of Monro. Those arising within the pituitary gland itself are classified as macroadenomas if more than 10 mm in diameter, and microadenomas if smaller. Classification by cell type is now realized to be less useful than by the effect on hormone secretion, whether reduced or increased. The relationship between endocrine effect and histology is quite variable; for example, both acromegaly and Cushing's syndrome may each be produced by tumours which are reported as 'chromophobe'.

Hypersecreting tumours

It is now realized that prolactin is the hormone most commonly produced by pituitary tumours, but it is also released when there is hypothalamic suppression. *Prolactin-producing tumours* are usually microadenomas and are an important cause of infertility in women, often associated with amenorrhoea, less often with galactorrhoea. They occasionally cause infertility in men.

Growth hormone in excess results in gigantism if occurring before the epiphyseal closure, and acromegaly in adults. These tumours, although hormone-secreting, may not present until chiasmal compression develops.

Adrenocorticotrophic hormone (ACTH)-producing microadenomas are the commonest cause of Cushing's disease; other causes are associated with basophil hyperplasia of the pituitary or result from primary adrenal disease.

Gonadotrophin and thyroid-stimulating hormone (TSH)-secreting tumours are extremely rare.

Hyposecreting tumours

These are the minority of tumours, presenting either with chiasmal compression or hypopituitary symptoms – often with both. Their growth tendency varies widely. Most begin within the pituitary fossa and remain confined to it, ballooning up the diaphragm and enlarging the bony outlines of the sella. Others escape from the sella and some spread far, perhaps because the anatomy of the individual allows this, but more likely because some tumours have a disposition to spread. Extrasellar extension alters the symptomatology. About 40% of these tumours are cystic, usually containing < 10 ml of clear yellow fluid. Occasionally a tumour outstrips its blood supply and undergoes necrosis or haemorrhagic infarction; this may be manifested clinically as pituitary apoplexy (p. 117). Craniopharyngiomas, that cause hypopituitarism and hydrocephalus, are dealt with later (p. 124).

Clinical syndromes

Acromegaly consists in a coarsening and enlargement of the facial features and the extremities and the typical appearance is immediately obvious. Soft tissue and bony components of this change can be recognized:

SOFT TISSUE

1.   Thick coarse skin and hair.
2.   Deep voice with big tongue (causing slurred speech).
3.   Huge hands and feet.
4.   Carpal tunnel compression giving numbness and pain in fingers.

Patients with acromegaly also have an increased incidence of hypotension, diabetes, arthritis and bronchitis. It also seems that they have reduced life expectancy.

BONY

1.   Huge frontal sinus.
2.   Prognathic mandible with separation of teeth.
3.   Broadening and flaring of terminal finger phalanges.
4.   Thoracic kyphosis secondary to osteoporosis (causing backache).

Cushing's syndrome is due to excessive production of cortisol, either due to adrenal tumour or to adrenal hyperplasia secondary to excessive production of ACTH by the pituitary. Three-quarters of cases are pituitary-dependent and three-quarters of these have a pituitary tumour; the rest are presumed to have hyperplasia. Obesity, skin striae, hypertension and a variety of other features occur, and 50% of untreated cases are fatal in 5 years. Following adrenalectomy for Cushing's syndrome some patients develop marked skin pigmentation with melanocyte-stimulating hormone over-production associated with a pituitary adenoma (Nelson's syndrome). In both this condition and in pituitary-dependent Cushing's syndrome ACTH levels are abnormally high. These levels usually fall in response to dexamethasone when due to hyperplasia of the pituitary but not when due to adenoma. When Cushing's syndrome is due to a primary adrenal disorder ACTH levels are very low.

Some degree of *pituitary insufficiency* is common with several types of macroadenoma of the pituitary. But it may be produced by other tumours adjacent to the sella which affect the pituitary stalk or the hypothalamus, through which the activities of the pituitary gland are controlled. It is an important feature to recognize because an endocrine crisis can readily be precipitated by various manoeuvres in hospital if the precaution of prophylactic intramuscular hydrocortisone treatment is not given.

The normal pituitary secretes trophic hormones and the clinical and biochemical aspects of pituitary deficiency derive mainly from the secondary deficiencies in target organs.

Gonadotrophic deficiency before puberty tends to retard the development of secondary sex characteristics: adult men have poor beard growth, women amenorrhoea, and both sexes loss of libido and deficient pubic and axillary hair. Oestrogen and androgen production is low, with reduced urinary 17-ketosteroids.

Decrease in thyrotrophic hormone leads to myxoedema and of growth hormone to dwarfism and infantilism. Because hypopituitarism is so insidious and its separate components readily produced by many other conditions, a pituitary tumour is rarely suspected in the early stages before chiasmal compression develops. Gonadotrophins usually fall first in adults and growth hormone in children; ACTH and TSH secretion are affected only later, and the deficiency is rarely as complete as in Simmond's syndrome.

Pituitary apoplexy, due to sudden necrosis or haemorrhage, begins with abrupt headache, followed by rapid visual loss and/or diplopia due to ocular palsies. Confusion and even coma follow, and an endocrine crisis is precipitated. Lumbar puncture may show bloody or xanthochromic CSF and, with the neurological findings, suggest subarachnoid haemorrhage from a rapidly enlarging internal carotid aneurysm. Angiography may need to be performed to exclude this possibility, but a CT scan usually suffices.

Chiasmal compression

This used to be the main cause bringing the patient to the surgeon, and it signifies suprasellar extension. Vision has commonly been failing for a year or more and a characteristic bitemporal hemianopia may already have developed; it is usually first evident in the upper quadrant of one side and progresses variably (Fig. 1.4): one eye may lose sight altogether before the other is affected at all. In 5% the hemianopia is homonymous, implying compression of the optic tract rather than the chiasm; this tends to occur when the chiasm is prefixed, i.e. the optic nerves are unusually short. Early field defects are best detected by testing in detail on a screen. Primary optic atrophy indicates long-standing compression which may fail to recover after operative decompression of the chiasm. Patients still present unduly late with pituitary tumours because further investigations are not pursued for visual failure for which no refractive error or ocular cause can be found. In most cases a lateral skull X-ray would suggest the diagnosis.

It is important to recognize *extrasellar extension* because of its implications for management. Spread *upwards* affects vision but occasionally blocks the foramen of Monro, produces hydrocephalus and invades the hypothalamus;

or *forwards* into the frontal lobes gives mental symptoms and anosmia; or *laterally* into the cavernous sinus causing palsies of cranial nerves 3, 4, 5 and 6 (Fig. 6.5); or *subtemporally*, epilepsy, hemiplegia and even dysphasia.

The differential diagnosis, apart from other pituitary tumours, includes arachnoiditis and the empty sellar syndrome; of the many other conditions the most common can be grouped as follows:

1. *Suprasellar* meningioma, optic nerve glioma and epidermoid/dermoid tumours, which less often produce endocrine features. When these do develop they are usually of recent onset, in contrast to the many years history typical of adenoma.
2. *Infrasellar* masses, chordoma, mucocele of the sphenoidal sinus, and optic nerve glioma are distinguished by radiological appearances: widespread destruction with chordoma, bulging back of the anterior wall of the sella with mucocele.
3. *Parasellar* masses, carotid aneurysm, inner third spheroidal wing meningioma, and dysgerminoas may be distinguished by MRI or angiography.
4. *Distant* tumours cause obstructive hydrocephalus, the dilated third ventricle invading the sella and eroding its bony margins.

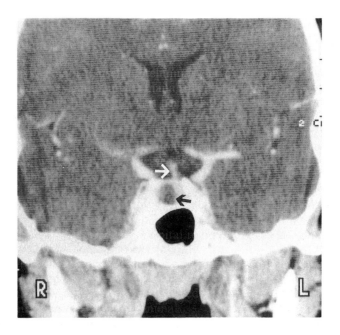

Fig. 6.8 Pituitary microadenoma. Coronal CT scan shows a low-density region within the gland (black arrow) and stalk deviation to the opposite side (white arrow).

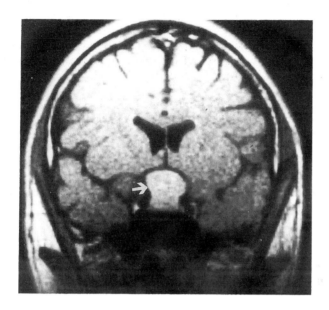

Fig. 6.9 Pituitary macroadenoma with suprasellar extension (arrowed) demonstrated with a proton density-weighted MRI.

Endocrine

Assessment of hormonal function has now become so complex that it is the preserve of the endocrinologist, and a detailed account would be out of place here. The investigations recommended vary from laboratory to laboratory, as do the normal values for various estimations. Elevated *growth hormone* levels should be suppressed with hyperglycaemia and elevated *ACTH* levels with dexamethasone. Failure to do so supports the presence of an adenoma. *Prolactin* levels above 4000 mu/l suggest prolactinoma rather than a functional cause, as does a failure to increase with thyrotrophic—releasing hormone (TRH) injection and metoclopropamide.

Hypofunction is tested with the combined pituitary stimulation test. Low hormone levels in themselves provide little diagnostic value but a failure of levels to rise to a specific stimulus – insulin (increasing growth hormone, ACTH and cortisol levels), gonadotrophin-releasing hormone (increasing luteinizing hormone (LH) and follicle-stimulating hormone (FSH) levels) and TRH (increasing TSH and prolactin levels) indicates impaired secretion.

Radiology

Plain skull X-ray may show enlargement of the pituitary fossa, which varies enormously according to the growth character of the particular tumour. The earliest sign is usually a double contour to the sellar floor in the lateral view. Usually there is equal increase in both the depth and anteroposterior diameter of the fossa with thinning of the floor; the dorsum may be levered back and the posterior clinoids isolated by erosion of the dorsum below them. These changes may be mimicked to some extent by most of the conditions which may

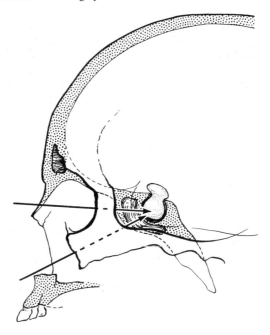

Fig. 6.10 Transsphenoidal approach to the pituitary. Either ethmoidal (solid line) or nasal (dotted line) routes to the sphenoid sinus may be used.

be confused clinically with pituitary adenoma, and no single radiological sign is diagnostic. Cone views and tomography can be used to increase the diagnostic accuracy.

CT scanning will show an enlarged pituitary fossa and suprasellar extension. High-definition slices taken in the coronal plane with the head extended may reveal microadenomas as low-density regions within normal pituitary tissue, but tumours under 5 mm diameter are difficult to detect. Deviation of the pituitary stalk gives indirect evidence of the presence of tumour (Fig. 6.8).

MRI is particularly useful in demonstrating suprasellar extension in the sagittal plane (Fig. 6.9). High magnetic field strength imagers can identify microadenomas more readily than CT. MRI also helps to exclude an aneurysm projecting medially towards the fossa. If unavailable, angiography may be required before operation.

Treatment

Operation

Most pituitary tumours are treated by surgery, using the *transsphenoidal route* (Fig. 6.10). This was originally introduced by Cushing to avoid the then considerable hazards of craniotomy; it still has a lower mortality and does not carry the risk of epilepsy. By this route, using the operating microscope, it is often possible to achieve selective removal of a microadenoma with preservation (or restoration) of normal pituitary function. It can also be used for tumours causing chiasmal compression, even when there is a large suprasellar extension. Through a small sublabial incision one side of the nasal septum is dissected clear and cracked off at the keel of the sphenoid. The sphenoidal sinus is entered and removal of the downward bulging floor reveals the pituitary. A less frequently used route to the sphenoidal sinus is through the ethmoid, using a skin incision at the side of the bridge of the nose. Postoperative CSF rhinorrhoea rarely lasts more than a few days, and infection is rare.

The frontal approach is now seldom used and is usually reserved for tumours with large lateral or frontal extensions. It involves turning a right-sided flap, opening the dura and retracting the frontal lobe. The trans-sphenoidal approach carries a mortality of less than 1%, but this is higher with an approach through a frontal craniotomy and there is an additional risk of epilepsy. Risks are increased when there is marked extrasellar extension. Although replacement hormone therapy (see below) has reduced the risk of postoperative endocrine failure, fatal hypothalamic crisis from manipulations too near the third ventricle remains a hazard which only surgical skill and restraint can prevent; for giant prolactin-secreting tumours, bromocriptine therapy combined with regular visual monitoring and followed with irradiation may be the safer option.

When there has been chiasmal compression, vision should improve in 90% of patients, half of them regaining a full field. Vision often returns immediately after operation, but may be delayed for several months. In the remaining patients blindness is avoided, even though there is no improvement.

Radiation

This is now mainly used for postoperative treatment when surgery is known to have been incomplete, and it reduces the 5 years recurrence rate to 5–10%. It is now seldom used as primary therapy, but might be appropriate in the old or frail in whom surgery was considered unwise. Although improvement is usually obvious in 3 or 4 weeks, the beneficial effects of radiation may be delayed for months. Without prior decompression, sight may even deteriorate temporarily, probably due to reactive swelling of the tumour. However, most tumours are radiosensitive, as witnessed by improving visual fields, by reduced tumour size on repeated CT scan and by the occasional post-radiation exploration which reveals no tumour at all. A trial of treatment is probably reasonable provided that the facilities allow weekly reviews of the visual fields and acuities, and there is agreement to accept surgery as soon as it is obvious that radiation is not proving effective. Some centres report that almost 90% of chromophobe adenomas have been adequately treated by radiation without recourse to surgery. Large doses of radiation can be obtained locally with isotope implants, but this is of no value in chiasmal compression.

If vision is rapidly failing radiation is clearly unsuitable because it does not act quickly enough. Large extrasellar extensions pose problems for the therapist and force him or her to disperse one dose over a wider area with diminished effectiveness. Cystic and acutely necrotic tumours are probably resistant. The risk of late effects of radiation on the hypothalamus and optic chiasm cannot be ignored if radical dosage is employed, because these vulnerable areas are in the field of treatment when the target is the pituitary. The only solution is to reduce the dose to safer but less effective levels. A strong argument against using radiotherapy initially in non-secreting tumours without preliminary surgical exploration is that the diagnosis is never confirmed. The differential diagnosis of chiasmal compression and of sellar enlargement is quite wide, and most of the alternatives are radioresistant, some of them very suitable for surgery (aneurysm, meningioma, mucocele). Only exploration will confirm beyond doubt that the diagnosis is a pituitary adenoma.

Drug treatment

Bromocriptine works by mimicking the action of prolactin-inhibiting hormone, which is probably dopamine.

In some centres bromocriptine is used as the treatment of choice in prolactinomas. It can certainly produce normal pituitary function and allow pregnancy. Reduction in tumour size occurs in up to two-thirds of patients. Whether it is better than selective removal of the adenoma is not yet known and its use depends on both patient and centre preference. Bromocriptine therapy, however, in the presence of visual impairment requires very careful monitoring of visual fields and acuity. Any deterioration indicates the need for urgent surgical decompression.

Somatostatin is the natural inhibitor of growth hormone release from the pituitary. Somatostatin therapy can reduce tumour size and growth hormone levels in patients with acromegaly, but its use as an alternative rather than a precursor to surgery requires further evaluation.

Management of endocrine failure (all types of tumour)

Treatment may be required for acute or chronic deficiency and prophylactically to cover operation.

Acute deficiency results from sudden withdrawal of pituitary function due to *haemorrhagic necrosis* in a pituitary tumour, to *hypophysectomy* or to *infarction* from obstetric haemorrhage and subsequent prolonged hypotension. When there is already chronic deficiency an acute crisis may be precipitated in a number of ways, and these constitute the majority of cases of hypopituitary coma and collapse. Infection or subjection to surgical or radiological procedures causes stress to which the adrenal would normally react by producing cortisone in response to pituitary stimulus, and the failure to do so results in *hypotensive collapse*: vomiting or diarrhoea leads to salt depletion which the hypopituitary patient less readily restores and a sequence of *metabolic imbalance* follows: cold weather may precipitate *hypothermic* coma if secondary hypothyroidism is a prominent feature of the deficiency state, whilst starvation and vomiting can precipitate *hypoglycaemia*.

Prophylactic cortisone should always be given before a hypopituitary patient undergoes surgery or a major neuroradiological procedure. What factor constitutes the stress is unknown; general anaesthesia is one, aggravated by preoperative starvation and by premedication with opiates or barbiturates, to which these patients are unduly sensitive; but collapse can also follow angiography under local anaesthesia. Nor is the severity of the pituitary deficiency, as indicated by laboratory tests, a reliable guide to the likelihood of a crisis; and it is wise to give 100 mg hydrocortisone succinate intramuscularly an hour before any procedure to a patient who has clinical evidence of deficiency. Cortisone is rapidly metabolized; even if 50 mg is given twice daily for a few days to cover stressful procedures, there is no risk of permanent adrenal suppression, if these glands should still be active, nor any danger of delayed wound healing.

Collapse or coma requires immediate treatment. Hydrocortisone succinate 100 mg should be given intravenously without delay and 50 mg intramuscularly 6-hourly. Plasma volume expansion and inotropic support may be needed and fluid and electrolyte balance restored.

A source of infection should always be sought and treated in otherwise unexplained crises.

Chronic deficiency, such as normally persists after operation in patients who had hypopituitarism before surgery, calls for replacement therapy. How much will be needed by any patient is not predictable – even after hypophysectomy some patients can be weaned from cortisone completely. Most benefit from cortisone 25–50 mg daily and thyroxine 0.05–0.3 mg daily. Men may report improvement in impotence and the return of beard growth with testosterone. Women concerned about loss of libido and dyspareunia from genital atrophy may benefit from cyclical oestrogen therapy. Patients on replacement therapy should be warned of the risks of operations, infections and gastrointestinal upsets; like diabetics they require increased replacement at such times when they are liable, possibly through ignorance or default, to have their vital drugs withdrawn.

Diabetes insipidus is more of a nuisance than a danger, although if coma supervenes, severe dehydration can result from the continued passage of large

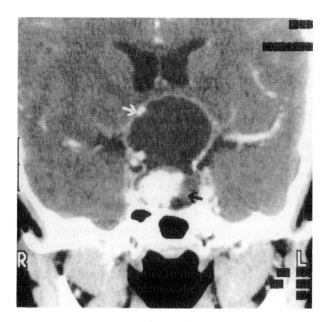

Fig. 6.11 CT of craniopharyngioma. The coronal view with contrast enhancement shows a dilated fossa containing calcified tumour (black arrow) and a large suprasellar cystic component with further calcification in the wall (white arrow).

volumes of urine with inadequate intake. Polyuria may become evident only when cortisone replacement is begun; preoperatively it can be distinguished from hysterical or compulsive water drinking by measuring the inability to produce concentrated urine, after 16–24 hours without fluid, which is rectified by a single dose of vasopressin. Specific gravity is an unreliable guide and the osmolality of the urine should be assessed; but in the first week or two postoperatively, when intake is controlled, a low specific gravity (<1002) is diagnostic.

Diabetes insipidus may be treated by lypressin nasal spray, 3–8 applications daily, thus avoiding the inconvenient injections of vasopressin tannate. Some patients respond well to a thiazide diuretic, e.g. bendrofluazide 5 mg daily, which may act by producing sodium depletion and stimulating formation of renin and angiotensin.

Hypophysectomy (removal or destruction of the normal pituitary gland) is now employed less often for hormone-dependent carcinomatosis (e.g. breast) than for diabetic retinopathy. Indications are florid retinopathy, associated with rapid new vessel formation, especially in juvenile diabetes.

Craniopharyngioma

These arise from a remnant of the buccal ectoderm of the pharyngeal pouch which forms the pars anterior of the pituitary. About 90% are cystic, at least in part, lined with squamous epithelium and containing dark brown fluid like engine oil, which is full of cholesterol crystals that shimmer in the light. Small intrasellar tumours do occur, but 50% are wholly suprasellar, causing no enlargement of the fossa, and growing mainly upwards towards the hypothalamus and third ventricle where they may cause hydrocephalus from obstruction of the foramen of Monro. Dumb-bell tumours, part in and part above the sella, also occur. They are thin-walled and insinuate themselves into their surroundings, making total surgical removal difficult.

Although congenital in origin, only half of these cysts present clinically under the age of 20; some declare themselves only in old age, when mental symptoms predominate due to arteriosclerotic changes superimposed on chronic hydrocephalus. In children, in whom this is one of the commonest non-gliomatous tumour, pressure symptoms tend to overshadow chiasmal compression; the combination of papilloedema and bitemporal hemianopia, when it occurs, is almost diagnostic. Failure to grow quickly enough, or delayed puberty, may be the only complaint or may accompany other syndromes. Both thin (Lorraine pituitary dwarfs) and fat (Fröhlich's adiposogenital syndrome) clinical types occur and many teenage age boys with unbroken voices harbour one of these tumours. Some develop diabetes insipidus.

But serious visual loss can also occur, sometimes complete blindness, from a combination of primary and consecutive optic atrophy. The sella is normal radiologically in 50%; 75% have suprasellar calcification on straight X-ray (Fig. 4.lb). CT scan shows a tumour of mixed density with both solid and cystic components and calcification is evident in 90% (Fig. 6.11). MRI will also show the tumour, which gives a higher signal than surrounding brain except for the region of calcification.

Treatment

Operation is essential to confirm the diagnosis and if possible the tumour should be removed. Whether a direct attack on the upward extension of the tumour is advisable depends on the nature of the tumour. Craniopharyngiomas tend to be closely adherent to the anterior cerebral arteries and their vital branches to the hypothalamus; if the cyst wall is calcified and unyielding, safe dissection may be impossible and subtotal removal is accepted as the safest course. Cyst drainage alone is the simplest procedure but has the highest chance of recurrent problems. When removal has been incomplete radiotherapy is necessary. When hydrocephalus is present and even if a large cyst has been successfully aspirated, it is best to bypass the block by performing a short-circuit or shunt.

Long remissions are the rule but even after apparent complete removal up to 50% may recur within a 10-month period. Most feel that attempted radical or even subtotal removal gives better results than simply cyst drainage combined with radiotherapy but there is no doubt that this comparatively simply manoeuvre, avoiding the hazards of attempted removal, may give long periods of remission, and in some instances this may be the most sensible approach.

Neuroma (schwannoma)

Any cranial or spinal nerve may give rise to one of these circumscribed tumours, but most intracranial neuromas are on the acoustic nerve, a few on the fifth at the Gasserian ganglion. Various synonyms exist (neurilemmoma, neurofibroma, neurinoma) but it is now becoming generally accepted that the proliferating elements in these tumours are derived from Schwann cells. There is no evidence that they originate in the nerve fibres themselves, although fibres may be found running through some tumours. The cells tend to form palisades in a reticulin network with xanthomatous change and fat-filled foam cells giving the gross appearance of yellow, buttery material in many tumours.

Families with generalized neurofibromatosis (von Recklinghausen's disease) tend to develop bilateral acoustic neuromas, often at a younger age than is common with the solitary tumours which occur in middle age. Tumours associated with von Recklinghausen's disease are often more fibroblastic in their stroma, more neurofibromatous, than solitary tumours.

Acoustic neuroma

The early diagnosis of acoustic neuroma is of concern to the neurosurgeon because the smaller the tumour, the less hazardous the operation. Operative mortality and morbidity increase steadily as the tumour grows in size.

Pathology

The growth arises on the vestibular division of the eighth cranial nerve, where the neuroglial sheath gives way to a neurilemmal one. This is just inside the internal auditory meatus (porus acousticus) which thus becomes enlarged to a funnel shape. These tumours are extremely slowly growing and although pea-sized tumours may be diagnosed and removed, this is unusual. More often, by the time the surgeon sees the patient the tumour has expanded into the cerebellopontine angle. Larger tumours burrow ventral to the midbrain and pons which are indented and distorted. Tumour may also grow up through the tentorial hiatus into the middle cranial fossa to involve the third and fifth nerves, and down to the foramen magnum where it impinges on the lower cranial nerves passing to their exit foramina. The seventh nerve is almost always carried up on to the anterosuperior surface of the tumour, intimately adherent to the capsule. Very often an arachnoid cyst develops on the surface of the tumour and adds to the amount of space taken up in the posterior fossa. Less often the tumour itself is mainly cystic.

Clinical

The development of the classical signs and symptoms is such a slow business, spread over several years, sometimes as many as 20, that each new feature tends to be treated as a new condition, and the relationship between the separate components of the cerebellopontine syndrome may escape notice. Deafness, tinnitus and vertigo commonly take the patient to the ENT surgeon; vestibular symptoms may be only temporary whilst unilateral deafness may not impress itself on a patient until he or she chances to rely on one ear, perhaps on the telephone. The differential diagnosis at this stage is wide, if there are no other signs, but by a variety of neuro-otological investigations it can usually be established that there is an eighth nerve lesion rather than disease in peripheral structures. Auditory and vestibular function are separately tested, although both are often affected.

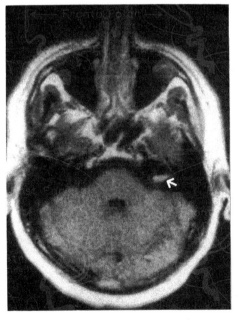

(a)

Fig. 6.12 Acoustic neuroma. (a) T1-weighted MRI with gadopentetate enhancement showing tumour restricted to the internal auditory meatus.

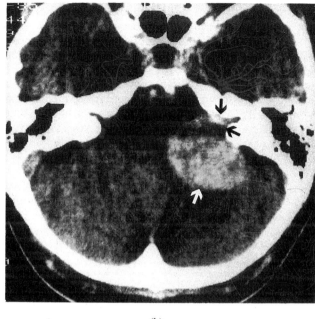

(b)

Fig. 6.12 (*cont*) (b) CT with contrast showing tumour in the cerebellopontine angle with widening and splaying of the internal auditory meatus.

Loss of hearing is crudely tested by the ability to hear the whispered voice at a certain distance, with the other ear masked. Sensorineural deafness can be detected by finding impairment of both air and bone conduction on tuning fork tests (Rinne); pure tone audiometry enables the degree of hearing loss for different frequencies to be charted in quantitative terms (decibel loss), and again bone and air conduction can be compared. Speech audiometry speaks for itself; nerve lesions commonly impair appreciation of speech more profoundly than of pure tones.

Vestibular function is tested by examining spontaneous and induced nystagmus. This may be directly observed, or recorded electrically; this (electronystamography) is a much more sensitive detector of nystagmus but an even greater advantage is the possibility of recording nystagmus with the eyes closed or in a dark room – that is, without fixation. This manoeuvre aggravates vestibular nystagmus but largely obliterates both central nystagmus (due to lesions of the nerve, brainstem or cerebellum) and congenital nystagmus. Nystagmus may be induced by rotation, by static position change or by caloric stimulation of the semicircular canals. These caloric tests enable the vestibular function on the two sides to be distinguished. Both hot (44°C) and cold (30°C) water may be used, and either increments of 0.2 ml are used or a continuing flow of water; in the latter case the time till onset of nystagmus is recorded. Acoustic neuroma is usually associated with a dead labyrinth (no reaction) from a fairly early stage.

Cerebellar ataxia and nystagmus, sometimes with early cranial nerve palsies (5,7,9,10,11), next appear. Diminished corneal sensation is the most constant sign. Facial weakness is rarely marked before operation, but slight weakness may be detected by delayed or absent blinking on the affected side. Facial pain, which may take the form of trigeminal neuralgia, sometimes occurs. A persistent suboccipital ache with a stiff neck is a frequent, if somewhat non-specific, complaint. Raised pressure may lead to neurosurgical investigations before the typical syndrome has evolved. Chronic hydrocephalus with marked mental changes and no clear history of eighth nerve or cerebellar disorder is a frequent presentation in the elderly.

Other less common tumours which grow in the cerebellopontine angle may closely mimic an acoustic neuroma. Epidermoid, meningioma and laterally placed intrinsic cerebellar tumours such as haemangioblastoma or ependymoma may all be equally indolent on occasion. Deafness is seldom the first symptom in patients with these other tumours and when present is often mild, despite the presence of other cranial nerve palsies or raised ICP.

Wherever neuromas occur in the nervous system they commonly cause a great increase in CSF protein (often over 100 mg per 100 ml), sometimes accompanied by xanthochromia. But a normal CSF protein level does not exclude the diagnosis, especially in the early stages.

MRI is the investigation of choice. Since the bone produces no signal, even tumours restricted to the internal auditory meatus, i.e. intracanalicular, can be demonstrated (Fig. 6.12a).

Either CT scan or MRI will detect larger tumours extending into the cerebellopontine angle, but intravenous contrast is essential for CT (Fig 6.12b; without this, acoustic neuromas are often isodense with brain and likely to be missed. These tests will also demonstrate any associated obstructive hydrocephalus due to compression of the fourth ventricle. If these investigations are unavailable, tomography of the internal auditory meatus may show erosion and widening on the affected side. Positive-contrast encephalography, using oily media, suggests a diagnosis of acoustic neuroma if the internal meatus fails to fill with contrast.

Treatment

Delaying operation serves only to increase the risks. Conservative treatment is only applicable to those few patients who harbour bilateral tumours, and then operation is still usually advised on one side.

Different operative approaches are available and selection of the most appropriate usually depends on the size of the tumour and the hope of preserving some residual hearing as well as facial nerve function.

The *translabyrynthine approach* is usually reserved for small or medium-sized tumours (>2.5 cm) in patients who have lost all hearing. The seventh nerve is encountered early in the dissection and the chance of preserving function is high. Inevitably, hearing is sacrificed with this route. Some protagonists advocate the removal of even large tumours by this method.

The *suboccipital approach* remains the standard approach for large tumours. In patients with small tumours with some preservation of hearing, this route may also be the most appropriate in the hope that some hearing may be retained. A paramedian incision halfway between the midline and the mastoid brings the surgeon directly on to the tumour (Fig. 5.3). Some prefer to improve access by resecting the lateral third of the cerebellar hemisphere, and this does not appear to add to the postoperative disability. If the arachnoid of the cisterna magna is purposely opened CSF will escape during the operation from the fourth ventricle, and the pressure in the posterior fossa will remain low. The tumour is collapsed by removing its soft interior, and the slack capsule is then dissected free from its surroundings, taking care not to drag on the pons or on the vessels entering it from the tumour. Drilling out the internal auditory meatus and removal of tumour tissue within the canal allow early identification of the facial nerve. This nerve is then identified on the medial aspect as it exits from the brain stem and dissected off the tumour capule.

If difficulty is encountered in dissecting tumour capsule from brainstem, it is wise not to persist in this direction but to work on another part of the tumour. Later, when more of the bulk of the tumour has been removed, it may be safe to return to the previous danger zone.

The total removal of a large tumour is sometimes done as a staged procedure, in order to reduce the hazards. The bulk of the tumour is removed at the first operation, and the remaining capsule on the second occasion. When a tumour spreads far up through the tentorial hiatus, or anterior to the pons, a second stage may be facilitated by division of the tentorium (Fig. 5.3b)

The *middle fossa approach* exposes the tumour from above. Although a less popular route, more surgeons are now attempting this for very small intracanalicular tumours in the hope of preserving hearing.

With all approaches the use of microsurgical techniques is essential; this has considerably reduced the frequency of cranial nerve and brainstem damage. Peroperative electrical stimulation aids detection and thereby protection of the facial nerve. Auditory evoked potentials may help when trying to preserve hearing. Permanent facial palsy is now usually avoided in small and medium-sized tumours, although recovery may take many months. For very large tumours (>4 cm) the risk of permanent facial nerve damage remains high (80%) and the mortality approaches 5%; if facial palsy does occur faciohypoglossal anastomosis done within the first year after operation, will improve tone in facial muscles at rest and patients may learn to initiate simple movements. With large tumours, neuroparalytic keratitis is a risk, due to the combination of facial palsy and corneal anaesthesia and preventive measures are begun immediately after operation (p. 89). A temporary bulbar palsy may necessitate naso-oesophageal feeding for some weeks after operation, and during this time, there is a risk of aspiration pneumonia. Ataxia may be aggravated by operation, though this too is usually only temporary.

In the elderly, debilitated patient with a large tumour, *subtotal (intracapsular) operation* may avoid these complications, and the immediate result can be very satisfactory, provided that sufficient tumour is removed from the tentorial hiatus to allow CSF to circulate freely and restore normal ICP. However, in 10–15%, tumour remnants rapidly regrow, and eventually in most patients recurrence of local symptoms or raised ICP occurs. Having survived an initial intracapsular removal, a patient requiring a second operation for recurrence faces a greater risk than that of the initial removal. Therefore, unless life expectancy is less than a few years, total removal is usually recommended.

Metastatic tumours

Pathology
In the brain itself these tumours arise by haematogenous spread through the arterial system or the valveless vertebral veins. They comprise the majority of intracranial secondary neoplasms, and make up 20–30% of all brain tumours recorded by pathologists, but only 5% of surgical series. Almost 1 in 5 of all cancer deaths has intracranial metastases at autopsy, a fifth of these having diffuse carcinomatosis. Three-quarters of those affected have major cerebral symptoms. Carcinoma of the bronchus is the commonest source of origin; a quarter of patients dying with this growth have brain metastases at autopsy; in a third the intracranial deposit is solitary, although this is seldom the only secondary in the whole body. Breast cancer and hypernephroma, and less commonly carcinoma of the gut and malignant melanoma, also metastasize to the brain, sometimes producing symptoms years after the removal of the primary growth. In some 15% the primary site is never discovered.

Blood-borne metastases form discrete tumours in the cerebral or cerebellar hemisphere; most supratentorial deposits are around the posterior end of the Sylvian fissure, in the region of supply of the terminal branches of the middle cerebral artery. Solitary tumours are normally firm and well-circumscribed, though there may be widespread oedema causing greater pressure effects than would be expected from the size of the tumour itself. Although the bulk of the mass is firm and may at first resemble a meningioma, the centre is frequently soft and necrotic; thick creamy fluid aspirated from this is easily mistaken for pus. On smears a metastasis may be distinguished from a glioblastoma only with difficulty; less often it looks like a sarcomatous meningioma. On the other hand it may be possible to recognize the type of carcinoma, even to hazard a guess as to the site of the primary.

Invasion of the dura, usually of the skull base, is a less common form of secondary intracranial neoplasia. Ordinarily the underlying bone is first affected with later spread to the dura. *Bone involvement* may be by blood stream spread (carcinoma of the breast or stomach, multiple myeloma) or by the direct extension of regional carcinoma (nasopharynx, paranasal air sinuses, middle ear; rodent ulcer or epithelioma of scalp). A dural carpet is formed which may spread over a wide area and become haemorrhagic; clinically this is reflected in progressive multiple cranial nerve palsies without raised pressure; plain X-rays may reveal erosion of the skull. Dural deposits *without bone change* occur in reticulosis (Hodgkin's disease) and leukaemia but are rarely the result of distant carcinoma.

Carcinomatosis of the meninges is a different entity arising from the dissemination of cancer cells in the subarachnoid space from a small deposit under the ventricular ependyma, in the choroid plexus or in the subpial part of the cerebral cortex. Although the arachnoid is infiltrated it looks only faintly opaque, or even quite normal to the naked eye. Cells may be recognized in the CSF.

Clinical
Carcinoma quite commonly declares itself first by intracranial invasion, sometimes at a stage when exhaustive investigation reveals no evidence of the primary tumour. Carcinoma of the bronchus by blood spread, and of the

nasopharynx by direct extension, are the tumours which most often behave in this deceptive way. Apart from this type of presentation patients with known primary malignancies, already treated or not, sometimes call for neurosurgical aid if intracranial extension is causing distressing symptoms.

Cerebral metastases usually give a short history of well-circumscribed focal signs, paralysis or focal epilepsy confined to one limb, and raised pressure. *Cerebellar* deposits cause distressing vertigo, vomiting and ataxia, usually with severe headache from obstructive hydrocephalus. Although a rapid course is the rule, intermittent symptoms may occur over a period of months. Sometimes clinical evidence of more than one tumour is found, and this is always suggestive of metastatic disease.

Carcinomatosis of the meninges produces a confusing clinical syndrome which frequently escapes recognition: dementia, epilepsy and scattered cranial and spinal nerve lesions suggest a disseminated pathological process; meningism does not always develop although there is usually a lymphocytic response with low sugar in the CSF, raising the suspicion of tuberculous meningitis. Malignant cells may be identified in the fluid by special staining of the deposit after centrifuging (p. 71).

Non-metastatic manifestations of malignant disease form an ill-understood group of disorders which may mistakenly give rise to suspicion of metastatic deposits in the brain (or spinal cord). Cerebellar disorders, dementia, myelopathy, peripheral neuropathy and neuromuscular disorders (myopathic and myasthenic types) all occur, and the unusual combination of such syndromes in the absence of tumour on imaging may suggest the diagnosis.

Metastases can arise in quite young patients, even in the teens; a preliminary chest X-ray, as well as thorough clinical examination, should therefore be carried out in every case of suspected brain tumour, however unlikely it may seem that the tumour is a secondary deposit. A skull X-ray may give the diagnosis (Fig. 4.3). CT scanning is usually the intracranial investigation of first choice, but MRI is even more sensitive in detecting small tumour deposits.

Treatment

When a metastatic brain tumour presents in patients who are otherwise well, with no evidence of primary tumour, treatment is along the same lines as for any other intracranial tumour. It may be recognized as secondary only when necrotic material is discovered at operation, or later on histological examination.

When a brain metastasis develops in a patient who has previously had malignant disease (commonly a radical mastectomy or lung resection) it is less easy to decide about treatment. If there is no evidence of secondary spread to other parts of the body and no recurrence of the primary, a brain lesion which is accessible and causing distressing symptoms is best removed. When an unsuspected primary tumour is discovered in the course of investigating a brain tumour the question of priority of treatment arises. As the patient has come to a neurosurgeon it is likely that CNS symptoms are predominant; if the metastasis is readily accessible it is probably best to operate without delay as a palliative measure. Although it may seem more logical to defer craniotomy until the primary tumour has been proved operable, it may be more helpful to the patient to relieve the immediate symptoms; histological examination of the cerebral specimen may confirm the diagnosis more expeditiously than investigating the suspected primary.

The palliation afforded by the removal of intracranial metastases is often very satisfactory. The tumour is frequently circumscribed, and can be shelled out completely and with less difficulty than any other brain tumour. About 10–15% of patients die within a month of such an operation. Occasionally patients survive for many years after the removal of a solitary brain metastasis, usually when a primary hypernephroma or breast carcinoma has been removed some years previously; but sometimes bronchial carcinoma declares itself long after removal of an intracranial deposit. In the absence of any systemic cancer, median survival is 2 years; this falls to 8 months if other evidence of systemic disease exists.

Chemotherapeutic agents are of little value unless given directly into the theca or ventricle for carcinomatous meningitis. The use of monoclonal antibodies as carriers of these agents may improve delivery of the drug to the tumour deposits. Radiation may improve the survival time of rather more than half the patients.

Vascular tumours

Haemangioblastoma occurs almost exclusively below the tentorium where it is as common as meningioma. Occasionally it is indistinguishable from angioblastic meningioma; the few cases reported above the tent are of this type. In the cerebellar hemisphere it usually forms a cystic tumour, a red mural nodule like a cherry in a cyst full of clear yellow fluid, somewhat resembling the cystic astrocytoma of childhood. A leash of vessels may be identified on the surface of the cerebellum (often the superior aspect), and these run to the nodule. Less often the vermis or the floor of the fourth ventricle is involved, usually by solid tumour.

These tumours may be multiple and sometimes run in families. When they do there may be angiomas in the retina and cysts and tumours of the pancreas and kidneys (Lindau's syndrome). Another associated feature, of single as well as of multiple tumours, is polycythaemia. Erythropoietin is produced by the tumour and the blood count returns to normal after removal.

Most patients present with raised ICP and cerebellar signs. Unsteadiness and vertigo may have been complaints for months or years, perhaps intermittently. Dementia or raised pressure due to obstructive hydrocephalus may predominate and overshadow cerebellar signs.

Cystic tumours are readily dealt with, for only the nodule need be removed. Solid tumours are formidable, for they are too vascular for piecemeal dissection; if the tumour should burst during dissection from the surrounding cerebellum, rapid enucleation is probably the safest course. Preoperative angiography should provide useful information about feeding vessels.

The outlook for cystic tumours is excellent, but the remnants of solid tumours may grow again and may even invade dura and muscle along the tissue planes opened at operation. Recurrence occurs in about 10–20 %, most often in familial cases and due to the growth of a second tumour. CT scanning is the best method for investigating a patient with suspected recurrence; ventriculograms are difficult to interpret after a previous operation, while an angiogram may show that there is more than one tumour present and their exact sites.

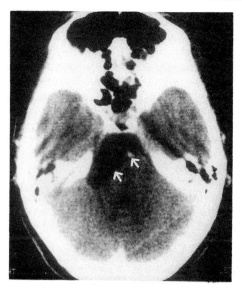

Fig. 6.13 CT showing a low-density epidermoid tumour within the cerebellopontine angle displacing the pons and the basilar artery (right-hand arrow).

Angiomas are really angiomatous or arteriovenous malformations, and although they may increase in extent they cause compression only when rupture leads to an intracerebral haematoma. They commonly declare themselves by producing subarachnoid haemorrhage and are discussed in Chapter 7 (p. 159).

Congenital tumours

Teratomas and *germinomas* most frequently occur in the *pineal region*, the former containing multiple tissue types, including epithelial elements, smooth muscle, bone and cartilage; the latter resembling seminoma of the testis, and frequently disseminating through CSF pathways. Ependymomas and astrocytomas are also prevalent types of tumours in this region. Tumours of the pineal gland itself – the benign *pineocytoma* and the malignant *pineoblastoma* – rarely occur.

These tumours can grow to a large size before detection. A haemorrhagic and polycystic mass expands bilaterally above the tentorium, and presses below on the dorsal midbrain. All produce obstructive hydrocephalus, often with dilated pupils and impaired upward gaze with ptosis due to midbrain pressure. Many of the tumours discussed above occur in young boys; a number of these develop precocious puberty which was at one time ascribed to endocrine activity in the tumour, but is probably due to involvement of the tuber cinereum by tumour which has seeded across the third ventricle.

Many pineal-region tumours are radiosensitive, and are therefore treated by shunting to deal with the hydrocephalus, followed by radiation. By serial CT scanning the response of the tumour can be monitored, and if it does not reduce in size then operation will be justified.

Epidermoids (cholesteatoma, pearly tumour) consist of epithelial debris accumulating inside a thin capsule lined with flattened cells to form white glistening flakes of material resembling mother-of-pearl.

Most occur in the basal subarachnoid cisterns, usually near the sella but sometimes in the cerebellopontine angle. Typical neighbourhood symptoms are produced but with a very long history. The capsule penetrates into every nook and cranny, making complete removal impossible, although the tumour is non-invasive. Occasional epidermoids are related to the lateral ventricles, sometimes wholly intraventricular. These intradural tumours can be diagnosed by CT scan which shows a characteristic low-density, even fat-density, lesion (Fig. 6.13). They are also associated with aseptic or chemical meningitis after operation, pleocytosis and pyrexia persisting intermittently for months. Although reports of organisms isolated from these tumours at operation may explain the meningitis, it is difficult after numerous lumbar punctures to exclude secondary infection when frank bacterial meningitis does develop.

Diploic epidermoids cause a lump on the skull and may indent the brain; erosion of the vault with a scalloped, dense margin is diagnostic. Another bony site is the petrous temporal where a circular erosion, obvious on X-ray, gives rise to slowly progressive facial palsy. Although some patients have had previous ear disease, this seems to be an entity distinct from infective cholesteatoma found with active otitis media. Early evacuation of this intrapetrous non-infective cholesteatoma through the middle fossa, using an extradural approach, may save the facial nerve from total destruction.

Dermoids also result from defective ectodermal closure, but the capsule includes dermal elements and the contents sebaceous material, hairs and oily fluid. Pericranial dermoids erode the bone near the anterior fontanelle in children. Orbital dermoids grow slowly from the lateral roof, causing painless proptosis and bone erosion.

Posterior fossa dermoids are both more dangerous and more variable in their presentation. All are in the midline; those which are wholly extradural have a skin sinus leading to a dimple just above the external occipital protuberance; often there is a subcutaneous lump in addition. Intradural cysts in the fourth ventricle may occasionally extend through the foramen to cause spinal compression. A sinus to the surface will predispose to recurrent meningitis or a posterior fossa abscess; without a sinus the cysts may cause obstructive hydrocephalus with cerebellar signs of varying degree. Careful study of the back of the head may reveal the sinus. CT scan usually shows a cystic appearance but the density is variable, ranging from very low (fat) to high, depending on the contents.

Chordoma arises in notochordal remnants in the basisphenoid or basiocciput to form a malignant and locally invasive tumour, which begins in the midline. Extensive bone destruction follows with the spread of tumour into the dura, paranasal air sinuses and ear. Clinical progression is very slow and may be intermittent; parasellar syndromes are more common than posterior fossa symptoms, usually without increased pressure. Dense calcification often occurs, and although the tumour may be in part myxomatous, it can be rock hard and cannot be removed completely.

Orbital tumours

The bony orbit is formed above by the floor of the anterior fossa, and the posterolateral orbital wall is the sphenoidal wing. This is also the anterior wall of the middle fossa, perforated by the optic foramen and the superior orbital fissure. Neurosurgeons are concerned with orbital disease because this has often spread from, or is liable to spread to, the intracranial cavity. Surgical exploration of the orbit for tumour may call for simultaneous exposure of the anterior or middle cranial fossae.

Orbital tumours are uncommon, but the main symptoms they cause are not; whenever proptosis or visual disturbance is found an orbital mass must be considered in the differential diagnosis.

Pathology
A wide variety of tumours have been reported in the orbit but only the most frequent will be mentioned. They arise in one of three situations:

1. *The optic nerve and its sheath* are most often affected by a *glioma (pilocytic astrocytoma)*. This tumour is almost confined to children, many of whom have von Recklinghausen's syndrome (p. 125). It begins some 10 mm behind the globe, and the enlargement of the optic nerve may cause expansion of the bony optic foramen which can be detected on plain X-rays. Spread backwards may result in involvement of the chiasm and the opposite optic nerve, or of the third ventricle with subsequent hydrocephalus. Such spread is not inevitable, however, and this tumour can be very indolent; it may show little or no obvious progression for many years, with or without any treatment, or after only incomplete removal.

    Meningioma of the sheath is much less common and occurs in adults. It is liable to cause pain and oedema in addition to proptosis and visual loss, which are the usual symptoms common to it and glioma.

    Retinoblastoma is a highly malignant familial glioma, occurring under the age of 4 years, often affecting both eyes and (exceptional among gliomas) metastasizing to lymph nodes and distant organs.

2. *Other orbital tissues* may become tumorous and the commonest condition of all to cause proptosis is the *orbital granuloma (pseudotumour)* which affects all the orbital contents. This is an unexplained condition in which the orbital fat, muscles and adventitia of vessels are infiltrated with lymph cells and plasma cells; spread of low-grade infection from neighbouring air sinuses has been suggested as a cause but is unproven. The affected tissues are firm and swollen, and local masses may be felt through the intact skin. This is a self-limiting process which normally responds dramatically to steroid therapy. Orbital exploration is only required if diagnostic doubt persists.

    Lacrimal gland tumours mostly resemble mixed salivary gland tumours and tend to recur locally, sometimes years after excision. Both *angiomas and lymphangiomas* occur and give rise to proptosis which may vary spontaneously or may be temporarily aggravated by the patient bending forwards, and reduced by pressure on the globe.

3. *The bony orbital walls* may be affected by tumours which project partly

into the orbit and partly either externally or into the surrounding cavities of the sinuses or cranium. Simple tumours include *dermoid cyst*, which often causes a palpable swelling at the outer upper angle of the orbit and a translucency on X-ray; *mucocoele* of the sinus, usually frontal, which is often associated with chronic or recurrent infection; *meningioma* of the sphenoidal wing, which gives rise to long-standing proptosis and visual loss, sometimes with a temporal swelling: and *osteoma* of the sinuses, usually frontal, which may also grow intracranially and breach the dura giving rise to rhinorrhoea or spontaneous aerocele. *Malignant* tumours may be primary, most often carcinoma of the ethmoid, or secondary, from distant carcinoma, sarcoma or melanoma.

Clinical

Proptosis is the most constant feature and the globe may also be displaced downwards or laterally, occasionally upwards. In doubtful instances the eyes should be viewed from above. *Intermittent* proptosis suggests a vascular, infective or granulomatous condition, whilst if the protrusion is *pulsatile* there is either an arteriovenous fistula in the orbit or a carotico-cavernous fistula (p. 230).

Marked *oedema* of the lids and conjunctiva suggests either endocrine exophthalmos, carotico-cavernous fistula or orbital granuloma.

Visual failure is gradual and may not be noticed until the eye is totally blind. Because of the visual loss diplopia may never be complained of although the visual axes of the two eyes are far from parallel.

Ocular movements are surprisingly well preserved even when the globe is markedly displaced; if there is marked ophthalmoplegia either endocrine exophthalmos or a lesion in the cavernous sinus should be suspected.

Anteriorly placed tumours (lacrimal gland or dermoids) may be *palpable*. The fundus is affected only by tumours on the nerve and sheath, and *optic atrophy* is more common than *unilateral papilloedema*.

Investigation

Measurement of the degree of protrusion, and serial clinical photographs document the progress of the condition, and can assess the result of treatment. Plain X-rays should include views to show the air sinuses, the skull and the optic foraminae. Thyroid function must be tested, and the possibility of a primary tumour elsewhere in the body excluded as far as seems reasonable. CT scanning gives the most information but carotid angiography may show up a vascular lesion within the orbit itself or a carotico-cavernous fistula. In some conditions MRI may provide additional information.

Treatment

Few orbital tumours can be diagnosed without surgical exploration. The aim is to make this as limited as possible in the first place. Some tumours are easily removed, some call for a major orbito-cranial approach, whilst other conditions are either inoperable or do not call for surgical measures beyond a biopsy to establish the diagnosis (e.g. the common orbital granuloma).

The surgical approach depends on the site of the tumour. For most tumours, i.e. those lying superior, lateral or inferior to the optic nerve, a lateral approach suffices. An incision is made in the eyebrow which is not shaved and the superolateral angle of the bony margin is turned back as a small flap. Tumours lying anterior and medial to the nerve can be removed through a medial ethmoidal approach. It is tumours lying posteriorly and medially, involving the nerve or extending intracranially, which call for a frontal craniotomy and deroofing of the orbit. This approach allows section of the nerve behind the posterior margin of an optic nerve glioma, if possible, to prevent backward extension. However, the indolent course of this tumour in many cases has led to controversy as to whether such drastic treatment is necessary or indeed justified; the need for a radical operation may depend on the extent of residual vision. Certainly the globe need not be sacrificed, even though the nerve is sectioned and the eye left sightless, because this tumour rarely extends forwards to the globe.

Endocrine exophthalmos

Not only does this form an important differential diagnosis when orbital tumour is under discussion, but it may call for neurosurgical intervention in its own right. The physiopathology cannot be fully discussed here. The link with overt thyroid disease may not be obvious; thyrotoxicosis may accompany the condition or have been treated months or years before, but some patients have no disturbance of thyroid function, even when this is tested by modern isotope techniques.

Women are twice as frequently affected as men. Both eyes are usually involved, but there may be a delay of up to 6 months before the second eye is affected. Oedema and ophthalmoplegia are obvious, much more so than for a similar degree of proptosis due to tumour. A coronal CT scan confirms the diagnosis, showing thickening of the extraocular muscles. Although the condition is commonly self-limiting, malignant cases occur in which vision is threatened by progressive protrusion and corneal ulceration. It is these cases that are sometimes sent to the neurosurgeon for decompression of the orbit.

Both this measure and such other treatment as is available are purely empirical. Correction of thyroid disorder by drugs or thyroidectomy may improve the condition or make it worse, or it may arise only when the treatment for thyrotoxicosis has been completed. Radiotherapy to the orbital tissues may be of value. Decompression does nothing to remove the cause, but may help to break the vicious circle of progressive oedema. As long as this involved a major frontal craniotomy (Naffziger's operation) the method was naturally looked on as a last resort, but several less drastic methods have been introduced in recent years. All involve a direct operation on the lateral wall of the orbit, with the removal of the orbital roof and lateral wall; the patient is left with a pulsating eye but this is not very noticeable nor subjectively troublesome. This lateral approach has proved successful and leaves an acceptable cosmetic scar. This relatively minor procedure can be considered for even mild cases, if symptoms are persistent and other measures fail to afford relief.

Suspected tumour recurrence

Once a patient has had a brain tumour he or she and the medical advisers are always alert to the possibility of recurrence. Almost any symptom, but especially headache or vomiting, however trivial, is apt to raise suspicion and the decision must be made whether to reinvestigate or not. Apart from irrelevant conditions, from influenza to hypertension, there are a number of intracranial events remotely related to the original operation which may mimic recurrence. Although most have been described already, they may conveniently be listed together here.

1. *Radionecrosis* is characterized by the sudden onset of focal signs, sometimes remote from the exact site of the previous tumour, without raised pressure as a rule, and often resolving spontaneously. This explanation should not be accepted for incidents occurring less than a year after treatment, and 2–5 years or more is the common interval.
2. *Obstructive hydrocephalus* due to postoperative adhesions may affect any part of the ventricular system. Reaction to the blood spilt at operation, or to low-grade postoperative infection, may lead to an adhesive arachnoiditis in the posterior fossa or at the tentorial hiatus, which causes a block at the outlet of the fourth ventricle or at the cisterna ambiens, resulting in total hydrocephalus. Occasionally the block is higher in the ventricular system, with dilatation of one lateral ventricle or of only one temporal horn. Obstructive hydrocephalus requires a ventriculoperitoneal shunt.
3. *Hypopituitary crises* (p. 122) have characteristics which should lead to early recognition, and the site of the original tumour will suggest the likelihood of this explanation for coma or collapse.
4. *Infection* may take the form of meningitis, usually in patients who have had a CSF leak, and this may first develop years after operation. An abscess in the tumour cavity more often declares itself within a few months as a recurrence of raised pressure and focal signs – too soon to be likely to be due to tumour regrowth.
5. *Local brain atrophy* can occur in areas adjacent to the site of tumour removal. The ventricle may dilate into an atrophic area to form a porencephalic cyst; or such a cyst can develop in relation to the subarachnoid space and indent the ventricle, with which it does not communicate. Local degenerative changes may be accelerated by vascular insufficiency, as arterial disease develops with advancing age; if a patient becomes arteriosclerotic, the area of brain surrounding the operation site, which has existed on a precarious blood supply for years, may be deprived more severely than the rest of the brain and focal signs and symptoms may then recur.
6. *Epilepsy* may occasionally be overlooked as a cause of relapse. A series of unwitnessed convulsions can leave a patient in coma or stupor for hours or days, during which tumour recurrence may be suspected. Intoxication with phenytoin causes ataxia and nystagmus which may mistakenly suggest intracranial mischief. Whether the development or recurrence of epilepsy should be taken as evidence of tumour recurrence is doubtful, but the sudden appearance of insistent focal epilepsy in a patient who has previously had a convexity or parasagittal meningioma is certainly suspicious. In general, however, patients can rightly be reassured that the occurrence of epilepsy does not mean renewed tumour activity.
7. *A second intracranial tumour*, developing in a patient who has already had one removed, will naturally first be regarded as a recurrence. This

possibility must be considered when the original tumour was a *metastasis*: or a *neurofibroma*, especially if the latter was in a patient with generalized von Recklinghausen's disease or a family history of this. *Meningiomas* are occasionally multiple, whilst most 'recurrences' of cerebellar *haemangioblastomas* are probably second tumours, again most often in patients with a family history. *Gliomas* which spread through CSF pathways (medulloblastoma, ependymoma and intraventricular astrocytoma) may recur at sites distant from the original mass.

8. *Recurrence of the original tumour* may be readily recognized because the symptoms and signs often closely resemble those which characterized the first illness. This is by no means the rule, however, and the issue may be further clouded by the absence of signs of raised pressure; not only are the fundi normal but the decompression often remains indrawn even when it has not become so firm as to be unyielding. CT scan or MRI is the best way to make the diagnosis. Shift of midline structures is difficult to interpret when there is a decompression, and perhaps also local atrophy, ventricular dilatation or porencephalic cyst.

Further reading

Tumours in general

Adams J.H., Graham D.I., Doyle D. (1981). *Brain Biopsy. The Smear Technique for Neurosurgical Biopsies*. London: Chapman and Hall.

Al-Mefty O., Kersch J., Routh A. *et al.* (1990). The long term side effects of radiation therapy for benign brain tumours in adults. *J. Neurosurg.*; **73**: 502–12.

Bullard D.E., Bigner D.D. (1985). Applications of monoclonal antibodies in the diagnosis and treatment of primary brain tumours. *J. Neurosurg.*; **63**: 2–16.

Choksey M.S., Valentine A., Showdon H. *et al.* (1989). Computerised tomography in the diagnosis of malignant brain tumours. Do all require biopsy? *J. Neurol. Neurosurg. Psychiatry*; **52**: 821–5.

Edwards M.S.B., Hudgins R.J., Wilson C.B. *et al.* (1988). Pineal tumours in children. *J. Neurosurg.*; **68**: 689–97.

Galicich J.H., Sundaresan N., Thaler H.T. (1980). Surgical treatment of single brain metastasis. *J. Neurosurg.*; **53**: 63–7.

Henk J.M. (1981). Orbital tumours. *Hosp. Update*; **7**: 439–50.

Jeffreys R. (1975). Clinical and surgical aspects of posterior fossa haemangioblastomas. *J. Neurol. Neurosurg. Psychiatry*; **38**: 105–11.

Leibel S.A., Sheline G.E. (1987). Radiation therapy for neoplasms of the brain. *Neurosurgery*; **66**: 1–22.

Ojemann R.G. (1992). Skull base surgery: a perspective. *J. Neurosurg.*; **76**: 569–70.

Russell D., Rubenstein L.J. (1989). *The Pathology of Tumours of the Nervous System*; 5th edn. London: Arnold.

Sundaresan N., Galicich J.H., Beattie E.J. Jr. (1983). Surgical treatment of brain metastasis from lung cancer. *J. Neurosurg.*; **58**: 666–71.

Thomas D.G.T., Graham D.I. (1980). *Brain Tumours. Scientific Basis, Clinical Investigation and Current Therapy*. London: Butterworths.

Thomas D.G.T., Nouby R.M. (1989). Experience in 300 cases of CT directed stereotactic surgery for lesion biopsy and aspiration of haematoma. *Br. J. Neurosurg.*; **3**: 321–6.

Acoustic neuroma

Bentivoglio P., Cheeseman A.D., Symon L. (1988). Surgical management of acoustic neuromas during the last 5 years. *Surg. Neurol.*; **29:** 197–204, 205–9.

Hardy D.G., MacFarlane R., Baguley D. *et al.* (1989). Surgery for acoustic neuroma: an analysis of 100 translabyrinthine operations. *J. Neurosurg.*; **71:** 799–804.

King T.T. (1988). Surgical approaches to acoustic nerve tumours. *Br. J. Neurosurg.*; **2:** 433–8.

King T.T., Morrison A.W. (1980). Translabyrinthine and transtentorial removal of acoustic nerve tumours. Results in 150 cases. *J. Neurosurg.*; **52:** 210–16.

Symon L., Pell M. (1992). Surgical management of acoustic neuroma and meningioma of the posterior cranial fossa. In: Teasdale G.M., Miller J.D. (eds.) *Current Neurosurgery*. Edinburgh: Churchill Livingstone.

Embryonic and maldevelopmental origin

Fischer E.G., Welch K., Bell J.A. *et al.* (1981). Treatment of craniopharyngiomas in children 1972–81. *J. Neurosurg.*; **62:** 496–501.

Hoffman H.J. (1985). Craniopharyngiomas. *Can. J. Neurol. Sci.*; **12:** 348–52.

King T.T., Benjamin J.C., Morrison A.W. (1989). Epidermoid and cholesterol cysts in the apex of the petrous bone. *Br. J. Neurosurg.*; **3:** 451–62.

Logue V., Till K. (1952). Posterior fossa dermoid cysts with special reference to intracranial infection. *J. Neurol. Neurosurg. Psychiatry*; **15:** 1–12.

Packer R.J., Sutton L.N., Godwein J.W. *et al.* (1991). Improved survival with the use of adjuvant chemotherapy in the treatment of medulloblastoma. *J. Neurosurg.*; **74:** 433–40.

Wold L.E., Laws E.R. (1983). Cranial chordomas in children and young adults. *J. Neurosurg.*; **59:** 1043–7.

Yasargil M.G., Curcic M., Kis M. *et al.* (1990). Total removal of craniopharyngiomas: approaches and long-term results in 144 patients. *J. Neurosurg.*; **73:** 3–11.

Gliomas

Flarell R.C., MacDonald D.R., Irish W.D. *et al.* (1992). Selection bias, survival and brachytherapy for glioma. *J. Neurosurg.*; **76:** 179–83.

Garcia D.M., Latifi H.R., Simpson J.K. *et al.* (1989). Astrocytoma of the cerebellum in children. *J. Neurosurg.*; **71:** 661–4.

Gjerris F., Klinken L. (1978). Long-term prognosis in children with benign cerebellar astrocytomas. *J. Neurosurg.*; **49:** 179–84.

Kyritsis A.P., Levin V.A. (1992). Chemotherapeutic approaches to the treatment of malignant gliomas. *Adv. Oncol.*; **8:** 9–13.

Lindegaard K.-F., Mork S.J., Eide G.E. *et al.* (1987). Statistical analysis of clinicopathological features, radiotherapy and survival in 170 cases of oligodendroglioma. *J. Neurosurg.*; **67:** 224–30.

Loeffler J.S. (1992). Radiotherapy in managing malignant gliomas: current role and future directions. *Adv. Oncol.*; **8:** 14–20.

Nazzaro J.M., Neuwelt E.A. (1990). The role of surgery in the management of supratentorial intermediate and high-grade astrocytomas in adults. *J. Neurosurg.*; **73:** 331–44.

Salazar O.M., Castro-Vita H., Van Houtte P. *et al.* (1983). Improved survival in cases of intracranial ependymoma after radiation therapy. *J. Neurosurg.*; **59:** 652–9.

Walker M.D., Alexander E. Jr., Hunt W.E. *et al.* (1978). Evaluation of BCNU and/or radiotherapy in the treatment of anaplastic gliomas: a cooperative trial. *J. Neurosurg.*; **49:** 333–43.

Whittle I.R. (1992). The biology of glioma. In: Teasdale G.M., Miller J.D. (eds.) *Current Neurosurgery*. Edinburgh: Churchill Livingstone.

Whittle I.R., Gregor A. (1991). The treatment of primary malignant brain tumours. *J. Neurol. Neurosurg. Psychiatry*; **54:** 101–3.

Meningioma

Adegbite A.B., Khan M.I., Paine K.W.E. *et al.* (1983). The recurrence of intracranial meningiomas after surgical treatment. *J. Neurosurg.*; **58:** 51–6.

MacCarty C.S., Taylor W.R. (1979). Intracranial meningiomas: experiences at the Mayo Clinic. *Neurol. Med. Chir.*; **19:** 569–74.

Mirimanoff R.O., Dosoretz D.E., Lingood R.M. *et al.*, (1985). Meningioma: analysis of recurrence and progression following neurosurgical resection. *J. Neurosurg.*; **62:** 18–24.

Pituitary tumours

Cooper P.R. (ed.) (1991). *Contemporary Diagnosis and Management of Pituitary Adenoma.* Park Ridge, IL: A.A.N.S.

Kohler P.O. (1987). Treatment of pituitary adenomas. *N. Engl. J. Med.*; **317:** 45–6.

McGregor A.M., Ginsberg J. (1981). Dilemmas in the management of functioning pituitary tumours. *Br. J. Hosp. Med.*; Apr: 344–52.

Teasdale G. (1983). Surgical management of pituitary adenoma. *Clin. Endocrinol. Metab.*; **12:** 789–823.

Teasdale E., Teasdale G., Mohsen F. *et al.* (1986). High resolution computed tomography in pituitary microadenoma: is seeing believing? *Clin. Radiol.*; **37:** 227–32.

Tindall G.T., Herring C.J., Clark R.V. *et al.* (1990). Cushing's disease: results of transsphenoidal microsurgery with emphasis on surgical failures. *J. Neurosurg.*; **72:** 363–9.

Wass J.H., William J., Charlesworth M. *et al.* (1982). Bromocriptine in the management of large pituitary tumours. *Br. Med. J.;* **284:** 1908–11.

Chapter 7

Surgery for vascular lesions

Haemorrhagic strokes

    Subarachnoid haemorrhage
    Intracranial aneurysms
    Arteriovenous malformation (AVM)
    Cerebral haemorrhage

Ischaemic strokes

In a significant number of patients suffering from cerebrovascular accident or stroke, radiological investigations can indicate the underlying lesion, which may be suitable for surgical treatment. These include many patients with subarachnoid haemorrhage due to aneurysm or anteriovenous malformation; some with primary intracerebral haemorrhage; and a few with ischaemic strokes. Radiology has taught that clinical criteria are unreliable in distinguishing between even the broadest categories of strokes.

These categories can be readily identified on a pathological basis as follows:

1.   Haemorrhagic strokes.
    (a) Subarachnoid.
    (b) Intracerebral.
2.   Ischaemic strokes.
      Vascular occlusion.
      Perfusion failure.

Haemorrhagic strokes usually cause headache, and often clouding of consciousness or even coma, at the onset; ischaemic strokes are frequently painless and, if due to local vascular occlusion, cause focal signs related to the deprived area – a blind eye, a weak arm or dysphasia. Swelling of a large infarct may lead to headache and depression of consciousness after 24 hours or so, due to raised ICP leading to midbrain shift and distortion.

Haemorrhagic strokes

Subarachnoid haemorrhage

Cause

Subarachnoid haemorrhage is a fairly common condition, affecting 12 per 100 000 of the population each year. Two-thirds result from rupture of an aneurysm on a major vessel; in 5% an arteriovenous malformation (AVM) has bled, and occasional cases are due to tumour, bleeding diathesis or anticoagulant therapy. Even after complete angiography no cause is found in up to a quarter of cases, most of whom have had a small haemorrhage and recover completely with little risk of recurrence.

Clinical

There is seldom an obvious precipitating cause for the haemorrhage, which is as likely to happen during relaxation as at the height of physical activity. When there is a considerable escape of blood, consciousness is lost rapidly and the patient may die in minutes or hours. If the patient recovers it is often only a matter of minutes before consciousness is regained. Smaller leaks give less dramatic symptoms, severe headache being the most usual complaint. This is almost always followed within minutes or hours by vomiting, and later by neck stiffness. Suspected meningitis may result in admission to a fever hospital. Consciousness is often clouded but the illness may be so mild as to be mistaken for influenza or migraine. When a patient presents with a major haemorrhage, careful enquiry sometimes reveals a minor incident in the previous few weeks that in retrospect is suspicious of a 'warning' initial haemorrhage. When patients remain ambulant, leg pain may develop due to the irritant effect of blood that has settled around the lumbosacral nerve roots in the subarachnoid space.

Headache is usual but not invariable. Commonly it comes on suddenly, and is either generalized or felt in the back of the neck, but occasionally it begins in one area and rapidly spreads. Pain limited to one eye suggests an ipsilateral carotid aneurysm. *Vomiting* almost always occurs. *Neck stiffness* is also usual but may not appear until the second or third day and occasionally not at all; photophobia commonly develops sooner.

Reactive arterial hypertension for 24–48 hours after subarachnoid haemorrhage is quite frequent, probably due to catecholamine release. Electrocardiogram (ECG) changes similar to those of myocardial infarction are sometimes seen.

Focal neurological signs are frequent but do not always provide a reliable pointer to the site, or even to the side, of the primary lesion, especially when there has been a severe haemorrhage. Minor signs, such as an extensor plantar response on one side, are of little value; even hemiplegia may be due to intracerebral haematoma which has extended far from the ruptured vessel. Misleading signs may also derive from ischaemia related to spasm in vessels some distance from the site of the bleeding, but a marked hemiplegia is often related to a middle cerebral artery aneurysm. In an alert patient with subarachnoid haemorrhage, an isolated third nerve palsy suggests direct nerve involvement from a posterior communicating artery aneurysm. In a patient in coma or with deteriorating conscious level, a third nerve palsy may result secondarily from tentorial herniation.

Clinical grades were proposed by Botterell as a means of indicating the overall state of the patient with recent subarachnoid haemorrhage due to

Table 7.1 The World Federation of Neurosurgeons (WFNS) subarachnoid scale

WFNS grade	GCS score	Motor deficit
I	15	Absent
II	14–13	Absent
III	14–13	Present
IV	12–7	Present or absent
V	6–3	Present or absent

GCS = Glasgow Coma Scale.

ruptured aneurysm, particularly in regard to assessing suitability for surgery. Since then, various alternative schemes have been used, based on data about severity of symptoms, meningism and focal deficit, combined with level of consciousness. However conscious level was not well-described within these systems and the World Federation of Neurosurgeons (WFNS) has proposed a new scale using the Glasgow Coma Scale (Table 7.1). These scales indicate the prognosis either with or without surgery and provide a basis for decision-making about individual patients. Categorizing patients immediately after admission makes it possible to assess and compare results of patients managed by different methods.

Diagnosis

The recognition of a small initial haemorrhage is by no means always easy, but the abrupt onset of headache, soon followed by vomiting, should always arouse suspicion. A number of patients with a major bleed report a less dramatic incident within the previous 2 or 3 weeks which was regarded as migraine or flu – sometimes even after admission to hospital. Confirmation of the diagnosis in the past was invariably obtained by lumbar puncture, but this carries a risk of precipitating tentorial herniation in the presence of an intracerebral or intracerebellar haematoma. Lumbar puncture should be

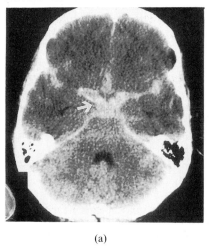

(a)

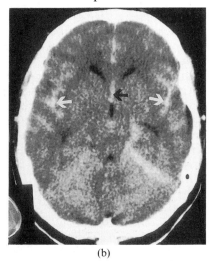

(b)

Fig. 7.1 CT scan after recent subarachnoid haemorrhage (from an anterior communicating aneurysm). (a) Blood in the basal cisterns; (b) blood in the anterior interhemispheric fissure (black arrow) and in both Sylvian fissures (white arrows).

Table 7.2 Natural history of subarachnoid haemorrhage due to ruptured intracranial aneurysm

	Mortality %	Cumulative mortality %
Die without recovering		
Before hospital	15	
After admission	28	43
Rebleed and die		
<1 month	14	57
1 month–1 year	7	64
1 year–10 years	10	74

Of those alive at 10 years, 8% are disabled, leaving only 18% alive and well.

avoided in patients with an impaired conscious level, papilloedema or focal signs. *CT scanning* is now the preliminary investigation of choice; this usually shows blood in the basal cisterns and/or fissures and will exclude the presence of a mass lesion (Fig. 7.1). If CT scanning is not available and the patient is alert, oriented and without papilloedema or focal signs, lumbar puncture carries little risk and when the history is atypical, may save an unnecessary transfer or investigation. If the CT scan shows no abnormality, then lumbar puncture is required to confirm or refute the diagnosis. If the CSF is heavily bloodstained, doubt may still exist as to whether the needle punctured a blood vessel rather than the theca; no matter how heavy the contamination, blood pre-existing within the CSF does not clot. Red blood cells normally disappear in 9 days, but may go sooner after a small bleed. Centrifuging the CSF and examining the supernatant for xanthochromia confirms the pre-existence of red blood cells in the CSF and is important evidence in favour of a genuine haemorrhage as against accidental contamination with blood. Red cell lysis takes time and xanthochromic staining of the CSF may not appear for 6–12 hours after the haemorrhage. CSF spectrophotometry is the most sensitive method for detecting the pigments which produce xanthochromia (oxyhaemoglobin, methaemoglobin and bilirubin). This technique will detect red cell breakdown products in 70% of patients 3 weeks after the haemorrhage.

Once subarachnoid haemorrhage has been confirmed, angiography is usually arranged without delay to establish the cause; some surgeons may postpone this if they feel that the patient's clinical state would preclude surgical intervention. In about 1 patient in 10, angiography is negative and nothing more need be done; in such patients, the cause remains obscure, but the risk of further haemorrhage is extremely small and the outlook excellent.

Prognosis and natural history

If coma persists for more than a few hours after subarachnoid haemorrhage, the prospects are poor, irrespective of the cause. Death may occur from the intracranial effects of the initial bleed, from rebleeding, from delayed cerebral ischaemia, or from extracranial complications, including cardiac arrhythmias, myocardial infarction, pulmonary oedema or gastric haemorrhage. Nowadays most patients with cerebral aneurysms undergo operation to prevent rebleeding, but data from previous studies give the natural history of aneurysm rupture and show the immediate and long-term risks of adopting a conservative approach (Table 7.2).

A clear distinction should be made between the mortality and morbidity associated with subarachnoid haemorrhage in general and that of different lesions. Also between overall mortality, which includes deaths at home or in the primary hospital, and that quoted by specialist units, who may follow a selective admissions policy, only accepting potential candidates for surgery, sometimes several days after aneurysm rupture.

Intracranial aneurysms

Aetiology
Until recently, the saccular or berry aneurysm was referred to as a *congenital* lesion, in contrast to the less common fusiform *arteriosclerotic* dilatation and the rare mycotic aneurysm associated with inflammatory lesions such as subacute bacterial endocarditis and polyarteritis nodosa. Congenital defects or 'gaps' often exist in the rather poorly developed medial layer, but these defects appear capable of withstanding relatively high intraluminal pressures. It is now recognized that other factors, including degenerative change with damage to the internal elastic lamina, high blood flow and hypertension are likely to play a part. However, congenital factors may still contribute and an inborn error of type III collagen deficiency has been found in a proportion of patients with saccular aneurysms. Aneurysms are rarely found in children and the peak incidence lies between 40 and 60 years, supporting a degenerative rather than a congenital aetiology.

Degenerative change
In cerebral vessels all the elastic elements in the wall are concentrated in the internal elastic lamina. In some patients it appears that early degenerative change with intimal hyperplasia may lead to damage of the elastic layer and to aneurysm formation rather than to the formation of an atheromatous plaque. A link certainly exists. In one series of patients with ruptured aneurysms, the incidence of severe coronary atheroma was much higher than in a control group of similar age, suggesting a predisposition to premature arterial degeneration.

High blood flow
Aneurysms appear to form at sites of haemodynamic stress where blood flow is high. Anomalous development of the circle of Willis occurs more frequently in patients with aneurysms. Moreover aneurysms tend to form at sites with augmented blood flow, e.g. on the side opposite a hypoplastic anterior cerebral artery. About 8% of patients with arteriovenous malformations develop aneurysms, usually on feeding vessels where blood flow is significantly increased.

Hypertension
Hypertension might be expected to accentuate any vascular weakness but its link with aneurysm formation is harder to establish. Patients with coarctation of the aorta, who have high arterial pressure in the caroticovertebral system,

are liable to develop ruptured cerebral aneurysms at an unusually early age. The relationship with polycystic kidney disease appears to relate to fibrotic change within the vessel wall rather than to hypertension. Hypertension is certainly not a necessary causative factor either for the development or for the rupture of aneurysms. Only half the patients in a recent large series had a pressure of more than 160/90 mmHg and autopsy studies have failed to demonstrate a higher incidence of hypertensive changes in aneurysm patients compared to age- and sex-matched controls.

Site (Fig. 7.2)
The majority of aneurysms occur in a few constant situations on the circle of Willis, most on the anterior half of the circle. More than a third arise from the *anterior communicating artery* complex; they may derive their blood supply from either or both carotids and are so situated that rupture may occur into either frontal lobe. The *internal carotid artery* is the next most common site,

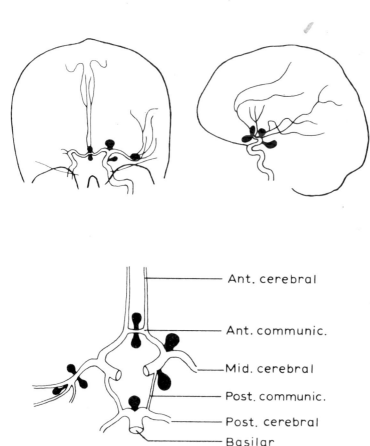

Fig. 7.2 Common sites for aneurysms.

usually at the origin of the *posterior communicating artery*, but also at the terminal bifurcation, at the origin of the anterior choroidal or ophthalmic arteries or in the cavernous sinus. *Middle cerebral artery* aneurysms account for about 20% and usually occur at the trifurcation, about 2 cm lateral to the origin of the internal carotid. Rarely the aneurysm develops on a more proximal branch, and so lies among the perforating arteries. *Pericallosal* artery aneurysms also occur, but are unusual. Half the posterior fossa aneurysms are on the *basilar artery*, most often at the terminal bifurcation into posterior cerebral arteries; some are on the *vertebral artery* on its last branch, the *posterior inferior cerebellar artery*, and these may pass undetected unless both vertebral arteries are demonstrated at angiography.

About 20% of patients have more than one aneurysm, sometimes symmetrically disposed. The first aneurysm displayed by angiography may not therefore be the only one, nor necessarily the one which has ruptured.

Dynamic pathology

Most aneurysms grow larger with time: serial angiograms leave no doubt about this. Adhesions develop, to neighbouring structures, to other arteries, and to the brain in which the aneurysm can become so buried that no part remains in the subarachnoid space. Secondary dilatations may develop and patchy thrombosis lays down layers of clot; the irregular lumen which still fills with circulating blood, and which is all an angiogram can show, then represents only a fraction of the whole sac and bears little relation to its external shape.

Aneurysms usually become clinically obvious only when intracerebral or subarachnoid *rupture* occurs. Most aneurysms rupture only when they are 5 mm or more in diameter and it is the fundus that gives way in most instances, the neck very seldom. If the aneurysm is buried in the brain the haemorrhage will be intracerebral, although blood may later reach the subarachnoid space via the ventricular system. Sometimes aneurysms become quite large without having ruptured, probably because stagnant blood near the edge of the sac thromboses and reinforces the wall. Local pressure effects may result.

Intracavernous aneurysms are protected as they enlarge by the dural walls of the cavernous sinus, and consequently they rarely rupture. Occasionally, when still small, one does burst into the cavernous sinus, giving rise to a caroticocavernous (arteriovenous) fistula, similar to that produced by trauma (p. 230).

Complications of aneurysm rupture

Rebleeding occurs in about 20% of patients not undergoing operation within the first 2 weeks and 60% within the first 6 months; of those, two-thirds die. Beyond 6 months, the risk of rebleeding falls to a level of 3.5% per year. If a patient survives a rebleed, there is a significantly greater risk of a further rebleed occurring than before. Balancing the risks of rebleeding against those of surgical intervention is often difficult and is discussed later (p. 157).

Cerebral infarction is the other major cause of mortality and morbidity after ruptured aneurysm, apart from the obvious effects of massive local damage from rupture. Patients who die within a few hours or days of the initial bleed without a mass lesion or rebleed frequently show evidence of patchy wide-spread ischaemic changes at autopsy. This may affect the distribution of major vessels (e.g. middle cerebral or its main branches); often there are small scattered areas of infarction and ischaemia in the central areas of the basal ganglia, hypothalamus and upper brainstem, reflecting reduced flow in the perforating and other small vessels.

Delayed cerebral ischaemia can cause deterioration in up to one-third of patients who survive the initial haemorrhage, whether or not there has been surgical intervention. Symptoms develop from 3 days to 3 weeks after the ictus, with a peak incidence occurring at about 8 days. Clinical features depend on the arterial territory involved but include hemiparesis, dysphasia, impaired conscious level, mutism and incontinence.

Delayed ischaemia was initially attributed to vasospasm or, more correctly, arterial narrowing on angiography, but not all patients with angiographic narrowing develop clinical evidence of ischaemia. This is perhaps not surprising as CBF depends more on the state of the small-resistance arterioles than on the larger vessels seen on angiogram. In many patients, autoregulation is impaired. Although an overall reduction in CBF often occurs, there are wide variations from day to day and no obvious correlation exists with the clinical state of the patient. The development of vasospasm and focal cerebral ischaemia correlates well with the amount and site of blood in the basal cisterns and fissures (as seen on CT scan). Vasoconstrictive substances appear in the CSF after subarachnoid haemorrhage, released either from the vessel wall or from the breakdown of extravasated blood clot; however, the narrowing is not merely due to vessel constriction, as arteriopathic change with myonecrosis occurs within the vessel wall and undoubtedly contributes to the angiographic appearances.

Vasospasm is not the only cause of delayed cerebral ischaemia; other factors are almost certainly involved. In up to 50% of patients, excessive renal secretion of sodium results in fluid loss and a fall in plasma volume; blood viscosity rises and leads to a reduction in blood flow. The presence of an intracerebral haematoma or hydrocephalus can raise ICP and reduce cerebral perfusion. Pre-existing arteriosclerosis may add to these acute problems and limit collateral flow, as may variations in cardiac output, blood pressure and blood gases.

Hydrocephalus occurs in two phases after subarachnoid haemorrhage, acutely within the first few days, or a more chronic type develops in the second week. Both forms probably result from blockage by blood of the pathways for CSF absorption. In most instances hydrocephalus is of the communicating type and may respond to lumbar puncture. Patients with blood clot obstructing the third or fourth ventricles require ventricular drainage. Although hydrocephalus occurs in over 20% of patients, less than 5% require permanent CSF drainage.

Intracerebral haematoma frequently follows rupture of a middle cerebral or anterior communicating artery aneurysms. Either frontal or temporal lobe haematomas may rupture into the ventricle; the distension of the third and fourth may contribute to the coma, mutism and hyperpyrexia which occur in some patients.

Syndromes due to unruptured aneurysm

Local neurological dysfunction from distortion of neighbouring structures by the sac is largely limited to aneurysms of the internal carotid. Those which arise within the cavernous sinus are most common in middle-aged women; the usual complaint is of pain, and later sensory loss, in one or more divisions of the trigeminal nerve, together with ocular palsies (3, 4, 6 cranial nerves). Although symptoms characteristically begin or increase suddenly, the onset can be insidious, resembling a tumour; erosion of the clinoid processes seen on X-ray may be indistinguishable from changes produced by a sellar or parasellar tumour.

Aneurysms at the bifurcation of the internal carotid artery are often directed forwards. They may then produce symptoms resembling a pituitary tumour with visual failure, field defects and optic atrophy. Endocrine deficiency is unusual, but the sella may be eroded on X-ray. Aneurysms arising at the point of origin of the posterior communicating artery are usually directed backwards and may cause pressure on the trunk of the third nerve. This leads to varying degrees of oculomotor palsy (dilated pupil, external strabismus and ptosis), sometimes accompanied by supraorbital pain but without trigeminal sensory loss. Rarely, aneurysms of the basilar artery, arising at the bifurcation or at the origin of the superior cerebellar artery, present with an oculomotor nerve palsy.

Investigation of suspected ruptured aneurysm

CT scan

Good-quality CT scanning can detect blood in the basal cisterns, fissures and subarachnoid space in 96% of patients with aneurysm rupture when performed within 48 hours of the bleed – but in only 50% of patients 7 days after the bleed (Fig. 7.1). Not only will it confirm the presence of subarachnoid blood but its location often indicates the likely site of the affected aneurysm. In addition, CT scanning may reveal an intracerebral haematoma or hydrocephalus, and indicate the need for urgent surgical intervention.

Angiography (Figs 7.3–7.5)

Angiography is usually performed when it is clear that the patient will survive the initial haemorrhage. With modern techniques, four vessel catheterization through the femoral route carries little risk. In this way as much information as possible is gained concerning the number and site of all aneurysms, and the relative contribution of blood flow from each of the major vessels. This can help in deciding about alternative operative tactics, for example by showing from which side an anterior communicating artery is mainly filled. By demonstrating the extent and distribution of vascular spasm, angiography may also influence the decision about the timing of surgery. When angiography reveals more than one aneurysm, the location of spasm, the size of the aneurysm and the regularity of its outline may point to the lesion responsible for the bleed, but localized blood clot on the CT scan is probably the best guide. Recent studies suggest that *MRI* may provide even more help than CT in locating the ruptured aneurysm, by demonstrating an increased signal from reactive oedema within brain tissue immediately adjacent to the site of the haemorrhage.

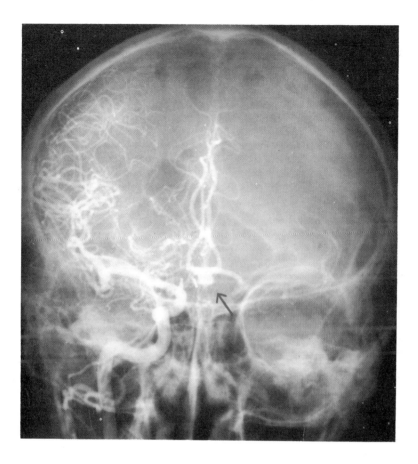

Fig. 7.3 Anterior communicating artery aneurysm. Sac projects downwards from an unusually large parent artery.

In the past, when CT scanning pointed to a specific site some surgeons restricted angiography to the corresponding vessel, only proceeding to examine other vessels if no aneurysm was found. With improved techniques and operative results, identifying incidental aneurysms as well as the responsible lesion is more relevant; in many instances prophylactic repair has become a realistic proposition.

Transcranial Doppler ultrasound (Fig. 7.6) provides a non-invasive method of examining the calibre of the intracranial vessels. Low-frequency pulsed ultrasound can penetrate the skull. The frequency shift of waves reflected from moving red blood cells at a specific depth indicates the flow velocity within the intracranial vessel under study. Results require care in interpretation. After subarachnoid haemorrhage, high velocity (e.g. above 190 cm/s) suggests significant vasospasm, but a generalized increase in CBF could produce similar findings.

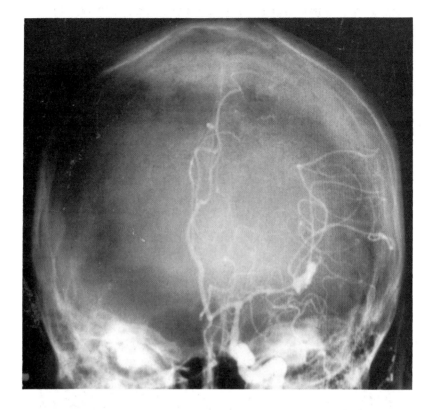

Fig. 7.4 Middle cerebral aneurysm with haematoma and spasm. Displacement of anterior and middle cerebral vessels indicates temporal lobe haemotoma. There is narrowing (spasm) of the terminal carotid segment and the horizontal part of the anterior and middle cerebral arteries; the distal anterior cerebral is of normal calibre.

Management

Patients in coma with suspected subarachnoid haemorrhage require urgent transfer to a neurosurgical unit, provided there is no factor which would absolutely contraindicate surgery. Such patients may benefit from immediate drainage of an associated hydrocephalus or from evacuation of an intracerebral haematoma. Others with suspected subarachnoid haemorrhage should be transferred within 12 hours in view of the trend towards earlier operation. On identifying a ruptured aneurysm on the angiogram, the main aim of treatment is to reduce the risk of rebleeding, both in the short term and in the long term, and to prevent cerebral ischaemia.

Non-operative measures

To reduce the risk of rebleeding

It is assumed that the main threat in the early days is from surges of blood pressure. It makes good sense to keep the patient quietly in bed, rising only for toilet functions, and to deal symptomatically with headache and photophobia. Some surgeons recommend active sedation to reduce anxiety, but there is no

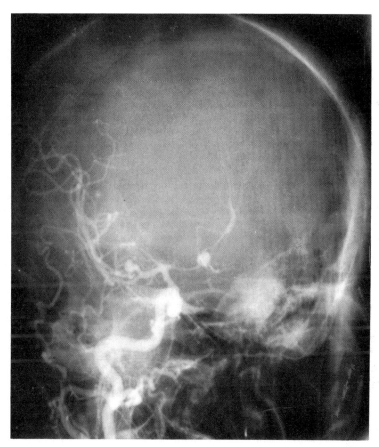

Fig. 7.5 Multiple aneurysms. Aneurysms on middle cerebral and anterior communicating arteries. There is marked narrowing of the anterior cerebral artery from just distal to its origin.

evidence that this has any beneficial effect. In the past some clinicians induced hypotension but studies have now shown that this does more harm than good; rebleeding is reduced but the incidence of cerebral ischaemia is significantly increased. Patients on medication for established hypertension should continue with previous treatment, but the clinician must resist attempts to treat the temporary reactive hypertension that follows subarachnoid haemorrhage. Antifibrinolytic agents, such as epsilon-aminocaproic acid and tranexamic acid, impede the breakdown of fibrin and can prevent or delay dissolution of the blood clot around the aneurysm fundus. Such agents do reduce the rebleed rate by about 50% but, as with antihypertensive therapy, the benefits of their use are offset by an increase in the incidence of cerebral ischaemic complications.

If pursuing a non-operative course (or if the angiogram is negative), the patient is mobilized as soon as symptomatically well. It is then important to encourage the resumption of normal life without restrictions because so little is known about factors likely to precipitate aneurysmal rupture.

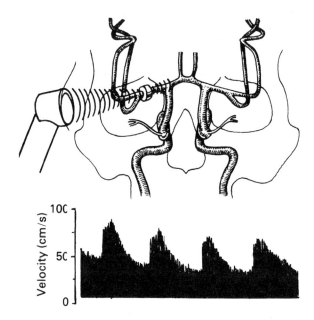

Fig. 7.6 Transcranial Doppler ultrasound measures flow velocity in the middle cerebral (as shown), anterior cerebral, posterior cerebral or basilar arteries. From Lindsay K.W., Bone I. and Callander R. (1992): *Neurology and Neurosurgery Illustrated*, 2nd edn. Edinburgh: Churchill Livingstone. Reprinted with permission.

To prevent cerebral ischaemia

Despite numerous trials of antispastic agents, none has prevented or reversed the arterial narrowing seen in up to 50% of patients on angiography. The presence of myonecrosis and thickening of the arterial wall rather than simple smooth muscle contraction probably accounts for their failure. The calcium antagonist *Nimodipine* was also introduced for its potential antispastic properties and trials have shown that this drug, given orally, reduces the incidence of cerebral ischaemia after subarachnoid haemorrhage by about one-third, and increases the number of patients making a good outcome. However, Nimodipine does not reverse the vasospasm; it probably either improves collateral blood flow or prevents the damaging effect of calcium influx into ischaemic cells. Nimodipine is now widely used and seems virtually devoid of side-effects.

Hyponatraemia develops in about 50% of patients after subarachnoid haemorrhage, but not as a result of inappropriate antidiuretic hormone (ADH) secretion. Erroneous treatment with fluid restriction almost invariably produces neurological deterioration from cerebral ischaemia. Studies have now shown that the low serum sodium does not result from haemodilution but from excessive renal secretion. This is accompanied by fluid loss, a fall in plasma volume and a rise in blood viscosity. The resultant impairment of cerebral perfusion in these patients may significantly contribute to the development of cerebral ischaemia.

Plasma volume expansion with colloid or fluids can reverse ischaemic neurological deficit. Patients should therefore receive at least 3 litres of fluid per day – even in the presence of hyponatraemia. Colloid (e.g. plasma protein, Haemacel) should be administered at the slightest hint that ischaemia is developing or given prophylactically in high-risk groups such as those with a large cisternal blood load on CT scan or with high Doppler velocities. A progressive fall in serum sodium requires *fludrocortisone* or *double-strength saline*. Whether expansion of the intravascular volume improves CBF by reducing blood viscosity, or by increasing cardiac output and blood pressure, remains uncertain. After aneurysm repair, if plasma volume expansion fails to reverse ischaemic signs, an inotropic agent to *induce hypertension* often succeeds. The risks of rebleeding preclude the use of this technique prior to operation.

Surgery for ruptured aneurysms

The surgical measures available are:

1. Occlusion of the neck of the aneurysm.
2. Reinforcement of the sac.
3. Ligation of one feeding vessel.
4. Trapping by occlusion of feeding vessel on both sides.
5. Induction of thrombosis in the sac.
6. Balloon occlusion of the sac.

Occlusion of the neck

The best method of permanent cure is to isolate the aneurysm from its parent vessel, generally with a clip. With modern techniques few aneurysms prove to be inoperable by this method, although some are simply too large to clip.

For an aneurysm to be safely clipped it should be accessible without sacrifice of either vital brain tissue or other vessels in the vicinity. The dissection of a recently ruptured aneurysm from surrounding vessels, and from brain which is swollen and friable as a result of haemorrhage, demands skill. The aneurysm may rupture during dissection and cause embarrassing bleeding; in these circumstances, control may risk occluding important vessels. Permanent hemiplegia or mental changes due to frontal lobe damage may occur after 'successful' clipping, or the patient may die from hypothalamic damage.

The hazards of operation in the acute stage have been reduced by various techniques. Control of respiration and blood pressure allows minimal brain retraction, especially when combined with spinal drainage. The operating microscope permits precise dissection of the aneurysm from vital adjacent vessels and with the bipolar coagulator and the use of sharp microdissection reduces the likelihood of thrombosis in adjacent vessels. Such careful techniques reduce not only mortality but also morbidity.

Aneurysms on the anterior part of the circle of Willis are exposed by the pterional approach: the carotid is identified lateral to the optic nerve and the dissection carried medially or laterally as required, with or without splitting the Sylvian fissure and retracting the frontal and temporal lobes. *Anterior communicating aneurysms* tend to be technically difficult, and serious side-effects may ensue if the anterior cerebral arteries or their perforating branches are damaged; permanent personality changes may be the price of occlusion.

Aneurysms at the trifurcation of the *middle cerebral* are so intimately adherent to their branches that clipping is sometimes impossible without sacrifice of a branch and the risk of hemiplegia, and on the left side of dysphasia. *Posterior communicating aneurysms* when they lie in a favourable position probably carry the least operative risk. *Basilar aneurysms* are approached either under the temporal lobe or via the pterion, splitting the Sylvian fissure and following the posterior communicating artery backwards. Aneurysms at this site carry the greatest operative risk, but most are clipped successfully, usually by surgeons who have developed special expertise with this relatively uncommon lesion. Aneurysms arising from the vertebral artery – usually at the origin of the *posterior inferior cerebellar artery* – require a suboccipital approach. Clipping risks damage to the lower cranial nerves which are often intertwined with the aneurysm sac.

In patients with *multiple aneurysms* the question arises as to whether or not those that have not ruptured should also be clipped. If they are on the same side as the one that has ruptured, and can be dealt with through the same approach, then the answer is probably yes. The additional risks are small and a further craniotomy is avoided.

Reinforcement of the sac

When dissection of an aneurysm reveals an anatomical arrangement which will not permit clipping, either because the sac is too sessile or the branches inextricable, an attempt may be made to reinforce the wall. The sac can be wrapped with muscle, muslin gauze or fibrin foam, or a combination of these agents. It is also possible to apply a rapidly solidifying polymer to the aneurysm which becomes closely invested with a non-yielding covering.

Proximal ligation

Improved techniques for directly clipping aneurysms have reduced the need for carotid ligation. However in patients for whom major surgery is contraindicated, or in parts of the world where experienced surgeons are not available, this provides a low-risk alternative. Its main proven value is in reducing the risk of rebleeding in the first 6 months after rupture. But beyond that period the risks revert to the expected natural history of a ruptured aneurysm, and there is no long-term protection. A cure may occasionally be effected by precipitating thrombosis in the aneurysm due to the reduced pressure. Angiography has shown that aneurysms do sometimes disappear after ligation. Local pressure signs (third nerve palsy from posterior communicating aneurysm) often resolve quite soon after ligation. Usually the *common* carotid is ligated; this is probably less effective than tying the *internal* carotid but the risk of hemiplegia is also smaller. The mortality and morbidity of this simple operation result from depriving one hemisphere of an adequate blood supply. Hemiplegia is often delayed in onset, and this limits the value of trial ligation under local anaesthesia as a means of detecting those at risk. Isotope studies of CBF (p. 67) have greatly extended understanding of intolerance to ligation, and can enable patients who are susceptible to be identified prior to permanent ligation.

Trapping
Aneurysms in certain situations lend themselves to trapping, that is ligation of the artery of supply on both the proximal and distal side. Those most frequently treated in this way are aneurysms in the cavernous sinus, including the caroticocavernous arteriovenous fistula. A clip is placed in the internal carotid artery immediately above the anterior clinoid and on the vessel in the neck just above the bifurcation. *Giant aneurysms* (more than 25 mm diameter) are difficult to deal with, although some can be clipped, when this is not possible they can be trapped as with middle cerebral aneurysms, generally after a superficial temporal – middle cerebral anastomosis.

Embolization
Advanced radiological techniques now permit the insertion of an arterial catheter through the neck of an intracranial aneurysm. Occlusion of the aneurysm fundus can be accomplished either by inflating a detachable balloon or by releasing multiple coils of platinum wire to induce thrombosis. The balloon technique, although ideal for high-flow fistulae, appears rather hazardous for aneurysm repair. Experience with coils is gradually accumulating; although long-term benefits remain uncertain, this may become a realistic alternative to clipping technically difficult aneurysms.

Timing of operation
Since the risk of rebleeding is highest in the first week after aneurysm rupture, it seems logical to attempt repair as soon as possible after the initial haemorrhage. When aneurysm surgery first become feasible in the early 1950s, surgeons operating within 2 weeks of the ictus reported high mortality rates. It soon became evident that the longer the operation was delayed, the better were the results. This set the trend for postponing operation to the second or third week, although as techniques improved, the period of delay gradually fell to about 7 – 14 days. But the longer the operation is delayed, the greater the chance of death from a further rupture. In the last decade surgeons, primarily in Japan, attempted operation within a few days of the bleed. In addition to preventing rebleeding, early operation can remove clot from around the vessel wall. Theoretically this might reduce the vasospastic stimulus and allow the use of induced hypertension to improve CBF in patients with incipient cerebral ischaemia. Impressive results with relatively low operative mortalities were reported, and the feasibility of operating within a few days of the ictus became established. But these results in themselves did not identify the optimum time for operation. It was first necessary to compare not just operative mortality and morbidity, but also management mortality and morbidity for patients undergoing operation in different time periods, taking into account those who died before surgery or who were not selected for surgery.

The recent publication of an International Cooperative Study involving over 3500 patients showed no difference in the overall outcome at 6 months between early surgery (0–3 days; 20% mortality), and late (11–14 days; 21% mortality). A planned operation between 7 and 10 days, at a time when cerebral ischaemia is at its peak, produced a worse outcome (28% mortality). As expected, surgical mortality improved if operation was postponed for more than 10 days. Early operation reduced rebleeding but did not alter the incidence of delayed ischaemia.

Table 7.3 Factors affecting patient outcome

Patient	Aneurysm	Haemorrhage	Brain damage
Age	Site	Interval since last	Conscious level
Blood pressure	Size	Number of bleeds	Focal signs
Arteriopathy	Side	Haematoma	Grade
	Shape	SAH density on CT	
		Vasospasm	

SAH = Subarachnoid haemorrhage.

Although administrative difficulties may prevent early operation in some centres, in most there appears to be a gradual drift in this direction, at least for patients in good clinical condition. If there is no evidence of any harmful effect of early surgery on patient outcome, then the savings in hospital costs alone make this a realistic approach.

Patient selection and surgical results

The interval between the last haemorrhage and the operation is not the only factor which affects patient outcome. Many other variables can influence the surgical results. *Clinical state*, whether described in terms of conscious level and focal signs or by one of the grading systems in current use, and age are the most important. Other factors are outlined in Table 7.3, which does not however include two important variables – the skill and experience of the surgeon and anaesthetist.

Although outcome significantly deteriorates with increasing age, improved surgical results over the last few years have resulted in a steady increase in the upper age limit for aneurysm surgery. Even in patients over 70 years of age, operative risks of aneurysm repair may be less than those of conservative management. Many surgeons restrict surgery to patients in 'good' clinical condition, i.e. WFNS grades I–III. In patients with impaired conscious level or focal signs, operation is often deferred until their condition improves. Others believe that early clipping, followed by treatment with hypertension, hypervolaemia and haemodilution, should be considered even in patients in grade IV and V. Most would postpone operation in the face of developing cerebral ischaemia and proceed only when the clinical state had improved, when vasospasm on angiography had resolved, or when Doppler velocities or hemispheric blood flow had returned to normal values. This is in accord with the finding that the longer the interval since the rupture, the lower the risk. But every day's delay runs the risk of recurrent haemorrhage. The international study indicates that there is no optimum time for operation, irrespective of the patient's condition. One exception is when an associated intracerebral haematoma causes deterioration from mass effect. The surgeon must then decide whether or not to proceed with haematoma removal, with or without clipping of the aneurysm. If the CT scan appearances suggest irreversible brain destruction, particularly of the dominant hemisphere, it is perhaps best to let events take their natural course.

Comparisons of surgical results between different clinics, during different years, or using different techniques are seldom valid, because data about one or more vital variables are usually missing or incomplete, and with outcome assessed in a variety of ways and at various times after operation.

Many clinics are now using the Glasgow Outcome Scale (p. 48) 6 months after surgery in order to standardize data, and to measure morbidity in survivors. This should include reference to mental function and epilepsy – sequelae that are easily overlooked when a superficial assessment is made.

Even when every attempt is made to match the variables, outcome varies considerably between different centres. In the international study, 2900 operated cases were admitted to 68 centres. Operative mortality ranged from 0% to 42% (median 8%), and good results from 100% to 25% (median 69%). Management mortality ranged from 0% to 66% (median 19%) and good outcome from 100% to 20% (median 59%). This study excluded patients deteriorating from an intracerebral haematoma.

Outcome was worse for vertebrobasilar and anterior communicating aneurysms, than for internal carotid and middle cerebral aneurysms. Of those patients who were alert on admission, 13% died, compared to 72% in coma.

Incidental aneurysms

On occasions angiography may reveal an asymptomatic aneurysm. The risk of rupture in a previously unruptured aneurysm is approximately 1% per year. This risk depends on size – the larger the aneurysm, the greater the risk of rupture. Paradoxically, for giant aneurysms over 25 mm in size, the risk appears lower, presumably due to the protective layers of thrombus which tend to line the inner walls. Since mortality from ruptured aneurysms approaches 50%, patients with a life expectancy of just 10–20 years would run a 5–10% risk of death from rupture. With an operative mortality risk for incidental aneurysms below 2%, surgery is a worthwhile proposition, provided the patient is prepared to accept the small immediate risk of death or morbidity.

Subarachnoid haemorrhage in pregnancy

The risk of aneurysm rupture increases as pregnancy develops and matches the expansion of blood volume and the increase in cardiac output. Surprisingly, rupture rarely occurs during labour itself. The risk of haemorrhage from arteriovenous malformations is also increased in pregnancy, but this risk remains relatively constant throughout gestation and labour. If subarachnoid haemorrhage occurs, then investigation and management should proceed as though the patient was not pregnant, other than the need for fetal protection during irradiation. If operative repair is not possible, then Caesarean section, although not essential, should provide the safest conditions for delivery.

Arteriovenous malformation (AVM)
(synonyms: angioma, angiomatous malformation)

These collections of abnormal vessels increase in size with time; despite the term angioma sometimes applied, they are not tumours, but congenital malformations. Malformed arterioles and venules form a vascular plexus within which lie varying degrees of fistulous communication. The veins progressively enlarge as they fill with arterial blood; eventually they appear as irregular aneurysmal type dilatations. In time the resistance in quite large vessels in the

AVM may be less than that offered by normal arteries in the surrounding brain; not only does the lesion enlarge, but as a result of a steal effect, adjacent brain tissue may fail to receive an adequate blood supply and chronic ischaemia may develop. AVMs vary considerably in size and in the extent in which arteriovenous shunting occurs.

Unusual forms exist – *capillary malformation/telangiectasis,* as the name implies, involves capillary dilatation; *cavernous angioma* is a raspberry-like dilatation of the capillary-venous system. The *Sturge-Weber syndrome* is a rare form consisting of a capillary angioma confined to the meninges in association with a superficial angiomatous malformation (port-wine naevus of skin or bucconasal mucosa, or uveal or conjunctival angioma). The cerebral cortex underlying the meningeal abnormality may suffer gliosis and calcification. Direct drainage of a midline arteriovenous fistula into the central veins forms the *giant aneurysm of the vein of Galen.*

Most AVMs (90%) occur in the cerebral hemispheres, the majority in the parietal or occipital lobes. About half reach the cortical surface, but may do so only on the medial aspect of the hemisphere. The brainstem and cerebellum are less commonly involved.

Most of these lesions eventually rupture. Intracerebral or subarachnoid *haemorrhage* is the initial symptom in about 50%, although AVMs account for only 5% of subarachnoid bleeds. The immediate and ultimate outlook is

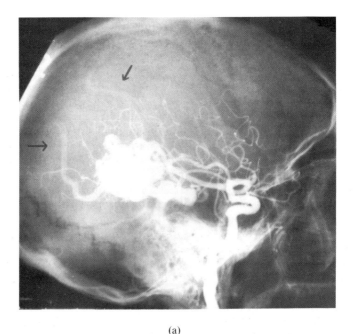

(a)

Fig. 7.7 Arteriovenous malformation (angioma) showing rapid circulation. (a) Arterial phase – contrast filling two large draining veins.

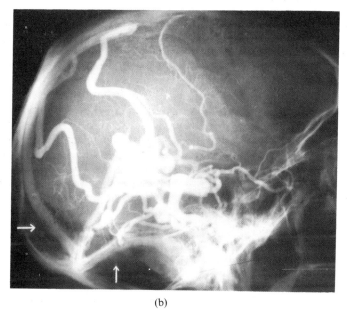

(b)

Fig. 7.7 (*cont*) (b) Capillary phase – contrast already in huge draining veins and in sagittal (horizontal arrow) and transverse (vertical arrow) sinuses.

considerably better than for ruptured aneurysm, and even after repeated haemorrhage many patients with an AVM have little disability. Large malformations seem less likely to bleed recurrently than small ones. *Epilepsy* is the initial symptom in a quarter of patients, and by the time the diagnosis is made, 50% have had one or more fits, which are usually focal, because AVMs are commonly situated in the posterior part of the hemisphere these are often sensory. *Migrainous headaches* occur in less than then a fifth of patients and are not always relieved by operative removal; a family history of migraine is common in patients with AVM, even in those who do not themselves suffer from headache. *Dementia* and slowly progressive *hemiplegia* are late developments due to ischaemia from diversion of blood into the lesion. A cranial *bruit* of a continuous to-and-fro type may be heard in about 25% and sometimes the patient is aware of this. Intracranial *calcification* is seen in 25% on plain skull film.

CT scanning shows up most AVMs, usually as patchy areas of mixed density due to the calcification. With intravenous contrast, enhancement is marked; even the smallest lesion may become apparent, with or without evidence of enlarged tortuous vessels. After recent rupture an accompanying haematoma is often seen.

Angiography shows the abnormal vessels which fill earlier than the normal arteries in the rest of the brain (Fig. 7.7). By the time the normal brain capillaries are filled, contrast is already seen in the veins draining the AVM. Some lesions are so tiny that they may easily be overlooked if an early enough film is not taken; in cases of doubt a second series should be done. All patients require four-vessel angiography; the anterior cerebral circulation may contribute feeding vessels to AVMs lying in the posterior half of the hemisphere and vice versa. Sometimes angiography reveals a coexistent aneurysm, usually lying on the proximal feeding vessel and presumably a result of 'high flow'.

The *prognosis* of arteriovenous malformations is more favourable than that of cerebral aneurysms. The risk of rupture of a previously unruptured AVM is 2–3% per year, but only 1 patient in 8 dies from rupture. Once rupture has occurred, the risk of further rupture is slightly increased in the first year, but thereafter the risk reverts to that of an unruptured lesion. Some patients live long with little disability, and this is a comfort for those with massive AVMs beyond the scope of operative treatment; but the threat of rupture remains, and if operation is possible it should be performed.

Excision is the method of choice, and modern methods make this feasible more often than previously. But the lesser threat of fatal haemorrhage and the availability of alternative techniques such as stereotactic irradiation/introduce a need for selection. Suitability for operation depends on lesion size and site – whether or not it lies in an eloquent region. At least 10% are inoperable by any standards.

Preoperative embolization may considerably aid operative removal and minimize blood loss, particularly with larger lesions. Cyanoacrylate 'glue' or particles of lyophilized dura or haemostatic gelatin foam (Gelfoam) are injected through a coaxial delivery catheter. To embolize high-flow vessels, balloons can be floated to the appropriate site, further inflated-with silicon, then detached from the catheter tip. Ligation or embolization of feeding vessels alone does not eliminate the AVM, nor does it prevent the risk of recurrent haemorrhage. Most use embolization as a preoperative measure to help control feeding vessels during operation.

Focused irradiation has been used for several years to treat arteriovenous malformations and this may prove useful for small, low flow, deeply seated lesions, where operative risks are high. This treatment utilizes either a focused portion beam or focused irradiation from multiple sources mounted on a stereotactic frame. Tissue destruction at the selected site takes up to 2 years to occur. Results suggest that complete obliteration occurs in about a quarter of patients; in the remainder, a reduction in size usually occurs but despite this, the risk of recurrence remains as before. This is a highly specialized technique of limited availability. In the UK, the equipment exists at only one centre.

Cerebral haemorrhage

Most patients suffering cerebral haemorrhage are hypertensive between the ages of 50 and 70. The site is usually in the region of the basal ganglia, and the result is hemiplegia associated with coma. Given modern nursing care about 50% patients survive, but two-thirds remain disabled. Surgery is of limited value in such patients, whose problem is the effect of the initial brain damage, not compression. Evacuation of the haematoma in a patient deteriorating from the mass effect may result in survival, but often with severe disability.

Sometimes the haemorrhage is more superficially placed, producing a different clinical syndrome with a good prospect of surgical relief. This *spontaneous subcortical haematoma* is commonly parietal, in the external capsule, but it may involve the frontal or temporal lobes. All ages can be affected, including children, and hypertension features in only a few. Focal signs may accompany headache and consciousness is seriously impaired only as a secondary development. In some patients the illness may be limited to sudden confusion without focal signs. CT scanning will show the clot, but angiography is necessary to exclude an aneurysm or AVM as the source of the haemorrhage. A proportion of these haematomas may result from rupture of a cryptic AVM, which is either obliterated by the lesion, or fails to fill on angiography due to compression from the haematoma mass. A repeat angiogram or CT scan with double-dose contrast after several months delay will exclude this possibility. Surgical evacuation can be carried out through a trephine or a craniotomy, and patients often make a very satisfactory recovery. Naturally there are patients who do not fall clearly into either of those two categories, and management decisions may be difficult.

Cerebellar haemorrhage may present acutely with rapidly developing headache, neck stiffness and posterior fossa signs, or subacutely with features resembling those of metastatic tumour. CT scan provides the diagnosis and may reveal hydrocephalus from compression of the fourth ventricle. If angiography excludes an underlying AVM, urgent evacuation of the clot usually relieves the symptoms and is followed by a good recovery.

Ischaemic strokes

Angiography has revealed that cerebral ischaemia is as often due to extracranial as to intracranial vascular occlusion; some patients have vascular lesions in both sites. It is now possible to carry out reconstructive surgery on the extracranial (neck) vessels and this is quite widely practised for patients with threatened cerebral ischaemia. The role of surgery is prophylactic and operation cannot revive infarcted brain tissue; however, the inclusion in some series of patients who are already hemiplegic makes it difficult to define clearly the value of this type of surgery. The following account emphasizes the neck vessels because at present it is only for these that surgery is of definite value.

Physiopathology of occlusive cerebrovascular disease

Severe disease of the neck vessels can be completely symptomless because of the efficiency of the anatomical and physiological arrangements in the circle of Willis for ensuring an adequate blood supply to the brain under even adverse circumstances. The resting total CBF is significantly reduced only when each of the four neck vessels is 70% obstructed, or three of the four are completely blocked or significantly stenosed, but the collateral reserve is compromised before this stage is reached. Although such severe disease is rarely found, half the patients with one carotid completely blocked do have at least one of the remaining three trunks affected to some degree. Although it is local defects in perfusion rather than alterations in total blood flow which produce symptoms, the potential total flow, or vascular reserve, is certainly important for establishing collateral circulation if further occlusions develop in extracranial or intracranial vessels. Apart from removing the embolic source, surgery contributes by improving the available reserve rather than by re-establishing local blood flow.

Many factors other than occlusion of main vessels are of importance in determining whether or when ischaemia will develop and how extensive or long-lasting it will be. Among these are the collateral channels available in an individual patient, variations in systemic blood pressure, alterations in blood viscosity, sludging in capillaries and the formation of cholesterol, calcific or platelet emboli. These latter may cause repeated transitory symptoms associated with occlusion of intracranial vessels, such as intermittent monocular blindness. However, this is controversial and fluctuations in perfusion may explain some of these events.

This multiplicity of factors influencing the cerebral circulation accounts in part for the difficulty in correlating clinical, angiographic and pathological findings in these patients. The inexact use of various terms contributes further to the confusion. *Stenosis* implies narrowing only, *occlusion* a complete block, while *thrombosis* describes a pathological state which may sometimes be the cause of an occlusion but is more often a consequence of obstruction. *Ischaemia* refers to inadequate perfusion of an area of brain with functional failure; only if it is sufficiently severe and prolonged does *infarction* develop. *Caroticovertebral insufficiency* is a useful term for symptomatic extracranial obstructive vascular disease, and emphasizes that the state of the quartet of neck vessels as a whole may be more important than the condition of any one of them alone.

Aetiology
Atheroma is the usual cause of stenosis and commonly affects the first 2 cm of the internal carotid artery above the bifurcation of the common carotid. *Thrombosis* may complete the block, or develop only secondarily when atheromatous occlusion becomes total. In either event it frequently spreads up the whole length of the internal carotid to its first intracranial branch (the ophthalmic). *Embolism*, associated with atrial fibrillation, is much less common than formerly, but embolism from an atheromatous plaque or a thrombus in a narrowed internal carotid may occlude cerebral vessels, often temporarily.

Trauma is an occasional cause of carotid thrombosis; this may be added to underlying atheroma, but can also develop in young individuals with healthy arteries. An intimal tear leads to dissection and occlusion. Up to 2 days after closed injury to the neck, or after head injury without overt neck injury, hemiplegia and impaired consciousness can develop. Most will present as a traumatic intracranial haematoma, and it is usually wise to exclude this before assuming that the carotid thrombosis is responsible. Rarely local *infection* may induce thrombosis, and so may involvement by local *carcinoma* in the neck.

Oral contraceptives have recently been suspected of precipitating arterial thrombosis in the cerebral circulation, but an association has not been statistically established. What the controversy has emphasized is that spontaneous occlusions both of the cervical internal carotid and of the middle cerebral artery are not uncommon under the age of 40, and even under 30. Moreover *pregnancy* considerably increases the risk of intracranial arterial thrombosis, and the mortality is significantly greater than in non-pregnant females or males of similar age. Postmortem in such patients often reveals primary arterial thrombosis without atheroma, but venous thrombosis is more common. Increased *blood viscosity* is increasingly recognized as a cause of reduced blood flow, and cerebral perfusion may improve if the haematocrit is lowered.

Clinical syndromes

Obstruction of the *carotid* had claimed most clinical attention because, since angiography has been available, carotid disease has frequently been recognized, and because almost all surgical endeavours have been directed to this artery. The *vertebral* is less often examined radiologically and is less accessible surgically.

Carotid occlusion can produce a wide variety of symptoms and of modes of onset, all of them manifestations of ischaemia of one cerebral hemisphere. Hemiplegia may be so severe and sudden as to suggest cerebral haemorrhage; or it may develop rapidly but remain incomplete, resembling the classical picture of cerebral thrombosis; or it may be so gradual and progressive that an intracranial tumour is suspected. All these types of stroke imply infarction and are therefore unlikely to be benefited by surgery. Of more interest to the surgeon is the patient who suffers *transient ischaemic attacks*. These temporary strokes may last a few minutes or a few hours, but recovery is complete within 24 hours; a limb may be weak or merely numb or there may be dysphasia. Occasionally transient blindness in one eye occurs, and the eye affected is ipsilateral to the affected carotid, whilst any signs referable to the cerebral hemisphere are of course contralateral. Emboli from a stenotic atheromatous plaque are commonly held responsible for these transitory attacks, and have been observed passing across the retinal vessels during the course of episodes. Other syndromes are *reversible ischaemic neurological deficits (RINDs)* that last longer (1-7 days) but are followed by complete recovery; and '*stroke in evolution*', progressing over several hours and then persisting. Any of this wide variety of ischaemic syndromes may be due to vascular abnormalities anywhere from the bifurcation of the carotid in the neck to the branches of the middle cerebral artery.

Vertebrobasilar occlusions cause episodes of vertigo, tinnitus and ataxia due to brainstem ischaemia; the syndrome of the posterior inferior cerebellar artery is most often a reflection of more proximal block, in a main vessel.

Physical signs related to the neck vessels, as distinct from those related to failure of cerebral function, are unreliable. A carotid bruit may be heard when there is stenosis (but not with occlusion), though this may be mimicked by a bruit transmitted from the thyroid or aortic arch and branches, or when there is severe anaemia. The absence of a bruit does not exclude the possibility of a stenosis; as a carotid stenosis progresses beyond 80% the bruit softens and eventually disappears.

Investigation

Clinical diagnosis is clearly difficult. It is much less easy to distinguish with certainty between cerebral haemorrhage, thrombosis and embolism than was formerly thought; indeed it is often impossible on clinical grounds to decide whether the primary causation is intracranial or extracranial. It is as unwise to try to decide the cause of haemoptysis without a chest X-ray as to attempt to guess the cause of stroke without visualizing the brain or its vessels.

CT scanning is the most reliable way to discover the cause of a persisting deficit. Haemorrhage is always evident, whereas infarction may take days to appear. With transient attacks the CT scan is often normal.

Ultrasound scanning with a probe directed at extracranial vessels in the neck detects the marked velocity changes occurring at the site of a stenosis (Doppler) or produces an image of the vessels under study (B-mode). *Duplex* scanning combines both modalities and gives most information. A negative ultrasound examination may avoid the need for angiography. *Transcranial Doppler* (p. 151) can also provide information about the intracranial vasculature.

Angiography is, however, the only way to make a definitive diagnosis of occlusion, stenosis or ulcerated plaque in the cervical carotid (Fig. 7.8) An arch aortogram via the femoral route is preferred, with selective catheterization showing in turn the extracranial and intracranial circulation. Angiography may reveal that the occlusion is of an intracranial vessel (Fig. 7.9).

PET and SPECT can both map out ischaemic areas within the brain. PET scanning, although available in only a few centres, also demonstrates oxygen utilization and extraction and can identify regions of *'luxury perfusion'* where coupling of blood flow and metabolism has failed and blood supply exceeds tissue demands.

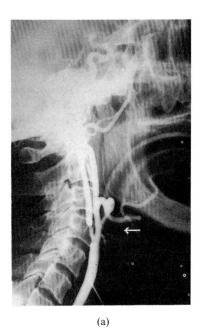

(a)

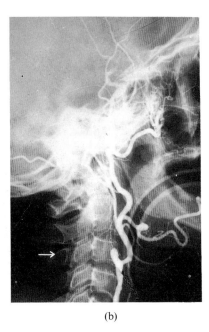

(b)

Fig. 7.8 Carotid disease in the neck. (a) Stenosis – segment of narrowing of internal carotid immediately above its origin. (b) Occlusion – a stump of internal carotid remains above the bifurcation.

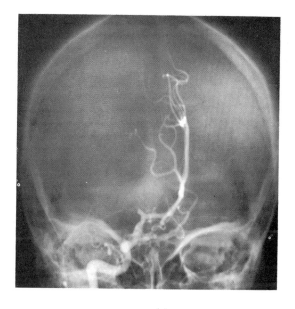

(a)

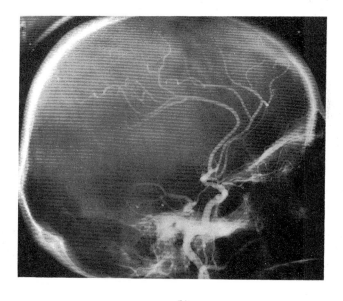

(b)

Fig. 7.9 Middle cerebral artery occlusion (postpartum). (a) The main artery is blocked immediately beyond its origin. Massive displacement of anterior cerebral branches due to swelling of the hemisphere containing a large infarct. (b) Complete absence of vessels in the middle cerebral artery territory. The posterior cerebral artery is displaced downwards by the transtentorial herniation.

Treatment

In past years most clinicians hesitated before using anticoagulants to treat patients with cerebrovascular disease. These carried the risk of converting an ischaemic lesion into a haemorrhagic infarct or of precipitating a fatal intracranial haemorrhage if given in error to a patient with a haemorrhagic lesion. Their use for established cerebral ischaemia has been largely abandoned.

Recent interest has centred around the administration of *thrombolytic agents* for thrombotic stoke. Recombinant tissue plasminogen activator (rt-PA) is infused intravenously as soon as possible after the onset of symptoms and preferably within 90 minutes. Pilot studies suggest that this may produce major improvement in up to one-half of treated patients. Such encouraging results indicate the need for a large randomized controlled trial.

The question of *operation* arises when carotid stenosis has been demonstrated angiographically and the patient has not yet developed a completed stroke. This will most commonly be when the patient has suffered one or more temporary strokes (transient ischaemic attacks or RINDs). Three distinct aims may be achieved as a result of surgery. The most important is the *prevention of complete occlusion* of the artery. It is of course well-known that occlusion of a single carotid vessel may be tolerated without any symptoms whatever and there are even cases with bilateral occlusion which are symptomless. However, in the background of atheromatous disease there is usually involvement of several vessels both extracranial and intracranial and the total circulation must be considered. Surgery for a narrowed carotid is more urgently needed if the opposite carotid is also narrowed or occluded, or if the vertebrals or basilar are also affected. Secondly, surgery may *remove a source of microemboli*, although, as indicated, anticoagulants may control this particular phenomenon fairly satisfactorily. The third, and most dubious, outcome of surgery is the *improvement of the circulation* to the brain; experiments suggest that narrowing is not important until the last 30% of the lumen is encroached on, but that is when all other vessels are normal. Radioactive blood flow measurements (p. 67) carried out immediately before and after endarterectomy show no significant difference in most instances, but the reserve of the cerebral circulation may be improved, as revealed by a greater response to increasing $PaCO_2$ after operation.

Surgery is therefore prophylactic and there is probably no case for emergency disobliteration of the carotid apart from the exceptional case of stroke in evolution when this occurs in the environs of a surgical unit and operation can be carried out within a matter of hours. A bypass may be put in place whilst endarterectomy is completed and a saphenous vein patch is usually employed in order to prevent stenosis developing as a result of suturing the arterial incision. Anticoagulants need only be given during the course of the operation. In the event of the circulation being extremely critical the operation may be made safer by hypothermia, or even by hyperbaric oxygen.

Despite the relatively widespread use of surgery for carotid stenosis, until recently it had never been established that operative treatment could improve outcome when compared to treatment with platelet inhibitors (aspirin or dipiridamole). Two large multicentre trials in Europe and North American have now shown that the risk of further stroke is significantly reduced when patients with more than 70% angiographic stenosis undergo operation. Those with less than 30% stenosis do as well with medical treatment alone. Optimum management in the intermediate group (30–70% stenosis) remains uncertain.

Although it has been widely practised for many years, a large international trial of extracranial – intracranial bypass showed no benefit in any patient subset, as a means of reducing the incidence of stroke. However STA-MCA (superficial temporal artery-middle cerebral artery anastomosis is still used when elective occlusion of the middle cerebral artery is planned, for example before trapping a giant aneurysm of this artery.

Further reading

Haemorrhage

Alvord E.C., Loeser J.D., Bailey W.L. *et al.* (1972). Subarachnoid haemorrhage due to ruptured aneurysms. *Arch. Neurol.*; **27:** 273–84.

Drake C.G. (1979). The treatment of aneurysms of the posterior circulation. *Clin. Neurosurg.*; **26:** 96–144.

Editorial (1987). Intracerebral haematoma from aneurysm rupture: operation in moribund patients? *Lancet*; **ii:** 1186–7.

Fisher C.M., Kistler J.P., Davis J.M. (1980). Relation of cerebral vasospasm to subarachnoid haemorrhage visualised by computerized tomographic scanning. *Neurosurgery*; **6:** 1–9.

Hasan D., Vermeulen M., Wijdicks E.F.M. *et al.* (1989). Effect of fluid intake and antihypertensive treatment on cerebral ischaemia after subarachnoid haemorrhage. *Stroke*; **20:** 1511–15.

Heiskanen O. (1981). Risk of bleeding from unruptured aneurysms with multiple cranial aneurysms. *J. Neurosurg.*; **55:** 524–6.

Heros R.C., Karosue K., Diebold P.M. (1990). Surgical excision of cerebral arteriovenous malformations: late results. *Neurosurgery*; **26: 570–8.**

Hunt W.E., Hess R.M. (1968). Surgical risk as related to time of intervention in the repair of intracranial aneurysms. *J. Neurosurg.*; **28:** 14–20.

Ingall T.J., Whisnant J.P., Wiebers P.O. *et al.* (1989). Has there been a decline in subarachnoid haemorrhage mortality? *Stroke*; **20:** 718–26.

Jane J.A., Winn H.R., Richardson A.E. (1977). The natural history of intracranial aneurysms: rebleeding rates during the acute and longterm period and implication for surgical management. *Clin. Neurosurg.*; **24:** 176–84.

Jane J.A., Kassell N.F., Torner J.C. *et al.* (1985). The natural history of aneurysms and arteriovenous malformations. *J. Neurosurg.*; **62:** 321–3.

Kassell N.F., Peerless S.J., Durward Q.J., *et al.* (1982). Treatment of ischaemic deficits from vasospasm with intravascular volume expansion and induced arterial hypertension. *Neurosurgery*; **11:** 337–43.

Kassell N.F., Torner J.C., Haley E.C. *et al.* (1990). The international cooperative study on the timing of aneurysm surgery. Part I: Overall management results. *J. Neurosurg.*; **73:** 18–36.

Kassell N.F., Torner J.C., Jane J.A. *et al.* (1990). The international cooperative study on the timing of aneurysm surgery. Part II: Surgical results. *J. Neurosurg.*; **73:** 37–47.

Lindsay K.W., Teasdale G., Knill-Jones R.P. *et al.* (1982). Observer variability in grading patients with subarachnoid haemorrhage. *J. Neurosurg.*; **56:** 628–33.

Ljunggren B., Brandt L., Kagstrom E. *et al.* (1981). Results of early operations for ruptured aneurysms. *J. Neursurg.*; **54:** 473–9.

Locksley H. (1966). Natural history of subarachnoid haemorrhage, intracranial aneurysm and arteriovenous malformation. *J. Neurosurg.*; **25:** 321–69.

Lunsford L.D., Kondziolka D., Flickinger J.C. *et al.* (1991). Stereotactic radiosurgery for arterio-venous malformation of the brain. *J. Neurosurg.*; **75**: 512–24.

McKissock W., Richardson A., Taylor J. (1961). Primary intracranial haemorrhage. *Lancet*; **ii**: 221–6.

Mattle H., Kohler S., Huber P. *et al.* (1989). Anticoagulant related intracranial extracerebral haemorrhage. *J. Neurol. Neursurg. Psychiatry.*; **52**: 829–37.

Maurice-Williams R.S. (1987). *Subarachnoid Haemorrhage.* Bristol: Wright.

Mendelow A.D. (1991). Spontaneous intracerebral haemorrhage. *J. Neurol. Neurosurg. Psychiatry*; **54**: 193–5.

Millikan C.H. (1975). Cerebral vasospasm and ruptured intracranial aneurysm. *Arch. Neurol.*; **32**: 433–49.

Nishioka H. (1966). Evaluation of the conservative management of ruptured intracranial aneurysms. *J. Neurosurg.*; **25**: 574–92.

Ondra P.L., Troupp H., George E.D. *et al.* (1990). The natural history of symptomatic arteriovenous malformations of the brain: a 24 year follow-up assessment. *J. Neurosurg.*; **73**: 387–91.

Pakarinen S. (1967). Incidence, aetiology and prognosis of primary subarachnoid haemorrhage. *Acta Neurol. Scand.*, **43** (Suppl. 29): 1–128.

Perret G., Nishioka H. (1966). Arteriovenous malformations: an analysis of 545 cases. *J. Neurosurg.*; **25**: 467–90.

Pickard J.D., Murray G.D., Illingworth R. *et al.* (1989). Effect of oral nimodipine on cerebral infarction and outcome after subarachnoid haemorrhage: British aneurysm nimodipine trial. *Br. Med. J.*; **298**: 636–42.

Robinson J.L., Hall C.S., Sedzmir C.B. (1974). Arteriovenous malformations and aneuryms and pregnancy. *J. Neurosurg.*; **41**: 63–70.

Saveland H., Hillman J., Brandt L. *et al.* (1992). Overall outcome in aneurysmal subarachnoid haemorrhage. A prospective study from neurosurgeons in Sweden during a one year period. *J. Neurosurg.*; **76**: 729–35.

Spetzler R.F., Martin N.A. (1986). A proposed grading system for arteriovenous malformation. *J. Neurosurg.*; **65**: 476–83.

Spetzler R.F., Martin N.A. Carter P. *et al.* (1987). Surgical management of large AVMs by staged embolisation and operative excision. *J. Neurosurg.*; **67**: 17–28.

Stehbens W.E. (1989). Aetiology of intracranial berry aneurysms. *J. Neurosurg.*; **70**: 823–31.

Van Gijn J., Van Dongen K.J. (1982). The time course of aneurysmal haemorrhage on computed tomograms. *Neuroradiology*; **23**: 153–6.

Vermeulen M., Van Gijn J. (1990). The diagnosis of subarachnoid haemorrhage. *J. Neurol. Neurosurg. Psychiatry,*; **53**: 365–72.

Vermeulen M., Lindsay K.W., Murray G.D. *et al.* (1984). Antifibrinolytic treatment in subarachnoid haemorrhage. *N. Engl. J. Med.*; **311**: 432–7.

Vinuela F., Dion J.E., Duckwiller G. *et al.* (1991). Combined endovascular embolization and surgery in the management of cerebral arteriovenous malformations: experience with 101 cases. *J. Neurosurg.*; **75**: 856–64.

Wiebers D.W., Whisnant J.P., O'Fallon W.M. (1981). The natural history of unruptured intracranial aneurysms. *N. Engl. J. Med.*; **304**: 696–8.

Wijdicks E.F.M., Vermeulen M., Ten Haaf J.A. *et al.* (1985). Volume depletion and natriuresis in patients with a ruptured cranial anaurysm. *Ann. Neurol.*; **18**: 111–16.

Wilkins R.H. (1980). Attempted prevention or treatment of intracranial arterial spasm: a survey. *Neurosurgery*; **6**: 198–210.

Occlusive disease

Brott T.G., Haley E.C.J., Levy D.E. *et al.* (1992). Urgent therapy for stroke: Part I. Pilot study of tissue plasminogen activator administered within 90 minutes. *Stroke*; **23**: 632–40.

Cross J.N., Castro P.O., Jennett W.B. (1968). Cerebral strokes associated with pregnancy and the puerperium. *Br. Med. J.*; **3**: 214–18.

European carotid surgery trialists' collaborators group. (1991). MRC European surgery trial: interim results for symptomatic patients with severe (70–99%) or with mild (0–29%) carotid stenosis. *Lancet*; **337**: 1235–43.

Haley E.C.J., Levy D.E., Brott T.G. *et al.* (1992). Urgent therapy for stroke: Part II. Pilot study of tissue plasminogen activator administered 91–180 minutes from onset. *Stroke*; **23**: 641–5.

Harrison M.J.G. (1980). Vascular surgery: surgery for ischaemic stroke. *Br. J. Hosp. Med.*; **23**: 108–12.

Jennett B., Miller J.D., Harper A.M. (1976). *Effect of Carotid Artery Surgery on Cerebral Blood Flow*. Amsterdam: Excerpta Medica.

NASCET Collaborators. (1991). Beneficial effect of carotid endarterectomy in symptomatic patients with high-grade carotid stenosis. *N. Engl. J. Med.*; **325**: 445–53.

Chapter 8

Intracranial infection

Intracranial abscess

Rare infective lesions of the nervous system

Meningitis

Encephalitis

    Herpes simplex
    AIDS

Osteomyelitis of the skull

Intracranial abscess

Origin

Intracranial abscess may develop due to direct spread from adjacent infection in the ear or sinuses, or following trauma. Alternatively infection can spread through the blood stream from a distant source.

Chronic suppurative otitis media can result in erosion of the tegmen tympani allowing infection to spread upwards into the middle of the temporal lobe; or it destroys the triangle of bone behind the middle ear, causing an abscess in the anterolateral segment of the cerebellar hemisphere. Temporal abscesses are twice as common as cerebellar; occasionally patients have both. Chronic ear infection may be relatively silent, with minimal discharge, causing only occasional pain and gradual deafness. Neither inspection of the infected ear nor study of X-rays of the petrous temporal bone enables a reliable prediction to be made as to whether a particular infected ear is potentially dangerous.

Infection probably spreads by infective thrombosis in small veins traversing the diploe to join venous sinuses, so that suppuration can occur within the brain without involving the superficial planes. However extensive extradural collections of pus are occasionally found in the course of performing mastoidectomy, even when there has been no reason to suspect an intracranial complication; the dura is remarkably resistant to infection.

In recent years the proportion of abscesses arising from an otogenic source has fallen; prompt antibiotic treatment of acute otitis has helped to prevent the development of chronic infection; if this does occur, early radical mastoidectomy should halt spread to the intracranial cavity.

Acute frontal sinusitis, like mastoiditis, now commonly responds to antibiotics without requiring surgical drainage; when frontal osteitis develops the risk of a frontal lobe abscess and subdural abscess is high. Less often extradural pus collects, usually when there is chronic infection of the sinus.

Haematogenous abscesses, due to blood stream spread from a distant focus usually occur in the distribution of the middle cerebral artery, either posterior frontal or temporoparietal. In the absence of overt lung infection, spread may result from infective endocarditis or cyanotic congenital heart disease. Infection probably begins at sites of small vessel occlusion, arising from a combination of hypoxia and thrombosis, secondary to polycythaemia.

Trauma, either accidental or operative, accounts for most of the remaining cases. Infective material may be carried directly into the cranial cavity, as in a penetrating injury, or superficial infection in scalp or bone may spread secondarily. Dural tears affecting the air sinuses or middle ear provide another route.

A number of abscesses occur for which no obvious cause is found; the presumption is that these are due to blood spread from insignificant primary foci, such as a tooth socket after extraction.

Intracranial pathology

Subdural abscess most often arises from acute sinusitis but may be otogenic. Pus spreads back over the convexity of the cerebral hemisphere, and also collects beside the falx on the medial surface of the brain. From here it may reach the opposite side and the superior surface of the tentorium; and it can then gain access to the posterior fossa through the tentorial hiatus. Eventually there is widespread pus producing a plethora of neurological signs, probably due to infective thrombosis in small vessels.

Parenchymal brain abscess usually goes through a stage of diffuse suppurative 'cerebritis' before liquefaction in the centre leads to a discrete collection of pus. A capsule then begins to form which eventually becomes quite tough and thick. Traumatic and haematogenous abscesses tend to become multilocular; if one loculus is sealed off from the main one, 'recurrence' may arise from persistence of this loculus after the other has been drained. Untreated abscesses prove fatal either by causing acute brain compression (and can do so in the early encephalitic stage when brain oedema may be widespread) or by rupturing into the ventricle or the subarachnoid space.

Bacteriology

Infections from the ear are usually mixed, and often include the anaerobic *Bacteroides fragilis* and *Streptococcus milleri*. *Strep. pneumoniae* and Gram-negative organisms, predominantly *Escherichia coli*, are often found. Sinus infections usually involve *Strep. milleri* and *Strep. pneumoniae*. Subdural abscess is nearly always due to these streptococci, whether coming from the sinus or the ear. *Strep. milleri, Strep. pneumoniae* or *Staphylococcus aureus* cause metastatic infection from either a cardiac or respiratory source. Infections from accidental or surgical trauma are usually due to *Staph. aureus*.

Occasionally coagulase-negative staphylococci are involved, particularly in the presence of a surgical implant. In the immunocompromised host such as patients with acquired immunodeficiency syndrome (AIDS; see p. 183), cerebral abscess may result from *Toxoplasma, Aspergillus, Listeria, Nocardia* or *Candida* in addition to the more common pathogens.

Nowadays it is unusual to fail to detect the responsible organism or organisms provided certain precautions are taken. Aspirated pus requires immediate aerobic and anaerobic culture, with prolonged incubation in microaerophilic conditions to detect *Strep. milleri.*

Clinical

Brain abscess is less dramatic, at least in its early stages, than is often imagined; and this is particularly true since antibiotics have been available. Eventually a picture of advancing brain compression with focal signs develops, but the diagnosis should be made before this. Suspicion should be roused whenever signs of intracranial mischief appear against the background of an infection known to predispose to brain abscess.

Otogenic abscess usually follows an acute recrudescence of infection in a chronically infected ear. A great deal of local pain in and around the ear gives way to headache, perhaps with some drowsiness and mild confusion. Not uncommonly, this is taken to be part of an acute mastoiditis, and brain abscess is only recognized a week or so after mastoidectomy when postoperative recovery is unexpectedly slow, and pyrexia and toxicity persist. In most such instances intracranial complications were probably already present when the mastoid was dealt with, rather than having developed as the result of this operation.

Temporal lobe abscess does not produce florid CNS signs. Epilepsy and hemiplegia are unusual presenting features, whilst patients seldom complain of the most constant sign – an upper quadrantic homonymous hemianopia. It will be detected only by the clinician who specifically looks for it. On the left side mild dysphasia may occur, but if the patient is ill and pyrexial this is readily mistaken for confusion or delirium. Papilloedema may develop but pressure can rise so rapidly with an abscess that there is not time for the fundi to become swollen.

Cerebellar abscess is more obvious because nystagmus, slow to the affected side, is almost constant, and some degree of ataxia usual; hydrocephalus may develop and lead to a rapid deterioration in conscious level.

Sinusitic abscess follows frontal osteitis which is associated with an oedematous swelling above the eye. Headache and pyrexia are accompanied by vomiting and some confusion. Epilepsy is very common, but marked hemiplegia is unusual (unless there is also subdural pus).

Abscesses of haematogenous origin are often more insidious, and there is seldom any recent acute infection to draw attention to the likelihood of intracranial mischief. A patient may be surprisingly well with 50 ml of pus in the middle of the hemisphere, apyrexial and with no neurological signs detectable. However, hemiparesis is common, as these abscesses occur in the middle cerebral distribution, and epilepsy may develop.

Subdural empyema produces more profound disturbance of function than pus in the brain itself because cortical thrombophlebitis and arteritis develop with resulting ischaemic lesions. Following sinusitis, headache and toxicity persist and epilepsy is common; this often begins as focal motor attacks which may progress to status. Hemiplegia or dysphasia suddenly develop, often following a bout of fits. The picture is of a gravely ill patient in danger both from spreading infection and persisting epilepsy.

Investigations

These should be carried out in a neurosurgical unit and if the clinical condition is at all suspicious of intracranial complications the patient should be transferred because an emergency burr hole may be necessary.

Lumbar puncture should be avoided if there is suspicion of cerebral abscess. An abscess is a rapidly developing mass lesion, and ICP may become dangerously high before papilloedema is evident, and the risk of precipitating brain shifts is considerable. In any event, apart from excluding meningitis, examination of the CSF is not crucial, because it is occasionally completely normal. Often the protein is raised to 60–100 mg, and there are about 100 cells, either polymorphs or lymphocytes or both.

CT scanning is the most useful investigation showing both the lesion and its mass effect. The abscess cavity appears as an area of reduced density surrounded by a capsule which enhances strongly with contrast (Figs 4.5 and 8.1). If the patient presents early in the course of the disease, 'cerebritis' may show as an area of low density. Any atypical appearance should raise the suspicion of human immunodeficiency virus (HIV) infection, especially in high-risk groups.

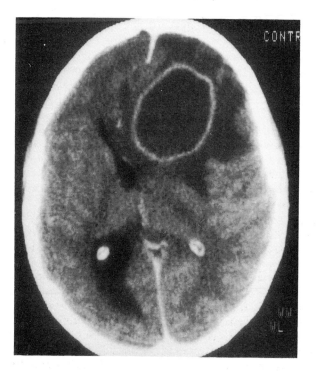

Fig. 8.1   Frontal lobe abscess with ring enhancement causing considerable mass effect.

MRI may detect the 'cerebritic' stage earlier than CT, but there are no specific features to distinguish infection.

In the absence of CT scanning an isotope scan will show an area of high uptake. Clinical signs should distinguish a supratentorial from a cerebellar lesion and angiography or contrast ventriculography respectively should identify the mass effect.

Subdural abscess is suspected clinically when there is a rapid onset of hemiplegia and focal epilepsy. CT scan is usually diagnostic showing a low-density extracerebral collection often with some enhancement on the inner surface. Occasionally these lesions are isodense on CT and, if bilateral, the absence of midline shift makes detection difficult.

Treatment
Whatever plane suppuration affects, the basis of management is the same: the establishment of local drainage, the administration of systemic antibiotics, and the treatment of the primary focus of infection.

Active mastoid or sinus disease should be treated surgically as soon as possible (usually within 72 hours) in order to avoid reinfection or fresh intracranial spread. Antibiotics will often have to be started on a best-guess basis, before cultures and sensitivities are available. Penicillin in large doses (1.2g every 2 hours) is the choice for possible aerobic streptococci, chloramphenicol for broad-spectrum cover and metronidazole (Flagyl) for anaerobes. All three antibiotics are given until a specific organism or organisms is identified, at which point treatment may be changed to the appropriate drug.

Methods of providing local drainage differ according to the type of abscess, but both parenchymal and subdural suppuration call for the utmost urgency. Once an abscess is diagnosed operation should proceed without delay. Compression can advance very rapidly with an acute lesion of this kind, and cerebellar abscess in particular is liable to produce sudden apnoea from medullary failure.

Burr hole aspiration
Most abscesses can be managed in this way. It is safer to make a clean burr hole than to attempt drainage through an existing incision (e.g. a mastoid wound) which could introduce fresh infection or allow brain to herniate.

If a blunt brain cannula is used the thickness and toughness of the capsule can be judged from the resistance felt. Regular postoperative CT scanning will monitor progress of the cavity, and indicate the need for further aspiration or excision. This and the clinical state will determine when a repeated tap is needed; most abscesses require two or three aspirations.

Early excision and decompression
Multilocular haematogenous and traumatic abscesses, from which often only small amounts of pus can be aspirated, and cerebellar abscesses are unsuitable for treatment by the above method. Excision under antibiotic cover provides a safe treatment and some recommend this method for all abscesses. Occasionally an otogenic temporal abscess yields very little pus, yet compression is acute with a tight brain; perhaps it is still in the stage of diffuse infection prior to the formation of pus in quantity, or it is multilocular with the needle draining only one cavity. In such circumstances it is unsafe to rely on the removal of a small

amount of pus, and an immediate decompression must be done. When the capsule is well-formed this provides an alternative method of treatment; often a single evacuation of the abscess cavity under direct vision is sufficient to prevent recollection. In eloquent areas, leaving the capsule intact minimizes damage to surrounding brain.

Stereotactic aspiration
Abscesses of haematogenous origin may present as small, deep, often multiple lesions. In these patients a stereotactically guided needle insertion is required to confirm the nature of the lesion and to identify the responsible organism. Long-term antibiotic therapy with the appropriate drug should result in gradual resolution, but this requires careful monitoring with regular CT scans.

Late excision
The aspiration method of treating abscesses was initially introduced as a temporary measure prior to excision of the abscess, but very often the response is so satisfactory that excision is never needed. However, there is some evidence that excision of a shrivelled frontal abscess may reduce the risk of subsequent epilepsy, in spite of the brain scar which such an operation must inevitably leave. Sometimes the cavity repeatedly fills; in such circumstances excision is essential.

Treatment of subdural abscess
This space is difficult to drain efficiently. Multiple burr holes are needed because tight brain plugs off each one so that it deals with only a limited area; at least three holes should be made on each side, one of which is parasagittal if plus lies alongside the falx. As when evacuating a subdural haematoma, the brain is depressed with a blunt instrument to allow pus to escape. Massive doses of systemic antibiotics must be given. Because the organism is usually streptococcus, which is always sensitive, the response is normally satisfactory, but there remains the dangers of loculated collections of pus, and of intractable epilepsy. Further burr holes will be needed if progress is arrested or new signs develop; satisfactory drainage may be effected only by turning a large bone flap. Some believe that a craniotomy should be performed at the outset to ensure complete evacuation of pus. This would certainly provide the safest method if burr holes fail to drain a significant amount of pus or if drainage fails to decompress a tight brain.

Extradural abscess is usually discovered when infected bone is removed, and the excision of the affected bone is all that is required to prevent recollection, providing the primary condition is adequately treated.

Mortality and sequelae
With antibiotics and improved imaging accurately locating abscesses and thereby aiding drainage, the mortality has fallen from about 50% to 10%. Early recurrences are due either to untreated loculi, or to inadequate antibiotic therapy (wrong drug, or too low a dose). Recovery is usually satisfactory after brain abscess, but subdural abscess may leave residual hemiplegia or dysphasia; occasionally ataxia persists after cerebellar abscess. Epilepsy is the most troublesome sequel, and follows in 80% of all abscesses above the tentorium; this risk is greater after frontal than after temporal lobe abscess and is common also after subdural suppuration.

Rare infective lesions of the nervous system

Tuberculoma is the least rare of these, but in the UK is very much less often seen than in countries such as Spain and South America where it forms one of the common intracranial masses. Frank tuberculous infection elsewhere is unusual. CT scan usually shows an irregularly enhancing lesion, often mistaken for tumour. The cerebellar hemisphere is the commonest site. Many become inactive and calcify, but others terminate by producing tuberculous meningitis (TBM). If the diagnosis is suspected preoperatively, antituberculous therapy should result in gradual resolution. If met unexpectedly at operation, immediate treatment with medication should help prevent TBM.

Hydatid cysts in the brain present as neoplasms. In areas where the disease is common, hydatid may be suspected if there are chest shadows in addition. CT scan shows a characteristic round, non-enhancing, low-density cystic lesion. Excision requires special care to avoid rupturing the cyst and spilling scolices which start fresh daughter cysts.

Meningitis

The neurosurgeon has many interests in meningitis. He or she must be ready to recognize it when it mimics intracranial tumour or abscess or subarachnoid haemorrhage; to deal with postoperative meningitis; to treat the primary lesions underlying secondary and recurrent pyogenic meningitis; and to manage certain complications of meningitis.

Classification

Bacterial meningitis
This is of most surgical interest, and is often secondary to another condition such as a *local abscess*, either intracranial or in the mastoid or air sinuses. Meningitis may precede or follow intracranial abscess, but the two sometimes develop together when infection spreads from ear or sinus disease. Organisms may spread *by the blood stream* from a more distant focus such as pneumonia or a boil.

Recurrent bacterial meningitis always raises suspicion of a dural defect, either *traumatic* following anterior fossa or petrous fracture (p. 222) bacterial due to a *congenital sinus* (indicated by a skin lesion over a spinal or posterior fossa dermoid), or due to one of the causes of *spontaneous* (i.e. *non-traumatic*) *rhinorrhoea or otorrhoea*. These include osteoma or mucocele of the air sinuses which erode locally; chronic hydrocephalus from any cause (p. 286); radiation hypophysectomy with simultaneous destruction of bone and dura over the sphenoidal sinus and the diaphragma sellae; and infective cholesteatomatous erosion of the petrous and overlying middle or posterior fossa dura.

Postoperative meningitis can develop after any neurosurgical procedure. Probably all wounds are bacteriologically contaminated when they are closed, but the body can deal with this in most cases. After prolonged procedures (>4 hours) contamination risks increase, whilst excessive blood clot or necrotic tissue, which have no power to resist active invasion, also predispose to infection. A particular threat exists when operation is followed by a CSF leak, either directly through the wound after the dura of the posterior fossa has been left open and ICP remains high, or as rhinorrhoea after operation on pituitary or basal anterior fossa tumours. Nasal polypectomy and mastoidectomy may occasionally cause dural damage and lead to meningitis.

The commonest organism (taking all cases of pyogenic meningitis) is still the meningococcus, which causes a disease entity that is readily recognizable and largely confined to children and young adults. *Strep. pneumoniae* infection results from otitis media, dural defects in the anterior fossa and from pneumonia. It can occur at any age but more often affects infants and the elderly. Staphylococcal meningitis is usually due to *Staph. aureus,* but *Staph. epidermidis* (coagulase-negative) from the skin surface most commonly causes meningitis complicating neurosurgical operative procedures; Gram-negative bacilli – *E. coli* and *Klebsiella* – are another frequent cause of postoperative meningitis. *E. coli* also causes meningitis in the early weeks of infancy, along with group B haemolytic streptococcus. *Haemophilus influenzae* infection is largely confined to children under 4, and the ear is the commonest primary source. Mixed infections, frequently including Gram-negative organisms and saprophytes of low virulence, characterize postoperative and otogenic infections; *Proteus* spp., *Pseudomonas aeruginosa*, diphtheroids, microaerophilic streptococcus and *Staph. aureus* and *epidermidis* are among those most often found. *Staph. aureus, Staph. epidermidis* and diphtheroids are the most common organisms to colonize shunt systems or other surgical implants.

Antibiotics are so commonly given for the preceding infection or for the preliminary symptoms of the meningitis that no organisms can be cultured from almost a quarter of patients with frankly turbid CSF teeming with polymorphs. In this group, antigen detection may identify pneumococcus, *Haemophilus* or meningococcus as the causative organism.

Viral meningitis
Enterovirus, mumps, herpes simplex, Epstein – Barr virus and, rarely, lymphocytic choriomeningtis may all cause a lymphocytic meningitis. The onset is usually less dramatic and the outcome often more benign than pyogenic infection.

TBM also produces a lymphocytosis in the CSF. It is an important condition to recognize since the results of treatment, if begun early enough, are good. When it complicates frank miliary infection or Pott's disease of the spine, the diagnosis is obvious, but most often it develops as an insidious illness.

Aseptic meningitis
This term is sometimes applied when a CSF pleocytosis, usually lymphocytic, is associated with a sterile culture. The possibility of this being due to TBM, a leptospiral meningitis, or to partly controlled pyogenic infection must always be considered carefully because these are treatable conditions. In contrast, carcinomatous meningitis carries a dismal prognosis. Most of those previously regarded as suffering from primary aseptic meningitis probably had some kind of virus infection.

Secondary aseptic meningitis is largely overlapped by the term chemical meningitis. Any foreign material introduced into the CSF pathways is liable to provoke a meningeal reaction which at times may be clinically obvious with meningism, pyrexia and pleocytosis. Air or positive-contrast medium injected for radiological purposes, intrathecal antibiotics, dural substitute, blood and necrotic tissue after operation, all may give rise to a sterile meningitis which must be distinguished from true infection.

Diagnosis

Meningitis is not always obvious. Infantile cases show few typical signs, but this diagnosis must be suspected whenever a child is drowsy and irritable for no obvious cause, or an infection responds poorly or relapses, or unexplained convulsions occur. TBM in both children and adults is insidious in onset; personality change, vomiting, constipation and headache make up the common complaints, none of which by itself might arouse suspicion of meningitis.

Pyogenic meningitis may strike so suddenly that coma supervenes within hours; but if infection is confined to the spinal meninges the CSF may be purulent without either disturbance of consciousness or even headache. Mild, aborted or arrested cases are common now that antibiotics are so freely given, and the possibility must be considered whenever an infection in the neighbourhood of the meninges unaccountably lingers or relapses.

Because of this inconsistency in clinical appearance, and the importance of instituting early treatment, lumbar puncture is required to establish the diagnosis, but patients in coma, with focal neurological signs or with papilloedema must first undergo CT scanning to exclude a mass lesion. If CT scanning is not immediately available for such a patient, it is best to commence antibiotics after removing blood samples for culture, rather than risk a significant delay in instituting treatment.

CSF pressure is usually raised, and the fluid, if containing more than 1000 white cells per millilitre, is turbid. Bacterial infection often leads to a polymorph count of several thousand. A few hundred lymphocytes suggests TBM, a viral meningitis, or a meningeal reaction to an intracranial abscess. Occasionally TBM also presents with a high polymorph count. The CSF sugar is abnormally low in bacterial meningitis. A very high protein suggests either TBM or a CSF block. An immediate Gram smear must be made and culture in aerobic and microaerophilic conditions with a carbon dioxide enriched atmosphere. A search for acid-fast bacilli is essential; this may take time but the discovery of just one bacillus clinches the diagnosis and saves considerable delay. Culture in Löwenstein – Jensen medium takes 6 weeks. New diagnostic techniques such as the polymerized chain reaction may speed this up in the future.

Although laboratory tests are essential for choosing the appropriate antibiotic, and for following progress, treatment must be started without waiting for bacteriological confirmation if the fluid is frankly turbid. Better treat an aseptic meningitis unnecessarily than reduce the chances of recovery from pyogenic or tuberculous meningitis by delaying treatment; hours may count in an acutely developing pyogenic case which deserves similar priority to a surgical emergency. Failure to improve indicates the need for a repeat lumbar puncture and monitoring of the CSF cell count. Organism resistance will require a change of antibiotic.

Treatment

Success depends on achieving a sufficient concentration of the correct antibiotic in the CSF without delay, on treating any primary focus of infection, and on recognizing and treating complications such as subdural effusions, spinal block and hydrocephalus.

Some antibiotics reach satisfactory levels in the CSF after systemic administration, particulary if high doses are given (e.g. 2g 2-hourly intravenously of penicillin). CSF levels are often higher than expected from experiments on normal tissues because the blood – brain barrier is altered by inflammation.

The initial choice of antibiotic must rest on the probability of a particular organism being responsible for the infection, having regard to the primary site incriminated. When there are no leads, penicillin systemically, with the addition of chloramphenical, probably provides the best cover with the least risk.

Postoperative infections tend to be low-grade with a relatively intact blood – brain barrier, thus decreasing drug penetration and making eradication more difficult. In this situation intraventricular antibiotics may be considered.

TBM calls for long-term treatment with antituberculous drugs, the combination of which requires specialist guidance.

Clinical improvement is the best index of response. If this does not occur, a repeat puncture and white cell count should be performed. The cell count in pyogenic cases should fall from thousands to hundreds within 48 hours; should it fail to do so, or rise again after an initial reduction, treatment must be reviewed. A different antibiotic may be indicated by *in vitro* sensitivity tests.

Persisting or recurring pleocytosis does not always call for change of antibiotic. In a few patients it seems that prolonged therapy irritates the meninges and maintains a high cell count; if the patient appears well by all other criteria it may be wise to stop all treatment and repeat the puncture after a few days.

Control of meningitis may depend on prompt treatment of the primary condition. Profuse leakage of CSF calls for early dural repair. A local source of infection, commonly mastoid disease or a brain abscess, may keep meningitis active by continually reinfecting the subarachnoid space, and this also calls for early surgery. Even if the meningitis is satisfactorily controlled without difficulty, surgery for any of these conditions should be delayed for only a week or so after recovery. No patient should go home with untreated mastoid disease or a dural defect after an attack of meningitis; he or she may decide not to come back for an operation, or defer it until a further and fatal attack of meningitis makes it too late.

Complications

Subdural effusions frequently complicate meningitis in children under the age of 4, and poor response to treatment or a bulging fontanelle calls for a subdural tap. The fluid is yellow with a high protein content, but is rarely infected and does not become purulent. Its effect seems to be mechanical, like that of an infantile subdural haematoma, and it requires the same treatment.

CSF obstruction, though characteristic of TBM, may occur with any organism, especially if treatment is inadequate and partly controlled infection persists. Exudate accumulates in the basal cisterns and in the spinal subarachnoid space and may produce hydrocephalus by obstructing CSF flow, making ventricular drainage necessary. A *spinal block* is suspected if the lumbar puncture pressure becomes low while the protein level rises out of proportion to the cells.

Epilepsy is particularly liable to develop in young children, and the outlook is considerably worse when this occurs. Not only do fits tend to develop in the more severely affected cases, but there is a risk of status epilepticus with its own considerable mortality. All epilepsy must therefore be treated vigorously (p. 227).

Late sequelae are unusual after acute bacterial meningitis. Complete recovery without any intellectual or physical impairment is the rule, because the brain is very resistant to infection from the surface. Danger arises chiefly from arteritis of superficial vessels causing infarction, the focal signs of which may persist. In the brainstem infarcts may be responsible for a fatal outcome. Deafness sometimes follows *Haemophilus influenzae* meningitis. Late hydrocephalus may develop due to permanent adhesions obstructing the various narrows – aqueduct, outlet of fourth ventricle or the basal cisterns. In TBM mortality ranges from 10 to 50% depending on how soon antituberculous therapy is commenced. In survivors sequelae persist in about 30% and include hemiparesis and cranial nerve deficits.

Encephalitis

Non-pyogenic encephalitis is a fairly common provisional diagnosis in patients admitted to a neurosurgical unit for investigation of acute illness. In over 40% this diagnosis proves to be mistaken and half of these patients prove to have intracranial conditions requiring surgery, such as abscess, tumour and haemorrhage. Of those finally diagnosed as encephalitis the causative virus is identified or strongly suspected in less than a third, herpes simplex being by far the commonest. Many of those in whom the diagnosis remains unconfirmed follow a mild course with complete recovery.

Herpes simplex

This is a severe form of encephalitis which still causes death despite recent advances in treatment. It selectively and asymmetrically affects the temporal and inferior frontal lobes and associated oedema may simulate a local space-occupying lesion. Headaches, confusion and pyrexia are constant findings; there is usually some degree of hemiparesis or dysphasia to indicate involvement of one hemisphere and seizures frequently occur. In the CSF the protein is raised, there is lymphocytosis and sometimes blood; occasionally atypical and primitive inflammatory cells are found. CT scanning shows irregular reduced density, most marked in the temporal lobes, and often lateral shift of the ventricles due to swelling. This swelling and shift can also be shown on angiography and ventriculography if CT scanning is unavailable. The EEG is always abnormal, showing generalized slowing with bursts of periodic high-voltage slow wave complexes over the temporal lobe. A firm diagnosis at this stage depends on brain biopsy. In severe cases the aspirate will reveal liquefied necrotic brain similar to pus. Immediate examination of the smears will show inflammatory infiltration with large mononuclears, lymphocytes and plasma cells; if any neurons are identified, necrosis may be obvious. Some laboratories are able to identify virus particles in the biopsy specimen. Some brain tissue should be sent to a virology laboratory in special transport medium; positive culture may be obtained in 48 hours or so. Confirmation may also come later from a rising titre of herpes antibody in the blood or CSF based on specimens taken at an interval of 10 days. Treatment with the antiviral agent acyclovir has reduced mortality from 70 to 20%, but 10% of survivors remain severely disabled. The earlier treatment is commenced, before necrosis becomes too advanced, the better the results. Since acyclovir is relatively non-toxic, most now advocate immediate treatment based on CT and EEG evidence without proceeding to biopsy, saving this for those patients in whom diagnostic doubt exists or who fail to respond to treatment.

Postinfectious encephalitis, occurring after common viral diseases such as measles and mumps, is probably an immunological type of response, causing demyelination. As a result recovery may be rapid and this may be accelerated or initiated by giving ACTH or corticosteroids. Measles is also incriminated as one of the causes of subacute sclerosing encephalitis, a chronic condition causing severe dementia and involuntary movements in children. It is associated with a very characteristic EEG pattern, all channels showing slowing and flattening but with repeated stereotyped high-voltage complexes. Biopsy will confirm the diagnosis.

AIDS

HIV has both neurotropic and lymphotropic properties. Seroconversion after exposure to HIV takes 4–12 weeks; a negative HIV test does not therefore exclude infection. About a third develop a persistent generalized lymphadenopathy after exposure; the remainder are asymptomatic. Months or years can elapse before the appearance of the AIDS-related complex – weight loss, lethargy, diarrhoea and minor opportunistic infections, preceding the development of full-blown AIDS. Once AIDS is established, death becomes inevitable, although zidovudine (AZT) may prolong survival.

Over 80% of infected patients develop CNS diseases either before or after the development of AIDS; 10% of AIDS patients present with diseases affecting the CNS. These include toxoplasmosis (5–15%), lymphoma (2–5%), cryptococcal meningitis (5%), cerebral infarction (19%) and AIDS-related dementia (35–50%).

The neurosurgical dilemma arises when patients who are known to be HIV-positive present with one or more intracranial masses. In the first instance biopsy or any other operative procedure should be avoided. In view of the likelihood of toxoplasmosis a trial of sulphadiazine and pyrimethamine is administered and biopsy is only performed if follow-up CT scanning shows no evidence of response. Similarly, patients in high-risk categories – homosexuals, intravenous drug users or haemophiliacs – should undergo HIV testing and if positive, biopsy should be deferred.

Risks to surgical, nursing staff and other health workers are extremely low, although full 'biohazard' precautions are required when operating on patients with known HIV infection. The risk of blood spread depends on the stage of activity and the extent of the viraemia. During an asymptomatic period the risk of transmission is far lower than when the patient has end-stage disease. Only 0.3% of staff receiving a needlestick injury have subsequently seroconverted. The recent detection of the virus in the aerosol spray produced by power instruments in the operating theatre has raised some alarm, but as yet there is no evidence of spread by this route.

Osteomyelitis of the skull

This most often results from the local spread of infection from the middle ear or frontal sinus. It gives rise to no particular clinical features distinct from those associated with infection in these sites.

Osteomyelitis of the vault may develop after trauma, either accidental or operative. The scalp may become infected first and the bone is secondarily involved. More often the wound heals by first intention but then a swelling develops followed by a discharging sinus in the line of the wound. The discharge of rather watery pus persists and granulations form round the mouth of the sinus; a probe leads directly on to bare bone. The patient remains well and the sinus may heal for short periods, only to break down again. For several weeks X-rays show no abnormality but eventually irregular rarefaction appears, perhaps with areas of dense bone where sequestra have formed.

Treatment consists of removing the affected bone; until this is done local and systemic antibiotics are of little avail. Postoperative osteomyelitis is seldom cured by nibbling the bone immediately under the sinus; it is best to remove the whole bone flap, which will usually be found irregularly eroded on its deep surface over a wide area (Fig. 5.4). Granulations cover the dura which itself is almost never breached. Once the bone flap is removed the wound usually heals quickly and the infection does not recur. The bone may be preserved in the deep freezing compartment of a refrigerator after it has been cleaned of granulations and sterilized, either by boiling or exposing to irradiation. Each of these procedures kills the bone by denaturing the proteins, but the flap may still be replaced after 3–6 months and will form a framework for the body to build up a new segment of skull.

Occasionally osteomyelitis of the vault arises after closed trauma, from blood-borne organisms infecting a pericranial haematoma. A tender boggy swelling then forms, known as Pott's puffy tumour. When a very wide area of the skull is involved it may not seem desirable to attempt to remove it completely; the contour of the skull may be preserved and the infection controlled if numerous burr holes are made, perhaps 10 or 20, to allow drainage of extradural pus. If the external table is more extensively involved it may be nibbled away between the burr holes, leaving open diploe.

Further reading

Beeden A.G., Marsen C.D., Meadows J.C. *et al.* (1969). Intracranial complications of middle ear disease and mastoid surgery. *J. Neurol. Sci.*; **9**: 261–72.

Editorial (1988). Treatment of brain abscess. *Lancet*; **i**: 219–20.

Feurman T., Wackym P.A., Grade G.F. *et al.* (1989). Craniotomy improves outcome in subdural empyema. *Surg. Neurol.*; **32**: 105–10.

Garvey G. (1983). Current concepts of bacterial infections of the central nervous system. Bacterial meningitis and bacterial brain abscess. *J. Neurosurg.*; **59**: 735–44.

Levy R.M., Pons V.G., Rosenblum M.L. (1984). Central nervous system mass lesions in the acquired immunodeficiency systems (AIDS). *J. Neurosurg.*; **61**: 9–16.

Miller E.S., Dias P.S., Uttley D. (1987). Management of subdural empyema: a series of 24 cases. *J. Neurol. Neurosurg. Psychiatry*; **50**: 1415–18.

Ommaya A.K., Di Chiro G., Baldwin M. *et al.* (1968). Non-traumatic cerebrospinal fluid rhinorrhoea. *J. Neurol. Neurosurg. Psychiatry*; **31**: 214–25.

Price D.J.E., Sleigh J.D. (1970). Control of infection due to *Klebsiella aerogenes* in a neurosurgical unit by the withdrawal of all antibiotics. *Lancet*; **ii:** 11213–15.

Raimondi A. J., Matsumoto S., Miller R. A. (1965). Brain abscess in children with congenital heart disease. *J. Neurosurg.*; **23:** 588–95.

Richards P. (1987). AIDS and the neurosurgeon. *Br. J. Neurosurg.*; **1:** 163–71.

Shearman C. P., Less P. D., Taylor J. C. (1987). Subdural empyema: a rational management plan. The the case against craniotomy. *Br. J. Neurosurg.*; **1:** 179–83.

Skildenberg B., Forsgren M., Alstig K. *et al.* (1984). Acyclovir versus vidaribine in herpes simplex encephalitis. *Lancet*; **ii:** 707–11.

Part III:

Head Injuries

Chapter 9

Frequency, causes and outcome

Causes and mechanisms of injury

Impact damage

Secondary damage

> Intracranial events
> Extracranial events

Effects of secondary events on the brain

Findings in fatal cases

Outcome in survivors of severe injuries

Assessment of outcome

Assessing severity of the injury

Head injuries are a major cause of death and disability, not only in westernized countries but also in the third world. Children and young adults are most often affected and that means many years of life lost or many years of disability.

Causes and mechanisms of injury

These vary from country to country and with the severity of injury. Only about half of fatal and severe head injuries are due to traffic accidents. Many victims are pedestrians, especially among children and the elderly, and their injuries are often more severe. Pedal cycles account for many injuries in childhood, often the result of falls during play rather than of road accidents. Falls account for more of the milder injuries than do road accidents, many of these occurring in and around the home. Assaults are a significant cause in deprived inner city areas. In the USA, firearms account for many head injuries due to interpersonal violence or to suicide attempts. Elsewhere fists and blunt instruments are the means of assault, with damage to the head often resulting from the victim falling on or against hard surfaces. Sport and work contribute to a relatively small number of head injuries. Alcohol is an important factor because not only are there drunk drivers and drunk pedestrians but falls frequently result from intoxication, while many victims and assailants involved in assaults are under the influence of alcohol.

The frequency of head injuries, as of accidents in general, varies from country to country and between urban and rural areas. Fatal head injuries are three times more common in North America, Australia, France and Germany than in the UK, Scandinavia or Japan. In the USA many more injuries occur among blacks in deprived urban communities than in white suburban or rural areas. In many countries head injuries are becoming less frequent due to the effectiveness of preventive measures. Some of these are designed to reduce the incidence of accidents – improved road design and the enforcement of laws relating to speed and alcohol levels. When an impact does occur, seat belts or air bags and better interior vehicle design can all reduce or prevent damage to the head. Helmets are very effective in motor cyclists and pedal cyclists, in industrial settings and several sports, including horse riding and mountaineering.

Mechanism of injury

Most civilian injuries (except in the USA) are *blunt*; either the moving head strikes a static surface (usually the road), or the static head is struck by a moving object. Rapid deceleration when the moving head suddenly stops, or the acceleration imparted when the head is struck, causes *diffuse* brain damage, usually evidenced by loss of consciousness. By contrast, penetrating injuries cause local damage, and consciousness may be retained. These are mostly due to low-velocity agents (sharp objects falling or fallen against, or used as weapons of assault). High-velocity ballistic missiles at close range cause extensive damage, but when nearly spent behave as low-velocity agents. Whilst penetrating injuries are always open, with the risk of infection, not all acceleration – deceleration injuries are closed, because the basal dura may be torn (see p. 222).

Impact damage

It is damage to the brain that matters and fatal brain damage can occur without a blemish on the scalp or a skull fracture. The importance of scalp injury and skull fracture is as evidence of head injury, of the site of impact, and of the possibility of open injury (p. 219) or of intracranial haematoma (p. 211).

Most brain damage from blunt injuries results from rotational acceleration causing widespread shearing strains in the highly compressible but easily deformed brain. When the brain moves within the skull these stresses are greatest at interfaces between structures of different density – grey and white matter, brain and blood vessels. More localized damage can also occur from the brain impinging on the free edges of the falx cerebri, the tentorium and sphenoidal wings, from bone fragments under a depressed fracture, and sometimes under the intact skull opposite the point of impact (contrecoup lesion). The ultimate mechanism of damage is deformation of nervous structures or blood vessels or both.

Severe and widespread shearing lesions of nerve fibres in the subcortical white matter of the cerebral hemispheres and in the brainstem are common in severe injuries that are followed by prolonged unconsciousness. In patients who die in the first few weeks, shearing lesions can be inferred at postmortem by the microscopic findings of retraction balls or microglial stars in the white matter. There are usually small lacerations visible to the naked eye in the dorsolateral quadrant of the rostral brainstem and in the corpus callosum after severe shearing injuries. In those who survive for months in a vegetative state (p. 49) the brain shows extensive demyelination of the corticospinal tracts from the subcortical region, through the brainstem to the spinal cord. After these severe lesions there is never a lucid interval but milder degrees of this diffuse axonal injury are found in some patients who have talked after initial unconsciousness but then lapsed into coma and died.

Since the discovery that even mild injuries can be associated with structural brain damage, which differs in quantity rather than in kind from that of severe injuries, the term concussion has taken on a new meaning. Whilst formerly used as a synonym for mild injury associated with only briefly altered consciousness, it is perhaps best abandoned, or at least reserved for injuries associated with a period of unconsciousness irrespective of duration, in which diffuse damage is presumed. Although its traditional use for mild injuries seems likely to continue and to cause confusion, it is better to describe an injury in terms of diffuse or local brain damage, and to qualify this by describing its severity (see below).

Contusion and laceration of the cortical surface are the most obvious lesions to the naked eye in the recently injured brain. Contusions are most frequent on summits of gyri, because these bear the brunt of the impact against the interior surface of the skull. They are most obvious in the tips of the temporal lobes and the inferior surface of the frontal lobes, no matter where the impact was. The pia is usually torn, leading to subarachnoid haemorrhage. The frequent disparity between the extent of contusions and the clinical severity has long made it obvious that the diffuse microscopic lesions just described are usually the most important component of impact brain damage.

Secondary damage

In patients who survive to reach hospital secondary brain damage due to subsequent intracranial and/or extracranial events is common. Some of these processes may begin within minutes of impact and it can then be difficult to distinguish clinically between the effects of impact and secondary brain damage.

Intracranial events

Haemorrhage in the subarachnoid spaces and into contusions and lacerations is a primary event. Secondary damage occurs due to cerebral compression by significant focal collections of blood in the extradural, subdural or intracerebral compartments (>30 ml). While such bleeding was probably initiated at the time of injury, the clinical effects may be delayed for hours or days. It is uncertain whether this is because bleeding continues or whether events such as brain swelling account for the later development of compression.

Brain swelling may be due to oedema (p. 26), to engorgement of blood vessels (p. 23) and this diffuse swelling, which may be unilateral, is much commoner in children. It may accrue in the underlying brain after removal of a compressing surface haematoma. The accumulation of blood in contusions and the subarachnoid space which does not amount to a discrete haematoma may contribute to local swelling.

Infection is a risk after all open injuries and may take the form of meningitis or intracranial abscess. Infection may be delayed by months or years, particularly after dural tears in the skull base.

Extracranial events

Hypoxia and hypercapnia resulting from respiratory insufficiency are common after head injury. Several factors can affect respiration – airway obstruction, chest injury, depressant drugs or delayed pulmonary complications. Airway obstruction also causes raised intrathoracic pressure which is transmitted to the intracranial cavity causing venous congestion, and this can aggravate brain swelling and perhaps also intracranial haemorrhage. Hypoxia can also result from depleted haemoglobin due to blood loss, usually from extracranial injuries and from systemic hypotension, possibly aggravated by blood loss during surgery and by some anaesthetic drugs.

Effects of secondary events on the brain

More than one of these secondary events frequently occurs at the same time and complex intracranial interactions can result. Most cause raised ICP which can aggravate brain shifts due to haematoma or local swelling. But the most important consequence of raised pressure is that cerebral perfusion pressure is reduced; systemic hypotension has the same effect. The net result is reduced CBF which threatens oxygenation to the brain, and this may be further impaired by systemic hypoxia (pp. 30 and 202). It is not surprising that a common secondary lesion at autopsy is hypoxic/ischaemic brain damage.

Findings in fatal cases

About half of fatal head injuries die before admission to hospital, almost all having either overwhelming brain damage or massive extracranial injuries or both. Common findings are a lacerated brainstem or hypothalamus or explosive damage to the brain as a whole, ruptured aorta or fracture-dislocation of the cervical spine. Two-thirds of deaths in hospital occur within 24 hours of injury but only some of these have irrecoverable primary brain damage. One third of hospital fatalities have talked at some time after injury – evidence that the impact brain damage had not been overwhelming. It is therefore unwise to assume that a death in hospital after head injury was inevitable, unless there is good autopsy evidence.

Common findings in hospital fatalities are a combination of impact brain injury and the consequences of secondary events. About 70% have evidence of raised ICP and about 60% an intracranial haematoma. Also common but less obvious is ischaemic brain damage, either distributed widely throughout the cortex and basal ganglia, or restricted to one major arterial territory. Local cortical ischaemia is often most marked in the boundary zones between adjacent arterial territories, suggesting underlying perfusion failure; or it may be in the territory of the posterior cerebral artery which is distorted by a tentorial hernia, resulting in medial occipital infarction.

Death after head injury is often largely due to associated injuries or extracranial complications. Preoccupation with the head injury may distract attention from the need to treat shock, and can lead to other serious injuries being overlooked (p. 198). These include chest injuries, ruptured internal organs with haemorrhage, and dislocation of the cervical spine. Late extracranial complications include fat embolism, gastrointestinal haemorrhage and oesophageal perforation.

A list of the autopsy findings does not define the cause of death. That depends on weighing both clinical and pathological evidence. It is helpful to consider the relative contribution to death of primary brain damage, secondary compressive lesions, other intracranial complications, and extracranial injuries and complications. Head injury mortality rates will differ according to whether all deaths are counted or only those in hospital. The patient mortality in hospital will depend on admission policies, and will vary from <2% in general hospitals to 20% in neurosurgical units that admit many severe injuries.

Outcome in survivors of severe injuries

Mental sequelae consist of personality change, memory disorders and reduced reasoning powers. Formal psychological testing is useful in defining the extent of memory impairment and cognitive loss. However, personality change is the most consistent and often the most damaging consequence of injury. It can occur without any marked abnormality in cognitive function. It may be obvious only to relatives or close associates of the patient and can easily be overlooked by the doctor who does not take the trouble to interview relatives and friends, and to ask them the right questions. The change usually takes the form of apathy or lack of drive, but sometimes disinhibition makes the patient talkative and tactless. Previously placid and pleasant people may become irritable and subject to temper tantrums. Whilst personality changes may be the most distressing feature for those around the patient, it is defective recent memory that often handicaps the patient most. These features of post-traumatic mental dysfunction create problems in rehabilitation, because the patient lacks motivation and the capacity to cope with therapeutic programmes without constant prompting.

Hemisphere sequelae consist of senorimotor hemiplegia and dysphasia. Patients with parieto-occipital damage may have persisting homonymous hemianopia. These features show a greater tendency to improve than do the mental features. Late traumatic epilepsy can be socially disabling, and it is most significant in patients who have otherwise made a good recovery (p. 226). Children are sometimes left with pontocerebellar disorders – bilateral motor spasticity, ataxia and dysarthria.

Cranial nerve palsies may result from injury of the central connections, or of the nerve trunks intracranially. Orbito-facial injuries may cause lesions of nerve branches in the absence of brain damage.

Anosmia is the commonest persisting complaint and occurs in almost 10% of patients admitted to hospital after head injury. It may result from fractures of the frontal base, involving the ethmoids and cribriform plate, and is then usually permanent. It is also frequent after mild injuries, often to the occiput, when recovery usually occurs within 3 months. Apart from the loss of pleasure, anosmia constitutes a hazard because the patient no longer recognizes the warning smells of escaping gas or burning.

The optic nerve is usually injured in the optic canal, frequently without fracture and sometimes after only mild concussion. Only visual field charting can determine the nature of incomplete lesions. If recovery is to occur it usually begins within a few days.

Lesions of the third, fourth and fifth nerves, affecting eye movements, are not uncommon. They may result from primary damage but third nerve lesions most commonly arise due to secondary compression from tentorial herniation; carotico-cavernous fistula may damage all three nerves. Dysconjugate gaze disorders indicate damage in the brainstem rather than to the nerves, except for the unusual case of frontal lesions causing the eyes to deviate to one side or the other. Persisting diplopia is sometimes due to a fracture of the floor of the orbit mechanically displacing the globe.

Facial palsy can occur with or without a demonstrated petrous fracture, but is usually associated with haemotympanum. Paralysis may be delayed for a few days and if so is almost always temporary; most immediate palsies also recover.

The eighth nerve is probably the most commonly damaged of all. However, neuro-otological tests may be required to detect milder degrees of trauma. Vertigo and nystagmus, from vestibular nerve or end-organ damage, may persist for months after even mild injury. Commonly the sensation of movement and unsteadiness is precipitated by sudden movement of the head, or placing it in certain positions. Nystagmus may occur only in these positions, but electronystagmography may be needed to reveal it. Caloric tests may show a reduced level in labyrinthine function on one or both sides. Deafness may be due to damage of the conductive system, of the end-organ, or of the nerve. Neuro-otological tests are necessary to distinguish these and to measure the amount of functional loss.

The features of the postconcussional syndrome, following mild injuries, are dealt with on p. 209.

Assessment of outcome

Apart from describing the various sequelae, it is important to evaluate the overall social outcome. The Glasgow Outcome Scale (Table 9.1) enables this to be done in a simple fashion, and can be used not only for brain damage from head injury but also for that due to other lesions.

Table 9.1 Glasgow Outcome Scale

Classification	Description
Dead	
Vegetative state	Sleep/wake but not sentient
Severely disabled	Concious but dependent
Moderately disabled	Independent but disabled
Good recovery	May have minor sequelae

Derived from Jennett and Bond (1975).

The *vegetative state* has been described (p. 49).

Severe disability defines a patient who is conscious but dependent. Dependence is defined as needing the assistance of another person for at least some activity during every 24 hours. This may apply to physical activity such as dressing, feeding or mobility. But impaired communication or mental disabilities can make it impossible for a patient without significant physical disability reliably to organize the day. Whilst severe disability is most often due to a combination of mental and physical handicaps, it includes some patients whose sole handicap is mental dysfunction.

Moderate disability covers a wide range of handicaps, both mental and physical. Most patients have persisting dysphasia or hemiplegia, or cranial nerve palsies, or epilepsy – but there will usually be some mental disability as well. These patients are able to cope on their own at home and to travel by public transport. Many are capable of undertaking work, although at a reduced level compared with their previous capabilities.

Good recovery indicates the capacity to resume previous work and leisure activities, but there may be mild residual sequelae.

Return to work is a poor indicator of outcome. Not only is it difficult to apply to housewives and children, but some disabled persons do return to their work, if this happens to be compatible with their particular disability. On the other hand many moderately or even minimally disabled patients find themselves unemployed after injury for a variety of reasons.

Studies on brain-damaged patients consistently show that mental disability contributes more significantly than does physical disability to the ultimate handicap. Almost all patients with physical handicap have some degree of mental disability, while the opposite does not apply. It is the combination of mental and physical disability that makes the overall handicap more serious than might be expected from either alone. The mental disability tends to interfere with rehabilitation, with family relationships, and with adapting to and coping with the overall disability.

There is no doubt that recovery after severe injury can continue for years. However, objective testing indicates that over two-thirds of patients have reached their final outcome category on the Glasgow Outcome Scale within 3 months of injury and that almost 90% have done so within 6 months. This is not to deny that improvements do continue, or that rehabilitation should be maintained for a year or more in severe cases. Whilst a few cases do change sufficiently to move up a category on this simple scale, late improvement in social functioning is usually due to patients and their families adapting to a relatively fixed disability, rather than to objective recovery of function.

Expectation of life in survivors with severe brain damage can be a matter of importance when assessing damages when legal liability for injury has been accepted. Severely disabled patients have little reduction in expectation, and as many are under the age of 30 they face some 40 years of dependent disability. Of patients who are vegetative 3 months after injury, about half will be dead by the end of the first year after injury, and a few will have regained consciousness and become very severely disabled. But those vegetative then may live for 10 or 20 years given basic nursing care and the provision of nutrition and water, usually by gastrostomy tube. It is increasingly accepted that such prolonged survival is worse than death and, particularly in the USA, it is now agreed by both ethical and legal authorities that it may be permissible after a year to withdraw life-sustaining treatment and let the patient die. This was agreed in Britain in a case that was decided on appeal by the House of Lords in 1993.

Whilst it is not easy to predict the ultimate outcome soon after injury, reports of remarkable recoveries can usually be attributed to failure to assess critically either the initial severity or the ultimate outcome. When these are carefully assessed it is found that outcome can often be predicted by the end of the first week, at least into the categories of vegetative or severe disability versus independence. These predictions depend on probability statistics applied to computerized databanks of clinical information from large series of patients. It is uncertain whether radiological and neurophysiological data can improve predictions based on clinical features such as duration of coma and evidence of focal brain damage.

Assessing severity of the injury

Discussions of early management, of the efficacy of alternative treatments, of outcome and of legal compensation all depend crucially on assessing the severity of injury. Several indicators of severity are available (Table 9.2) but not all can always be applied. The best picture of severity will emerge if reference is made to as many of these as possible.

Soon after injury conscious level is usually the best guide to severity of brain damage. The Glasgow Coma Scale (p. 47) is now usually used to classify head injuries, as a basis for triage and management decisions. A score of 8 or less indicates a severe injury, 9–12 moderate and 13 or more mild. The presence of a skull fracture should be noted, remembering that significant local damage

Table 9.2   Measures of severity

Initial features
    Conscious state[*]
    Fracture
    Focal neurological signs

Complication
    Epilepsy
    Haematoma
    Meningitis

Duration
    Coma
    PTA[†]

Sequelae
    Physical
    Mental

[*]Glasgow Coma Score (initial, after resuscitation): mild, ≥ 13 moderate, 9–12; severe, ≤ 8.
[†]PTA= Post-traumatic amnesia: Very mild, < 5 minutes; mild < 1 hour; moderate, 1–24 hours; severe, 1–7 days; very severe, > 7 days; extremely severe, > 4 weeks.

can occur without coma when there is a compound depressed fracture. Focal neurological signs occur in only a minority of injuries, and although their presence should be noted, they are not essential to classification of severity.

Once recovery has occurred the severity of the original diffuse brain damage is best judged by the duration of altered consciousness. That may be difficult to assess when the patient is first seen some time after injury. Notes made at the time of admission may be unavailable or uninformative. Fortunately the patient carries with him or her the information required, namely the duration of the post-traumatic amnesia (PTA) that can be ascertained by direct questioning. This is the interval between the injury and when the patient begins to have continuous ongoing memory. The patient will remember this as when he or she 'came to', realising where he or she was and what had happened to him or her. This is always some time after the patient has opened his or her eyes and begun to talk and to recognize relatives – which is when onlookers will have judged the end of coma. After severe injuries it may be weeks after that stage before the patient remembers events from day to day and is fully oriented – the end of PTA. An assessment of PTA is only required within broad time periods to assess severity.

It is important to distinguish between the severity of the primary injury and the ultimate severity, which may reflect the development of complications. This can be of consequence for certain legal purposes. The most obvious example is when an acute intracranial haematoma develops after a mild injury, and leads to death or severe disability. The seeming paradox of a mild injury with serious consequences and a good recovery after a severe injury can lead to legal arguments about the liability of whoever caused the original injury for the ultimate outcome.

For Further reading see Chapter 11 p. 232.

Chapter 10

Management of uncomplicated injuries

Is there evidence of diffuse or focal brain damage?

Is there a skull fracture, and is it an open injury?

Is the patient getting worse or better?

Primary care of mild injuries

Initial care of the unconscious patient

> Airway
> Fluid requirements
> Clinical observations
> Investigations

Management of raised ICP

Steroid drugs

> Osmotic agents
> Hyperventilation
> Cerebral metabolic depression

Care of continuing coma

> Chest complications
> Nutrition
> Pyrexia and infection
> Other problems

Recovery from coma

The less severely injured

Most head injuries are mild, and whatever is done the patients make a good recovery. Yet all who are unconscious, no matter how briefly, are at risk from respiratory obstruction, while a few of the mildly injured develop intracranial haematoma or infection. Patients in coma need immediate airway care, and continued intensive nursing. Some will require controlled ventilation and, if in shock, cardiovascular resuscitation and support.

About a third of head-injured patients from road accidents or falls from a height have an extracranial injury. The unconscious patient cannot draw attention to his or her injuries by complaining of pain, and a positive search must therefore be made. A swollen thigh suggests a fractured femur, haematuria a fractured pelvis, surgical emphysema fractured ribs. Shock usually indicates extracranial injury, as it is seldom due to head injury alone. Chest injuries need attention because they tend to aggravate the effects of head injury. Abdominal injuries may call for more urgent immediate treatment than most head injury problems require. Tyre marks or impression patterns on clothing on the abdominal wall indicate likely internal damage. The absence of bowel sounds supports this suspicion and indicates the need for investigation for peritoneal or retroperitoneal blood. Injuries to the cervical spine should be excluded by X-ray in all unconscious patients. Damage to the cervical cord or brachial plexus can cause inequality of the pupils from a Horner's syndrome, and a paralysed arm – which may give a false impression of intracranial injury. Flaccid paralysis of both legs immediately raises suspicion of spinal cord injury because brain damage alone seldom causes complete loss of tone.

All injuries must be adequately observed to detect complications, the aim being to ensure that the brain does not suffer secondary damage from hypotension or hypoxia. Initial assessment of the head injury should define its nature, the degree of brain damage and the risk of complications. This requires answers to a series of questions.

Is there evidence of diffuse or focal brain damage?

Altered consciousness indicates diffuse brain damage. Note whether or not the patient talks or has ever talked since injury. If talking, is he or she oriented in time and place? What can he or she remember of the accident and of what has happened since?

Focal neurological signs indicate local damage, but are found in only a minority of recently injured patients. The size and reaction of the pupils should be recorded as soon as possible before local swelling makes it difficult. Immediate abnormalities may indicate local damage to the optic or third nerve (Fig. 2.9) whereas subsequent change may signal a focal expanding mass. Hemiparesis may be overlooked if there are limb injuries, and dysphasia mistaken for mental confusion.

Is there a skull fracture, and is it an open injury?

Overwhelming brain injury can occur without skull fracture, whilst many patients with fractures have no clinical evidence of brain damage. Yet it is important to know soon after injury whether there is a skull fracture. In patients who are mildly injured and might be sent home a vault fracture indicates a greatly increased risk that an intracranial haematoma will develop (p. 214). These patients should therefore be kept under observation and some will be considered for neuroimaging. Even when CT and/or MRI are available in a hospital it is quite impractical, and indeed inappropriate, to use them for more than a few of the many head injuries that present at the emergency department. Skull X-ray is a useful triage tool for admission, for further investigation, and for neurosurgical consultation (pp. 214, 215). Skull X-ray may also provide evidence of open injury, indicating that a scalp laceration overlies a depressed fracture, or that a fronto-facial injury is associated with a fracture of the base of the anterior fossa. Awareness of the presence and site of a skull fracture can therefore contribute to the prevention and early recognition of the two most important complications of mild injury – intracranial haematoma and infection. Facial fractures may be obvious on the skull X-rays, but special views may be needed to show mandibular fractures.

Is the patient getting worse or better?

Alterations in the conscious level are the most reliable evidence of secondary intracranial events. It is vital to discover whether the level of consciousness has changed since the time of injury. Ambulance personnel, police and any other witnesses must be detained and questioned; if not available, they should be actively sought. The information obtained, with as accurate an account as possible of the timing of events, must be clearly recorded. Without such information a neurosurgeon may feel compelled to operate, because he or she is uncertain whether the present state represents severe impact injury or deterioration due to compression. Changes in the level of consciousness are most easily detected by serial recording of the Glasgow Coma Scale, which can be reliably used by a wide range of personnel (p. 47). If the patient is not talking, it is essential to discover whether he or she has ever talked since the injury. If talking, does his or her state of orientation or confusion represent improvement or deterioration? Alcohol can lead to misinterpretation of the clinical state (see later).

The development of abnormality of size and/or reaction in a pupil that was previously normal indicates cerebral compression on that side. Bilaterally fixed and dilated pupils in a patient whose motor response is flexion or localizing suggests the recent occurrence of an epileptic fit, or that homatropine drops have been instilled (to facilitate ophthalmoscopy). Small and fixed pupils raise the possibility of pontine injury or of the administration of morphine.

Alterations in vital functions occur as late features of brainstem compression. They include rising blood pressure, slowing pulse and periodic, stertorous breathing. Rapid shallow respirations usually indicate hypoxia, fat embolism or other pulmonary complications. Hyperpyrexia reflects upper brainstem or hypothalamic injury. Asymmetric deterioration in the motor response indicates either brainstem distortion or progressive damage or compression of the cerebral cortex on one side.

Primary care of mild injuries

Over 90% of patients coming to hospital after recent head injury are walking and talking and they recover uneventfully. Large numbers of these patients are admitted to hospital for a day or so in the hope that this may lead to early detection of the complications that affect only a small minority. Many need never have come into hospital if the risks had been more realistically assessed, whilst delayed diagnosis of complications still occurs. Sometimes this is because patients have failed to come to hospital soon after injury, particularly those who were assaulted or drunk, some of them having been in police cells. But in some the significance of the initial injury was underestimated at hospital, confused patients were regarded as fully conscious, or unconsciousness ascribed to alcohol or stroke. All patients with any degree of mental confusion, or PTA exceeding 5 or 10 minutes should be kept under observation, at least for a few hours. The same goes for those with severe headache or repeated vomiting. As many as a third of adult patients will have recently ingested alcohol but detectable mental confusion from alcohol alone occurs only when the blood level exceeds 200 mg/100 ml. The level falls by 10–15 mg/hour and coma lasting more than a few hours should not be ascribed to alcohol alone until other causes have been excluded. Facilities for keeping such patients for 6 hours or so may avoid the need for formal admission.

Although only 2% of head-injured attenders at hospital have a skull fracture, almost all the complications occur in these patients. It makes sense therefore to keep patients with a fracture under observation, no matter how well they seem. For indications for CT scanning, see Table 11.2.

Large numbers of mild injuries occur in young children, in whom haematoma is a much less common complication. Separation from parents by admission adds insult to injury, and it is reasonable to allow responsible parents to watch their children at home, having been given careful written instructions to contact the hospital immediately if drowsiness, abnormal behaviour, headache or vomiting should develop.

Scalp lacerations are a feature of a third to a half of all attenders – indeed this is what brings many patients who have no brain damage to hospital. A few are associated with an underlying depressed fracture (p. 219). This is more likely if the galea is torn or the laceration is longer than 5 cm. Unless there is a fracture, it is enough to shave the immediately surrounding scalp and to clean the wound before suturing, after having injected local anaesthesia. If the galea is lacerated skin sutures must include this, or a two-layer closure should be made. Adhesive strips may be enough for small lacerations, particularly in children.

Initial care of the unconscious patient

The main aim of management in more seriously injured patients is to minimize the risk of secondary brain damage from impaired cerebral oxygenation. This means maintaining systemic oxygenation and blood pressure and avoiding factors that raise ICP (Fig. 10.1).

Airway

Every unconscious patient runs the risk of swallowing his or her tongue or inhaling vomit or nasopharyngeal secretions. Blood may collect in the mouth and throat from fractures of the nose or jaws or base of the skull, whilst salivary and mucus secretions may be stimulated by local damage. The stomach is often full and vomiting can occur at any moment, with the risk of aspiration.

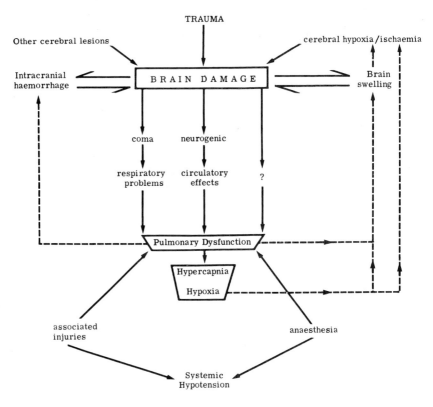

Fig. 10.1 Systemic sequelae of head injury threatening to accentuate brain damage. (See also brain-lung interactions, p. 76.)

When an unconscious patient is first seen the top priority is to ensure that the airway is clear, and then to maintain this during transport to the hospital, between departments there, and during transfer to the neurosurgical unit. Correct positioning of the patient is the simplest way to keep the airway clear. In the prone or semiprone position the jaw and tongue fall forwards, and any potential aspirate dribbles out rather than down the trachea. An oral airway can be helpful but should not be put in until the mouth has been cleaned out either by finger or mechanical suction. Aspiration of the stomach contents with a nasogastric tube should be done as soon as possible.

If the patient will tolerate an endotracheal tube one should be passed as soon as possible, because this will not only maintain the airway but also allow removal by suction of aspirate or secretions. It is doubtful whether patients whose protective reflexes are intact should be given sedative or paralysing drugs in order to allow a tube to be passed, although this is often done as soon as an anaesthetist is available. Whether once a tube is passed controlled ventilation should be established is also debatable, particularly if this will necessitate the need for sedative or relaxant drugs. No one disputes the need for these measures if there is an associated chest or major facial injury, or if there has been massive aspiration. The concern is that patients with less severe injuries who might recover quite soon are now sometimes unjustifiably treated in this way – treatment that is not entirely risk-free. One problem is in assessing the patient's conscious level. If ventilation is to be established there should be careful evaluation of the degree of responsiveness before this is done but after the airway has been cleared.

Fluid requirements

Most patients who are admitted unconscious are sufficiently recovered within 24 hours to take fluids. Head injury alone does not cause hypovolaemia. It is therefore unnecessary to institute intravenous fluid therapy in the first 12 hours unless there are associated injuries which call for this. If the patient is unable to take oral fluids after 12 hours intravenous dextrose saline should be started (2 litres in 24 hours for an adult); if coma continues the aim should be to change to nasogastric feeding as soon as possible.

Clinical observations

Having made an initial assessment, and decided whether the intracranial condition is improving, static or deteriorating, the situation is kept under constant review, particularly in the first 24–48 hours after injury. When a talking patient lapses into coma it is obvious that something is wrong. When the already unconscious patient becomes worse the change is less striking and its recognition depends on regular monitoring of the conscious level, of focal neurological signs, and of vital signs. It is in such cases that special investigations are essential.

Investigations

Skull X-ray may be deferred until an unconscious patient has been admitted, and resuscitation is complete. If, as is likely, CT is to be done, it may be unnecessary to do a skull X-ray.

CT scanning should be considered in any patient in coma, or whose level of consciousness is deteriorating. Not only is it effective in detecting and localizing, or excluding, an intracranial haematoma, but it may also show contusions, oedema, infarction, swelling and evidence of a severe white matter lesion (tears in the corpus callosum and midbrain, blood in the lateral ventricles, associated with minimal cortical contusion or shift). Effacement of the basal cisterns suggests an increase in ICP. However, about a third of serious head injuries, have normal or near-normal scans.

Angiography is now used only where (or when) CT scanning is not available. Displacement of vessels indicates a mass lesion, but not whether it is haematoma, swollen contusions or oedema.

ICP measurement is becoming more widely used in patients with severe injuries, seldom as a diagnostic test but usually to monitor the effect of treatment and to guide management. Various techniques are available (p. 28) and the method used will depend on local conditions.

Management of raised ICP

Various regimes of 'aggressive' medical therapy for comatose head injuries have been promoted during the last decade. Most rest on the assumption that raised ICP is a key factor leading to death or disability after severe head injury. However, the evidence for this is by no means clear-cut, and even those who strongly advocate such methods do not agree on what level of ICP should be regarded as requiring various degrees of intervention.

There is no doubt that very high levels of ICP, if sustained, may cause fatal brain damage. On the other hand such high levels are uncommon in the absence of an intracranial haematoma. After a patient with diffuse injury has been resuscitated and adequate ventilation and blood pressure established, elevations of ICP above 20 mmHg are uncommon. Even when these occur they may be a reflection or measure of the severity of damage rather than of a mechanism for producing further damage in a brain that would otherwise recover. When a rise in ICP is due to the swelling of a brain which is already damaged, various compensatory mechanisms often prevent a substantial increase in pressure until damage is very advanced. Therefore, when a patient has clinical evidence of diffuse brain damage and a moderate elevation of ICP a reduction of the pressure to normal levels may not result in improved outcome. This view does not preclude the possibility that the ICP may eventually rise sufficiently to result in cerebral circulatory arrest as an agonal event.

Under experimental conditions in animals many of the therapies now recommended for head injury management in humans do reduce the extent of brain damage produced in a number of ways. Usually, however, these interventions have been applied before or very shortly after the experimental insult, and are much less effective when applied later – as they have to be in clinical circumstances. Some methods have been translated from their clinical use in conditions other than trauma, and may not be so effective after head injury.

Steroid drugs

No one doubts the value of these drugs in producing rapid improvement in patients with brain tumours associated with oedema. However, CT scanning has shown that oedema is much less marked after head injury than had previously been believed. Several controlled trials as well as other studies have now failed to show any better results in patients treated with steroids, even in megadosage.

Osmotic agents

The most commonly used agent (20 % solution of mannitol) reduces ICP by withdrawing water from those parts of the brain that still have an intact blood – brain barrier. It is often useful as a method of buying time so that patients may be resuscitated and investigated before removing their intracranial haematoma. The dosage varies between 0.25 and 1 g/kg body weight given over 30 minutes. The effect of mannitol lasts for only 3–4 hours. After this time new intracellular osmoles are formed so that repeated doses become less effective and eventually systemic acidosis and renal failure can occur.

Other diuretics, such as frusemide, have been used in the management of raised ICP. It is not clear, however, whether their effects are due to increasing plasma osmolarity secondary to dehydration, or whether they have a direct effect on the transport mechanisms of the brain itself.

Hyperventilation

The benefits claimed for hyperventilation (to a $PaCO_2$ of 20–25 mmHg) lie mainly in the possibility of inducing cerebral vasoconstriction and so reducing ICP. Certainly the reduction in ICP lasts rather longer than after the administration of mannitol, but the change is still only temporary. Cerebral vessels readjust to maintained changes in $PaCO_2$ whilst extreme levels of hypercapnia may induce such severe vasoconstriction that cerebral hypoxia results. Monitoring jugular bulb oxygen saturation indirectly indicates the extent of the brain's demand for oxygen, and may identify which patients are likely to tolerate the vasoconstriction associated with hyperventilation. As yet there is no convincing evidence that the *routine* use of hyperventilation improves the outcome of severely head-injured patients who are otherwise adequately treated. Controlled ventilation may be important when there is clear evidence of respiratory disorder of some kind, and it may then result in a lowering of ICP.

Cerebral metabolic depression

Barbiturates in doses that produce burst suppression on EEG reduce CBF, because metabolism is reduced; consequently ICP also falls. However, this treatment carries a high risk of severe cardiovascular depression, which may be irreversible and until there have been adequate controlled studies there is no case for the use of barbiturates.

The improved results associated with more intensive treatment of severe head injuries have not been as marked as was at first thought. Where there has been benefit it seems likely to have been the result of more energetic resuscitation, earlier recognition and treatment of extracranial complications and of intracranial haematoma, rather than from specific medical measures.

Care of continuing coma

Patients still in coma 24 hours after injury may remain unconscious for several days, sometimes for a week or more. It then becomes important to take steps to prevent the complications of prolonged unconsciousness.

Chest complications

Depressed consciousness predisposes to aspiration which may result in a small area of infected atelectasis, diffuse bronchopneumonia or massive pulmonary collapse. The pointer to these chest complications is an increased respiratory rate; there may be cough and pleural pain, and with massive collapse obvious dyspnoea and mediastinal shift. If these complications are anticipated they can often be prevented; when they do develop the treatment is to institute, or intensify, the prophylactic measures.

As long as the patient will tolerate an endotracheal tube it should be assumed that he or she needs it. Modern tubes can be tolerated for over a week in adults, and for longer in children. Laryngeal damage is minimized by using low-pressure cuffs and small tubes (internal diameter 9–10 mm). Because of this, tracheostomy is now seldom required. Indications are fractures of the mandible or cervical spine which make it unwise to undertake intubation; or major chest injury or complications which require prolonged mechanical ventilation or repeated bronchoscopy or very frequent suction.

Tracheostomy is very rarely required as an emergency. Immediate crises are best dealt with by an endotracheal tube which is left in place until tracheostomy can be done under proper conditions. Indeed it is always safer to have an endotracheal tube in place before tracheostomy is performed. This reduces the venous congestion in the neck which occurs when there is partial respiratory obstruction. Adequate wound suction is an indispensable requirement, without which it is unsafe to operate.

Local anaesthesia is used, and the neck is slightly extended over a sandbag placed between the shoulders. A transverse incision below the cricoid cartilage gives the best cosmetic result. The isthmus of the thyroid is divided and bleeding controlled before the anterior parts of the second and third rings of the trachea are excised and stitched back to form an open trapdoor. If the first ring is interfered with, stenosis is liable to develop. Suction is applied immediately to prevent tracheal secretions from being inhaled deep into the lungs by the sudden inflow of air. Only then is the tube inserted. The wound does not usually need stitching and should never be tightly closed as surgical emphysema may then develop.

To prevent crusting and tenacious sputum, air should be delivered through a humidifier, at least for the first few days. Passive breathing exercises by the physiotherapist are supplemented by two periods a day of postural drainage during which the foot of the bed is elevated and chest percussion performed; no harm comes from the head-down position, which may indeed be maintained for most of the day, but the head should be up for half-an-hour after feeds.

Suction is needed to remove nasopharyngeal secretions, and if the catheter is passed through the nose no cooperation is demanded of the patient and he or she cannot bite the tube, which should be passed far enough down to stimulate coughing. No fluids should be given by mouth unless a good swallowing and cough reflex is present. Bronchoscopy may be needed for main bronchus obstructions, and should be available in the ward with a minimum of preparation; it may be done repeatedly, though if this proves necessary tracheostomy is probably called for. Antibiotics for chest complications are less important in treatment than establishing mechanical drainage and ensuring re-expansion of the lung. If there has been a definite aspiration then it is proper to give a 5-day course.

Pulmonary embolism may be mistaken for chest infection. Commonly occurring in the second week, in patients not specially predisposed to infection, a mild pyrexia due to the leg thrombosis may precede the chest symptoms by a few days; pleural pain, dyspnoea and small haemoptysis suggest the diagnosis.

The value of chest X-rays in ill patients soon after injury (or operation) is now seldom debated. If there is a main bronchus block calling for bronchoscopy the area of limited air entry can usually be detected clinically. The wedge-shaped shadow of pulmonary infarction does not develop until the clinical syndrome is obvious and treatment has already been instituted. When chest infection is recurrent or difficult to control, or the patient has a tracheostomy or a naso-oesophageal tube regular films may detect the development of an effusion or an abscess at an early stage. Soon after injury films can be helpful in detecting pneumothorax, lung contusion and collapse, and the response of these to therapy.

Nutrition

It is not enough to provide the theoretical requirements because the fluid and metabolic demands of the brain-damaged patient are variable. Not only may he or she expend energy in hypertonic muscles or in hyperactivity in bed, unlike other sick people, but damage to the hypothalamic pituitary region may cause specific metabolic disorders.

Water depletion can result from insufficient intake which can readily occur in a patient who is sufficiently cooperative to take sips but who is not given supplementary tube feeds. Even when the standard requirement of 2 litres in 24 hours is met, dehydration can develop if there is unsuspected diabetes insipidus due to the head injury. The conscious patient would demand more fluid but with impaired consciousness and incontinence the situation can rapidly get out of control. Uraemia can follow dehydration and may be exaggerated by too generous a diet, especially if proprietary protein concentrates are used too freely.

Altered salt excretion, resulting in either salt-hoarding or losing syndromes, is a specific post-traumatic metabolic upset which may be accentuated by excessive salt intake (too much protein or intravenous saline) or inadequate intake (dextrose in water by gastric tube or intravenously). Hyponatraemia may result from the syndrome of inappropriate ADH secretion, causing excess water retention and hypervolaemia.

The importance of all these complications is that they may cause increased drowsiness and vomiting, accounting for failure to improve and in some cases contributing to death. These disorders should be anticipated by careful attention to nutritional needs, and frequent checking of the blood electrolytes, urea and the urinary output.

Intravenous administration is unnecessary except when there is persistent ileus, and nothing is needed on the first day when the gut is often unreceptive in any event. After 24 hours 40 ml of water should be given by naso-oesophageal tube every hour, and if this is retained the amount can be rapidly increased to a litre or more a day (in 250 ml feeds). After 2 or 3 days a 2000-calorie high-protein diet must be introduced, gradually at first as diarrhoea may be precipitated. Either proprietary powders may be mixed or milk, eggs, sugar and vitamins are made up by a dietitian.

Pyrexia and infection

The commonest cause of pyrexia is probably chest infection. However, high temperature developing within hours of injury may indicate a lesion affecting the hypothalamic temperature-regulating centres. Heat-losing mechanisms are paralysed and the skin may be dry and even cool. It may be aggravated by the heat production associated with extensor rigidity or epileptic fits. Unless promptly controlled, central hyperpyrexia itself can be damaging. An axillary temperature of 38.5 °C is cause for removal of blankets, placing a fan by the bed and, in non-centrally heated wards, perhaps opening the window. These actions may have to be explained to relatives, who might otherwise regard them as possibly harmful to the patient. If there is no response, or the initial temperature is higher, tepid sponging is required; more effective still is sponging with Savlon (chlorhexidine) or alcohol or the application of icepacks. Chlorpromazine 25–50 mg intramuscularly every 6 or 8 hours is useful for controlling hyperpyrexia because it prevents shivering, the body's principal mechanism for increasing temperature.

After a few days, sudden pyrexia suggests urinary infection if the chest is not to blame. Parotitis rarely occurs with adequate nursing care but in the later stages when patients are recovering from coma and are being given solid food they may retain food in their mouths from one meal to the next unless carefully watched. Infection of a scalp wound may indicate the possibility of intracranial suppuration (abscess or meningitis). The latter may develop quite rapidly in a patient who was not hitherto suspected of having an open injury; pyrexia, stiff neck and further lowering of conscious level are the clues.

Septicaemia must also be considered, especially in patients with associated injuries or where intravenous therapy has been needed.

Other Problems

Skin excoriation readily occurs in restless patients in wet beds, and pressure sores in the quietly comatose. The unconscious, immobile patients must be turned in bed several times daily. Paul's tubing strapped on the penis is a useful way of collecting the urine and helps to keep the bed dry; in women an indwelling catheter is the only effective method, but the possibility of urinary infection and its sequelae must be remembered.

Corneal drying and abrasion are a danger in the unconscious patient who lies with the eyes wide open. The lids should be closed with thin strips of waterproof strapping, applied by a responsible person who will make certain that the strapping cannot itself rub against the cornea. Hypromellose drops should be instilled 4-hourly and a watch kept for infection. Care is taken to avoid damage from bed linen and observers should not repeatedly elicit the corneal reflex as a guide to conscious level.

Recovery from coma

All but the mildest injuries pass through a stage of restless, disorganized behaviour before regaining full consciousness. This lasts only an hour or so after milder injuries but several days of unconsciousness may be followed by many more days of cerebral irritation. As anxiety about survival abates, the family begin to worry about the patient's future sanity. Some patients become continuously restless and noisy, throwing bedclothes, feeders and urinals on the floor, swearing and shouting and trying to get out of bed. This can be disturbing to other patients and to nurses. There may be pressure to use sedative drugs or even to transfer the patient temporarily to an acute mental ward. However, the physical activity associated with this state is not harmful to the patient in most cases, indeed he or she may be exercising the chest and limbs better than physiotherapy can. By the time this behavioural pattern develops it is usually several days after injury, and the danger of a rapidly developing haematoma has by then passed. It may therefore be reasonable to give mild sedatives at night. Steps should be taken to ensure that agitation is not being aggravated by a full bladder, headache or pain from extracranial injuries. Restraints are to be avoided if at all possible but it may be necessary to put a 'boxing glove' bandage on the hands to prevent patients picking at wounds or splints or pulling out the nasogastric tube.

The less severely injured

Most patients admitted to hospital with a head injury have regained full consciousness within 24 hours of the accident. However, they still require sympathetic care if their recovery is to be as smooth and rapid as possible. A head injury is not only a bewildering experience in itself, but the thought of brain damage has sinister associations. Both the patient and relatives will be concerned to know whether the skull was fractured and whether the function of the brain will be affected in the future.

Headache is a common complaint and when severe may be due to subarachnoid haemorrhage and may be associated with neck stiffness. It should cause concern about the possibility of meningitis or an accumulating haematoma only if it is increasing and there is reason to suspect such complications. In most cases all that is needed is to keep the patient in bed and give aspirin or codeine tablets. Once the headache subsides the patient can begin sitting up, and if this does not cause a recurrence, he or she can get out of bed. Gradual return to normal activities is the secret of a smooth recovery. Recurrence of headache is common if a patient is suddenly got up and sent home after a few days in bed.

Recovery after mild injuries may take 3 or 4 weeks. During this time the patient often finds his or her power of concentration poor, that he or she lacks confidence, and that noise (e.g. of children) irritates him or her greatly. The patient may become anxious or even depressed because of these symptoms and begin again to complain of headache, but this is now described as pressure or heaviness or a band round the head. There may be dizziness or light-headedness, probably related to damage to the vestibular system or nerve (p. 194). Previous pleasures are no longer enjoyed, books bore him or her, television is annoying and libido is low. The remarkable consistency of the symptomatology of the postconcussional syndrome from one patient to another suggests an organic basis. However, there is a wide variation in its severity, or at least in the amount the patient complains about it. These variations seem to depend more on the individual patient than on the severity of injury. Indeed, often the most bitter complaints occur after the mildest injuries – perhaps because less care and consideration are extended to such patients. Certainly the most severely injured patients are quite oblivious of events during the period of unconsciousness and of subsequent cerebral irritation and confusion. These may distress the patient's relatives but his or her experience begins the day he or she comes out of his PTA. By this time the unpleasant meningism of subarachnoid haemorrhage had subsided, and he or she may never remember having suffered a severe headache. Once awake, little is expected of the severely injured patient for some time, while the mildly injured patient is expected to pull him or herself together in a few days.

For many years it was suspected that many of the symptoms of the postconcussional syndrome were in the patient's mind. However, tests show that impaired cognitive functioning occurs for several weeks after even mild injuries, while MRI studies leave no doubt that even mild concussion can be associated with definite organic brain damage. Not only has the damage done been underestimated, but so has the significance of the symptoms suffered. What is needed is to explain to the patient and family that, although he or she has fortunately escaped serious brain damage, it will take a few weeks before he or she is completely back to normal. The patient should be warned to expect headache and dizziness for some time, with some temporary limitation of mental capacity. For these reasons the patient should not resume stressful activities too soon, particularly those requiring mental concentration (e.g. studying or sitting examinations). Reports that athletes rarely suffer postconcussional symptoms have also been exploded. Although many of them resume work and even sport relatively soon after such an injury, direct questioning reveals that they have suffered the same symptoms.

Another problem is waiting for legal compensation for the personal injury. Lawyers quite legitimately press their clients to recall in detail all their complaints, many of which the doctor is trying to minimize. Symptoms sometimes resolve rapidly once a settlement is completed.

For Further reading see Chapter 11 p. 232.

Complications after head injury

Intracranial haematoma

    Chronic subdural haematoma in adults
    Infantile subdural haematoma

Open injuries

    Compound depressed fracture
    Basal dural tears
    Treatment of dural tear

Traumatic epilepsy

    Treatment
    Prophylaxis for late epilepsy

Fat embolism

Caroticocavernous fistula

Repair of skull defects (cranioplasty)

Intracranial haematoma

Many patients with head injury who die in hospital have an acute intracranial heamatoma that has caused cerebral compression. This complication may become evident in life but too late to be treated effectively; sometimes it remains unsuspected until revealed at autopsy. Some haematomas develop so rapidly, or in patients so distant from surgical care, that there is never a chance of saving their lives. These are exceptions, however, and if the criteria for diagnosing intracranial haematoma were more widely known, and/or more promptly heeded, many lives could be saved. Indeed acute haematomas are found in more than 75% of patients who talk and die.

    These comments, and the descriptions that follow, refer to haematomas that cause compression and require surgery. However, CT scanning and MRI often reveals small collections of blood that do not act as mass lesions. These radiological haematomas are mostly haemorrhagic contusions, frequently in cerebral cortex or basal ganglia; but thin collections in the extradural and subdural spaces are also frequently reported. More difficult to distinguish from surgical clots are sizeable collections in subcortical areas of the cerebral hemisphere, usually the frontal lobe. These are sometimes found a few days after injury in patients who are neurologically stable. If the clot volume is less than about 30ml and there is no marked brain shift, surgeons are usually reluctant to operate. Although some of these lesions progress, many resolve spontaneously.

Classification

Haematomas occurring within 2 weeks of injury are acute, half of them being evacuated within 24 hours. The only chronic heamatoma of any frequency is the subdural (p. 217).

Two-thirds of acute heamatomas in adults are intradural, the incidence increasing with age, peaking at 40–60 years. Often there is both subdural and intracerebral clot, associated with cortical lacerations and contusions – the so-called burst lobe. Most commonly this affects the temporal lobe, but the frontal lobe is sometimes involved, either on its own or together with the adjacent temporal lobe. A third of intradurals are solely subdural, over an intact cortex. Least common are pure intracerebral collections, most of them in the frontal lobe.

Extradural haematomas account for a third of the clots occurring in children but for only a fifth of those in adults, in whom more than a third have an associated intradural clot (which is unusual in children). Most often an extradural is temporal in site, related to bleeding from the middle meningeal artery. But a quarter are frontal, parieto-occipital or in the posterior fossa – probably from diploic vein bleeding.

More than a half the adults and two-thirds of the children operated on for acute haematoma have talked at some time after injury. However, in one large series less than half had the classical sequence of coma/lucid/coma; others were always conscious or unconscious, or went from unconscious to conscious or the opposite. None of these sequences reliably distinguished extradural from intradural clots.

Deterioration of consciousness is the most consistent clinical feature, but is less obvious in patients who have been confused or in a coma since the time of injury – which is often the case with intradural clots in adults. It is most reliably detected if frequent observations are recorded using a simple and tried method such as the Glasgow Coma Scale. Late detection is often due to regarding altered consciousness as due to alcohol or to stroke, and overlooking the history or suspicion of, or evidence for, head injury. It is vital to recognize that deterioration in verbal response from oriented to confused is as important as a deterioration in the motor response from localizing to flexion.

Pupillary dilatation on the side of the clot is a reliable sign, but it often develops late, sometimes not at all, and occasionally affects the opposite pupil first. Variation in pupil size for a few minutes during recovery from injury is not uncommon, but progressive dilatation with impaired reaction to light is always significant. It is important to know if the pupil has reacted normally since the injury, thereby excluding primary damage to the nerves; also to exclude drugs, local or systemic, that could affect pupillary size and reaction.

Hemiparesis and/or dysphasia are uncommon features, but an asymmetric response in the limbs to pain in an unconscious patient can be an important clue to compression or cortical damage.

Headache and vomiting may be early signs of cerebral compression in the awake patient, particularly if persistent, and are a common feature in children.

Autonomic signs of brainstem compression are late features – slowing pulse, rise in blood pressure and respiration that is stertorous and later slow and periodic.

The occasional posterior fossa haematoma can cause headache and vomiting without impairment of consciousness: respiratory abnormalities and even arrest can occur suddenly. Signs of occipital injury are usually a stiff neck and fracture; there may be an associated clot above the tent, adjacent to the clot below.

Detection and localization

Not all patients who deteriorate after injury have a haematoma; in those who do, surgery can be more effective if the site of the clot is first identified radiologically, using CT or MRI. The aim of an effective head injury service should be to ensure that most patients with this complication reach a neuro-surgical unit before they have reached an advanced stage of deterioration. That depends on efficient triage to identify the minority of patients at risk. They can then be kept under observation, and have radiological imaging when there is definite suspicion. CT and MRI are very effective in detecting and localizing intracranial haematomas (Fig. 11.1), but it is impractical to screen large numbers of mildly injured patients to discover the occasional one with a clot.

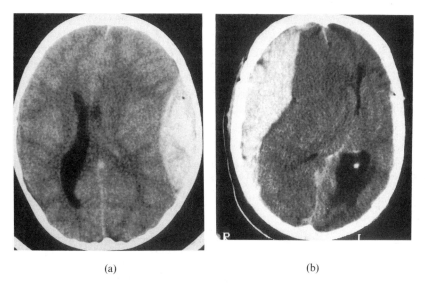

(a)   (b)

(a) Extradural haematoma. Note the displacement of the ventricle. (b) Pure subdural haematoma extending over the hemispheric surface, producing extensive midline shift, obliteration of the ipsilateral ventricle with dilatation of the contralateral occipital horn.

Fig. 11.1   CT of traumatic intracranial haematoma.

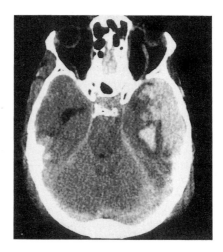

Fig. 11.1 (*cont*)   (c) Intracerebral temporal lobe haematoma with overlying subdural (i.e. burst temporal lobe).

Fortunately risk factors have been discovered and quantified that allow triage on a rational basis (Tables 11.1 and 11.2). Although adults are much more prone to acute haematomas, the same risk factors apply in children, namely a fracture of the skull vault and altered consciousness. Almost 90% of adults with an extradural have a fracture, as do 60% of those with an intradural clot. Although few mildly injured patients have a fracture, those who do are at much greater risk of haematoma. Patients without a fracture and fully conscious and well can safely be sent home. Skull X-ray therefore remains a widely available and low-cost triage tool. It is useful in providing evidence of injury in patients unable to give a history, especially those suspected of being drunk or having had a stroke, as well as in some who appear so well-recovered that they might otherwise be sent home. Those at high risk should have CT scan (Table 11.2).

Table 11.1   Absolute risk of acute intracranial haematoma developing in attenders at emergency departments ranges from 1 in 12 559 to 1 in 4 according to age, skull fracture and conscious state

		Children	*Adults*
No skull fracture			
	Fully conscious	12 559	7866
	Impaired	580	180
	Coma	65	27
With fracture			
	Fully conscious	157	45
	Impaired	25	5
	Coma	12	4

Derived from Teasdale *et al.* (1990), *Br. Med. J.* 300: 363.

Table 11.2   Guidelines for CT scanning and consideration of consultation with regional neurosurgical unit regarding possible transfer

Confusion or worse after resuscitation, even if no fracture
Any deterioration in conscious level since injury
Focal neurological signs or a fit
Fractured skull, even if no impairment of consciousness

Operation

This is seldom simple, even with the skills and equipment available in a neurosurgical unit. Most clots are intradural and associated with cerebral laceration; even if the clot has been found and evacuated, control of bleeding can be a problem. Although burr holes are sometimes enough to relieve pressure temporarily, craniotomy is invariably required for adequate removal of clot and haemostasis. In developed countries it is therefore seldom justified for general surgeons to open the skull. However, the increasing availability of CT scanning in general hospitals will make it possible to detect and localize intracranial haematomas there, and this might tempt some general surgeons to operate. If the patient can reach a neurosurgeon within an hour, he or she has a better chance of survival and reasonable recovery if moved to the specialist unit. Only if this is out of the question, and the patient's state is desperate, should an attempt be made to relieve pressure by whoever is available and willing to open the skull. Not all the clot may be removed, nor the bleeding adequately controlled, but the patient can be left with a packed open wound until the neurosurgeon can come, or the patient can be sent to the neurosurgeon.

En route to the neurosurgeon for primary surgery, temporary reduction of ICP can be achieved by giving mannitol (p. 204). Bleeding into the clot added to that during surgery can be substantial (particularly in children), and sudden relief of raised ICP can aggravate hypotension. Plasma volume expanders provide a temporary measure until cross-matched blood is available.

Operating without radiological localization of the clot should rarely be necessary. Blind burr holes often miss the lesion and valuable time is then lost rather than gained. Clinical clues to the site of a clot include a boggy scalp over a temporal extradural, the side of the first pupil to dilate, and the side and site of a vault fracture. This is a good guide to the location of an extradural, but less reliable for supratentorial intradural clots which may be remote from the fracture and sometimes on the opposite side.

Operation on a deeply unconscious patient may be started under local anaesthesia. If an endotracheal tube is not already in place one should be passed, to reduce cerebral congestion from partial airway obstruction.

After a partial head shave, a large bone flap should be turned, which for most clots will be frontotemporal (Fig. 11.2a). Blind burr holes for a suspected extradural should be sited over both anterior and posterior branches of the middle meningeal, using vertical scalp incisions that could be the basis of a flap (Fig. 11.2b). If only burr holes are made to begin with, they will need to be enlarged by nibbling bone in order to locate the clot or allow its evacuation, as well as to control bleeding. Almost always it is best to proceed to turn a flap once the clot has been found and some relief of

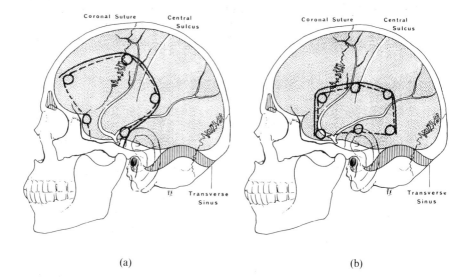

(a) Subdural/intracerebral haematoma ('burst' lobe) – the bone flap allows adequate exposure of the anterior poles of the frontal and temporal lobes. (b) Extradural haematoma – the bone flap usually overlies the anterior and posterior branches of the middle meningeal artery, but a preceding CT scan guides exact placement.

Fig. 11.2   Approach to traumatic haematomas.

pressure achieved. Arterial bleeding is controlled by diathermy, venous oozing by haemostatic gauze preparations, and that from bone with wax.

After removal of an acute intracranial haematoma some patients recover rapidly. But some develop oedema of the compressed hemisphere, and some reaccumulate clot and need a second operation. Where ICP monitoring is available it is usual to use this postoperatively in order to detect complications early; repeat CT scanning is the rule in patients not obviously improving satisfactorily.

Outcome after surgery

Increased awareness of the risk factors for haematoma, together with the availability of CT scanning, has improved outcome. However, this benefit is maximized only where there is a coordinated programme for the initial care of head injuries in all hospitals, based on agreed guidelines (Table 11.2). The mortality for extradural haematoma should be well below 20% in adults and less than half that in children, but more than 30% of patients still die with intradural clots after evacuation. This is partly because many of these patients have sustained severe initial injuries. Mortality is higher the deeper and longer the coma by the time of operation, and it climbs steadily with increasing age. At least 10% of survivors are left with severe disability, some others with moderate disability. In patients whose initial injury was mild, death and disability are usually due to delayed diagnosis and evacuation. Epilepsy is an important late sequel, more common after intradural lesions (p. 226). Some older patients are chronic alcohol abusers, and this can limit the chances of a good recovery. Few patients over 70 make a good recovery; those who do have had either an extradural or pure subdural, complicating an injury that was not severe.

Chronic subdural haematoma in adults

Only half the patients with this type of haematoma will admit to a head injury, and then it has often been mild. Some have reduced coagulability of the blood due to anticoagulant therapy or primary blood diseases. Many of the patients are elderly, having sustained a minor injury which they cannot remember.

The exact pathogenesis remains obscure. An outer and inner membrane are formed which can be cleanly stripped from the dura and arachnoid. Solid clot may fill some of the space between these membranes, but more often there is a collection of liquefied blood and CSF. It is uncertain whether the haematoma slowly increases in size due to recurrent bleeding, or by the attraction of CSF into the cavity by osmosis. Although the most extreme examples of tentorial herniation and midbrain distortion are seen with this condition, the CSF pressure is often low. Moreover at operation under local anaesthesia the haematoma may not be under pressure, and the brain may show little tendency to re-expand once the fluid has been removed.

Headache is the commonest complaint and can be severe and episodic, sometimes interpreted in children as migraine. Behavioural changes can lead to admission of older patients to a mental hospital, and as two-thirds are over 50 years of age, cerebrovascular disease or early dementia may be suspected. Drowsiness and apathy are the most usual features but confusion may be prominent. Dysphasia, if not recognized for what it is, may also suggest dementia. By this time the patient may be unable to give any account of an injury. A characteristic feature in some patients is variability in the conscious level – unrousable at one time and awake and talking and eating a few hours later, only then to relapse.

Signs of hemisphere dysfunction are common but are often slight, sometimes restricted to reflex change and minimal weakness. Due to severe brainstem shift and compression of the opposite cerebral peduncle against the tentorial edge, limb weakness is sometimes ipsilateral to the clot and is not therefore a reliable localizing feature. Only a fifth develop a dilated pupil. Epilepsy occurs in less than a tenth. Some patients are investigated as brain tumour suspects, the haematoma being discovered unexpectedly on CT scan.

Few patients show a fracture. A radioactive brain scan frequently shows an abnormality, but CT scan is now the basis of diagnosis. Care is needed to avoid missing an isodense bilateral clot which is causing no lateral shift of the ventricles.

Treatment
Chronic haematomas can be drained by making at least two burr holes and irrigating saline between them. One hole should be in the parietal region and

the other in the frontal or temporal area, according to where most haematoma seems to be located. The brain does not always re-expand immediately but unless the patient is in coma it can be left to come up slowly, encouraged by nursing the patient head-down.

Failure to improve may be due to persisting low pressure state with the brain failing to re-expand. The head-down position and attention to general hydration may be enough to improve the condition.

Re-accumulation of a haematoma is unusual but some of the original fluid, missed at the first operation, may appear on the surface and be released either by introducing a brain cannula through one of the burr holes or by opening this formally in the operating theatre. Sometimes the patient, who is often old and arteriosclerotic, simply takes time to recover, and needs only to be protected from developing fresh complications such as chest infection, retention of urine or bedsores until he or she is restored to normal. The ultimate recovery is usually satisfactory, although a few fail to regain normal mental alertness and some develop epilepsy.

Infantile subdural haematoma

Subdural haematoma or effusion in the first 2 years of life forms a clear-cut entity, in regard to presentation and management. Most of these infants are under 6 months and less than half have any history of trauma (including birth injury); however, evidence of trauma elsewhere is not uncommon and this, with denial of injury by the parents, usually points to the 'battered baby' syndrome. Vomiting and convulsions are the usual presenting symptoms, and a tense fontanelle with retinal haemorrhages the most frequent signs; the latter are almost pathognomonic and occur in more than half the cases. Many of these infants are anaemic.

The diagnosis is confirmed by CT scanning. The condition is treated by subdural taps, using a sharp needle inserted obliquely beneath the bone at the outer angle of the fontanelle. Both sides should always be tapped, but only 10 ml removed from each side on the first occasion as bleeding may be started again and brain shifts aggravated if too sudden a decompression is performed. The fluid is usually yellow with a variable amount of blood, but always a high protein content (over 1 g). Up to 1500 white cells are commonly found, both polymorphs and lymphocytes, but this need not cause suspicion of infection. However, a small number of effusions do form as a complication of meningitis, particularly due to *Haemophilus influenzae*.

Repeated tapping may show a diminishing amount of fluid and no further treatment is then required. More often the fluid keeps re-accumulating and the brain remains depressed more than 1 cm away from the skull. In that event membranes have formed on the dural surface (thick and vascular) and on the arachnoid surface (thin and transparent), and surgical intervention is required. The vogue for removing the inner membrane by craniotomy has given way to subdural shunting procedures, to peritoneal or pleural cavities; either no valve or a low-pressure valve is used in this system.

Open injuries

Compound depressed fracture

This results from impact with sharp objects of low mass which impart little acceleration to the skull as a whole. Any brain damage is usually localized with little or no concussional damage. As a result consciousness is often impaired only briefly, if at all. Without care, unless bone fragments or brain are seen in the wound, the damage underlying a simple scalp laceration may remain unrecognized. Puncture wounds due to pointed objects (fallen against or used in an assault, or an airgun pellet), are easily overlooked as penetrating injuries. Some injuries, on the other hand, look worse than they are, because even when brain in oozing out of the wound the patient may be fully conscious and without signs. Neurological signs occur only when an eloquent area is involved by the fracture (e.g. motor strip, speech cortex or visual cortex). The dura is torn in about half of compound fractures, creating the potential risk of intradural infection. About half of all depressed fractures are in children in whom most of the closed depressed fractures occur (no scalp wound). Even under a closed fracture the dura is sometimes torn and the cortex lacerated – but in these circumstances there is no risk of infection.

Diagnosis

Clinical examination may be misleading because the scalp laceration may not overlie the fracture, whilst an apparently intact outer table may conceal depression of the inner table (Fig. 11.3). X-rays are usually necessary for diagnosis and two views at right angles should be taken, because depression may be obvious on only one (Fig. 11.4). If CT scanning is relied on, care is needed

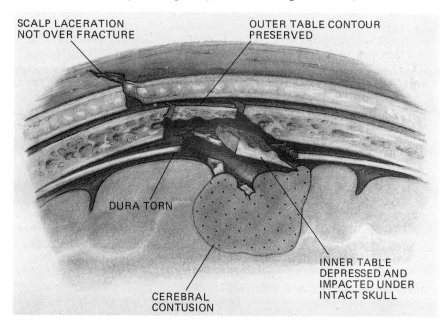

SCALP LACERATION
NOT OVER FRACTURE

OUTER TABLE CONTOUR
PRESERVED

DURA TORN

INNER TABLE
DEPRESSED AND
IMPACTED UNDER
INTACT SKULL

CEREBRAL
CONTUSION

Fig. 11.3 Depressed fracture, to illustrate how diagnosis may be missed. Note the splitting of inner from outer table, with only the inner fragment depressed. Double-density shadow (see Fig. 11.4) is produced by a fragment driven under intact skull.

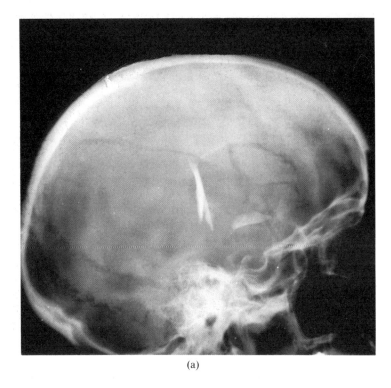

(a)

Fig. 11.4 Radiological diagnosis of depressed fractures. (a) Double density indicates depressed fragment although angulation is not directly seen.

to include the affected area of bone. If focal signs and an impaired conscious level coexist, a CT is necessary to exclude an associated intracerebral haematoma.

Treatment

The aim in treating compound fractures is to minimize the risk of infection. Compression of the brain by depressed fragments is not of particular significance, even in predisposing to late traumatic epilepsy. With closed fractures therefore elevation is only undertaken if there is thought to be a serious cosmetic problem – as in the forehead in young children.

Elevation and debridement of compound fractures should be done within 24 hours but there is no immediate urgency providing the wound is cleaned and the surrounding hair shaved. Treatment of associated extracranial injuries is often more urgent. Depressed fractures that are considered likely to involve one of the venous sinuses may be better left and antibiotic cover given, but if serious contamination makes operation essential, cross-matched blood should be available as blood loss can be considerable.

Debridement consists of removing devitalized tissue and foreign bodies and achieving primary skin closure. This may require some extension of the existing scalp laceration in order to make the scalp more mobile.

A burr hole made beside a depressed fragment combined with some bone nibbling will usually allow elevation of the fragment. Unless the dura is already torn it should not be opened. If already opened, badly bruised brain tissue

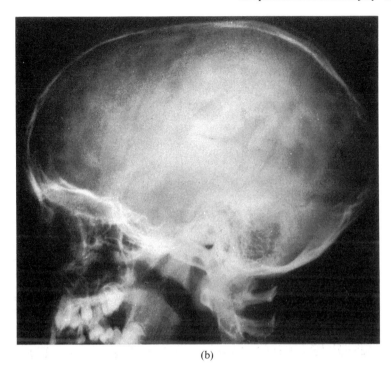

(b)

Fig. 11.4 (*cont*)   (b) Radiating and circumferential fracture lines (cartwheel), but no evidence of depression.

should be sucked away and bleeding controlled. Small dural tears can be sutured, and larger ones patched with a piece of pericranium. Providing the wound is clean and closure has not been delayed, large pieces of bone can be replaced in the form of a loose jigsaw and the pericranium stitched over to keep them in position. This avoids the need for later cranioplasty and carries little risk of infection. If cranioplasty is considered necessary it should always be deferred, as immediate implantation of foreign material runs a considerable risk of infection.

When the wound is clean and there is no marked depression or comminution, it may be safe to leave the bone fragments and simply carry out thorough cleaning and suture of the laceration. There have been several series treated successfully in this way, but it is probably safe only when closure can be done within 12 hours of injury.

Sequelae
Most patients make a rapid recovery if properly managed and few suffer from persisting sequelae. In contrast, inadequate initial treatment, usually due to failure to recognize an open injury, may result in meningitis and/or intracranial abscess, with possible death or disability. A small proportion of patients develop an intracerebral haematoma and this increases the mortality and morbidity. Epilepsy occurs in the first week in about 10%, and rather more than this will develop late traumatic epilepsy, the incidence of which varies according to various factors (p. 226).

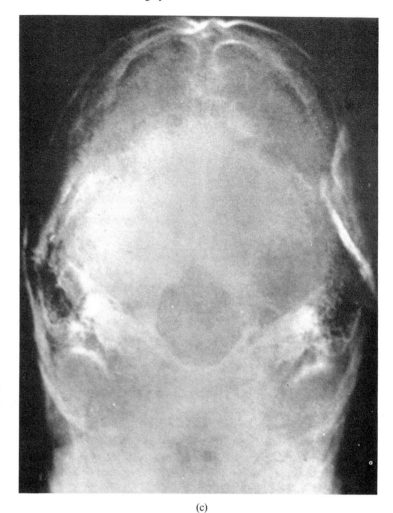

(c)

Fig. 11.4 (*cont*)   (c) Axial view of the same skull as (b), showing marked depression.

Basal dural tears (Fig. 11.5)

Meningitis still occasionally causes death after basal skull fractures, yet the means are available both to prevent this complication and for treating it effectively should it develop and be recognized in time.

A dural tear is presumed in the following circumstances:

1. CSF leak from nose or ear.
2. Intracranial air on plain X-ray or CT (Fig. 11.6).
3. Broad fracture lines or elevated fragments involving the roof of the air sinuses or the petrous bone.
4. Meningitis.

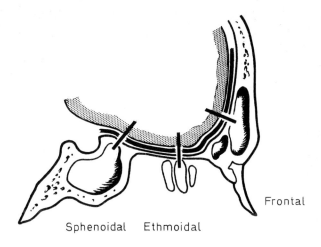

Frontal

Sphenoidal   Ethmoidal

Fig. 11.5   Dural tears into sinuses, associated with anterior fossa fractures.

CSF leak

Otorrhoea is usually profuse but short-lived and there is seldom any doubt about it. Once it stops, the risk of infection is small unless the patient already has chronic otitis media.

Rhinorrhoea is less obvious and even after careful observation there may be no certainty that the fluid is CSF. Injuries likely to cause rhinorrhoea are often associated with facial and nasal fractures. The nose is filled with blood that exudes serum, while the damaged mucous membranes of the sinuses secrete excessively, in each case simulating a CSF leak. If enough fluid can be collected to test for glucose its presence is diagnostic of CSF. Sometimes rhinorrhoea is reported by a nurse who finds a wet pillow in the morning. A recumbent patient may report a salty taste when positioned for radiological investigation.

Rhinorrhoea may first appear several days after the injury, probably because blood clot that has been filling a dural defect dissolves. More often rhinorrhoea noticed immediately after the accident dries up after a few days, probably because the brain plugs the dural defect. Although this stops the leak, it may not provide protection against ascending infection from the nose; moreover it may prevent dural healing. Meningitis may therefore develop many years after injury in a patient who does not remember having had rhinorrhoea. Allergic rhinitis or discharge from nasal polypi may simulate late CSF rhinorrhea.

Intracranial air

Air enters the cranium through a dural defect and mostly collects in the basal subdural and subarachnoid spaces. Occasionally air gains access to the ventricles and it may accumulate in the brain itself through a cerebral laceration. The resulting aerocele may develop tension – an unusual cause of brain compression after injury (Fig. 11.6).

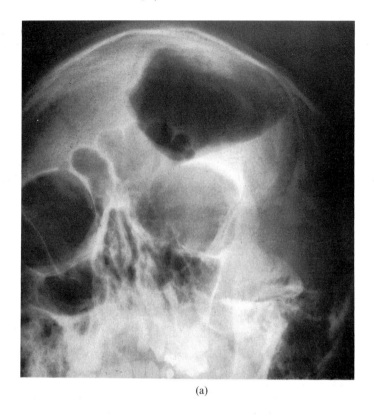

(a)

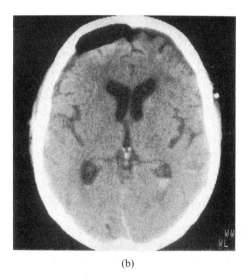

(b)

(a) Air above the frontal sinus on plain X-ray. (b) Air in frontal subarachnoid space on CT scan.

Fig. 11.6   Traumatic aerocele.

Fracture lines

Fractures through the skull base are notoriously difficult to detect on skull X-ray. CT is the optimal method of examination and, provided that suitable slice widths and window levels are selected, will clearly demonstrate fracture lines.

Meningitis

Infection can develop in the first few days, while the patient is still unconscious, and it can then be difficult to detect. Suspicion of meningitis is the one indication for lumbar puncture after head injury. If turbid fluid is discovered, treatment begins immediately with penicillin 4 MU q.i.d., chloramphenicol 1 G q.i.d. and metronidazole 500 mg q.i.d., the last to cover anaerobic infection from the ear. Identification of the responsible organism and its sensitivity permits selection of a specific antibiotic. Pneumococcus is the usual organism and, although always sensitive to penicillin, a delay of a few hours can still cost a patient his or her life.

Treatment of dural tear

In the first few days after injury it may be difficult to diagnose a dural tear with confidence. However, it should be suspected in any patient with bilateral orbital haematomas, a fracture involving the air sinuses or bruising over the mastoid. Such patients, as well as those with an obvious leak, should have prophylactic antibiotics. Detailed radiology is best deferred until the patient is sufficiently recovered to cooperate.

By the end of the first week the rhinorrhoea often stops and further treatment is not usually necessary. Most surgeons will recommend surgical repair if leakage persists beyond a week, or if there has been intracranial air, an attack of meningitis, or evidence of broad or angulated fractures in the roof of the sinus. Surgery is best delayed until the scalp is healed and recovery is underway – usually 2–3 weeks after injury.

The best guide to the site of the tear is fracture lines; if these and the rhinorrhoea are on the same side, unilateral exploration is adequate. Bilateral rhinorrhoea does not always mean tears on both sides, because a fracture of the bony septum may put the two sides of the frontal sinus in communication. When there is obvious bilateral damage, or no fractures are seen, it may be necessary to explore both sides of the base of the skull through a coronal skin-and-bone flap. To avoid this, an attempt may be made to recognize into which meatus of the nose CSF is escaping, by the use of radioisotope traces injected by lumbar puncture. Anosmia almost invariably indicates an ethmoidal tear whilst those in the sphenoid usually cause profuse and persistent rhinorrhoea. Occasionally rhinorrhoea results from a petrous fracture, the fluid running along the Eustachian tube to the nasopharynx. Petrous fractures are usually on the floor of the middle fossa and can be approached through a vertical skin incision and small craniectomy, as in the exposure of the fifth trigeminal root, or by a small temporal flap. Intradural explorations are most reliable in both the anterior and middle fossae, small hernias of the brain leading the surgeon to the dural defect. Small tears can be repaired using temporal fascia or periosteum, but large defects may require fascia lata from the thigh.

Traumatic epilepsy

Early epilepsy (first week)

A fit occurs 30 times more often in the first week after injury than in any of the next 7 weeks. Moreover, fits in the first week are often focal motor attacks that do not generalize, a type of epilepsy that seldom occurs later. These two features indicate that first-week epilepsy is a distinct entity, and it affects about 5% of hospitalized head injuries. Early epilepsy is more common after a compound depressed fracture, or injuries associated with > 24 hours PTA, or complicated by an acute intracranial haematoma. In children under 5 years of age, however, an early seizure not infrequently occurs after a trivial injury.

The first early fit occurs within 24 hours of injury in half the cases, and in half of these within the first hour. A third of patients have only one fit in the first week, but 10% develop status epilepticus. A generalized fit causes temporary deterioration in the patient's conscious level, and if the fit itself has not been witnessed, this may raise suspicion of an intracranial complication. Although early epilepsy is more common in patients with an acute haematoma, a fit is never the only sign of this complication. Only a tiny proportion of patients with early epilepsy are found to be developing a traumatic haematoma. Status is commoner in children and is a hazard that calls for urgent treatment (p. 227). The main significance of an early fit is that it greatly increases the risk of future (late) epilepsy. This applies to both children and adults, to both mild and severe injuries, and whether one or more early fits has occurred.

Late epilepsy (more than a week after injury)

Although only about 5% of non-missile injuries develop late epilepsy, it is a significant complication because it tends to persist. In patients who have otherwise made a good recovery it can be a considerable disability, mainly because it restricts eligibility to hold a driving licence and limits other activities associated with work or leisure. About half of those who develop late epilepsy have their first fit within a year of injury, but in a quarter the onset is delayed for more than 4 years. Prediction of the likelihood of late epilepsy rests on accurate clinical information about the nature of the injury and early complications. EEG is of little value in this prediction; not only do half the patients with established post-traumatic epilepsy have a normal record, but an abnormal record is a common reflection of brain damage in patients who never have a fit.

Three factors predispose to late epilepsy. It occurs in about 35% of patients who have had an acute intracranial haematoma evacuated, in 25% of those who have had early epilepsy, and in 17% of those with a compound depressed fracture. This compares with a risk of about 1% if none of these risk factors applies.

The risk after evacuating an intradural haematoma is about 40% compared with 20% for extradural; but with a sizeable intracerebral haematoma managed without surgery the risk of epilepsy is only about 20%. After compound depressed fracture the risk varies from 3 to 60% according to how many risk factors are operating – PTA over 24 hours, dural tear, focal neurological signs and early epilepsy (Fig. 11.7). In practice these risk factors are relatively uncommon and 70% of patients with depressed fractures can be reassured that the risk is less than 20%, whilst 40% have less than 5% chance of developing epilepsy. The importance of early epilepsy as a predictor is most significant in patients who have neither an intracranial haematoma nor a depressed fracture, because their risk of epilepsy is very small unless they have early epilepsy. These clinical predictors of late epilepsy are all available at the time the patient leaves hospital after injury. As the years pass without a fit occurring the original risk steadily decreases.

Treatment

Early epilepsy
When a fit occurs in the first few hours after injury, it is important to resist the temptation to give large doses of sedative drugs which, by depressing consciousness, can confuse clinical observation for intracranial complications. In a third of cases only one fit occurs; many of these are focal and constitute no immediate threat. If a fit occurs, phenytoin 200 mg can be given followed by

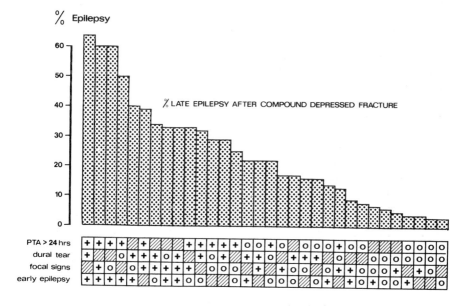

Fig. 11.7 Incidence of late epilepsy after compound depressed fracture in patients with different combinations of risk factors (where three of these are known).

200 mg 6 hours later, and daily thereafter. If more than one generalized fit occurs, the dose may be increased and if status develops urgent measures are needed (see below). Some neurosurgeons recommend prophylactic phenytoin in patients at high risk from early epilepsy (those with severe injury, intracranial haematoma or compound depressed fracture as risk factors).

Status epilepticus
This term is applied to a series of generalized convulsions without recovery of consciousness between attacks, and should be distinguished from continuing

focal fits without impairment of consciousness (p. 11). The ill-effects of status are cumulative and a vicious cycle may develop which becomes difficult to break. The sooner the fits are stopped, the greater the chance of recovery without secondary brain damage. Damage is related mainly to the venous congestion and hypoxia associated with respiratory arrest and straining at the height of each successive seizure. Children are particularly at risk of brain damage and even death can occur after trivial injury.

Status requires rapid control, aiming not only to stop the seizures but also to maintain adequate oxygenation by establishing a clear airway and by counteracting the effects which anticonvulsant drugs may have on respiration or blood pressure. As anticonvulsants may have to be given in doses which produce coma, in order to control seizures, the services of an anaesthetist or the facilities of an intensive care unit should be enrolled as soon as possible, together with laboratory monitoring to check $PaCO_2$, PaO_2 and metabolic acidosis.

Valium (diazepam) is the drug of first choice. An intravenous injection of 10 mg coupled with an intramuscular injection of 10 mg will often suffice; if fits either fail to respond or soon recur, an intravenous drip should be set up with a Y tube so that either Valium or glucose saline can be given (50–100mg in 500 ml); up to 40mg/hour is safe but hypotension should be watched for if other drugs have already been given to control the fits.

Phenytoin (epanutin, dilantin) should be given as a loading dose of 15 mg/kg intravenously at a rate of 50mg/min whilst monitoring ECG and blood pressure. If status persists, 200–300 mg of phenobarbitone is added intravenously at a similar rate (50 mg/min).

Paraldehyde is certainly effective and has a wide margin of safety; its drawback is the irritant nature of the intramuscular injection which must be deeply placed (10ml, repeated in 30 minutes if necessary). Although an intravenous drip can be used, cases requiring this are probably better treated with Valium.

Thiopentone (Pentothal) is the most reliable drug but as it may induce hypotension or laryngeal spasm it should not be used until safer drugs have proved ineffective, and an anaesthetist is available. After an initial dose of 25–100 mg intravenously a drip with a Y tube allows the dose to be titrated to the needs of the individual case (100 mg in 500 ml).

Heminevrin can also be useful and, as with thiopentone, the dose is titrated against the clinical response.

Of these drugs, only phenytoin and phenobarbitone have a lasting anticonvulsant effect, and it is important to establish a continuing regime, usually with phenytoin, once the immediate situation is under control.

Resistant cases of status are rare if really aggressive treatment is applied promptly, and care is taken to maintain adequate oxygenation by keeping the airway clear by position, suction and, if necessary endotracheal intubation. If epilepsy does persist it may require the ultimate deterrent of curarization and controlled respiration. Although convulsive movements will obviously cease as soon as the patient is curarized, full dosage of phenytoin should be continued; paraldehyde and phenobarbitone are best withdrawn so that spontaneous respiration will readily be re-established when the decision is made to allow it. This is probably worth trying after 12 hours. Once the vicious circle is broken by this method there is often no tendency for fits to recur but it may take longer than this; EEG may indicate when it is safe to discontinue curarization. If a case is resistant to conventional treatment, nothing short of the full regime of controlled respiration should be considered; giving small doses of pentothal without intubation is most unwise.

Prophylaxis for late epilepsy

The serious social consequences of even an occasional fit in a patient who has otherwise made a good recovery make it desirable to prevent epilepsy if at all possible. Whilst it might therefore seem prudent to offer prophylactic anticon-vulsants to all patients with a substantial risk of epilepsy, several reports in the last decade show disappointing long-term results from such treatment. Al-though epilepsy may be suppressed while drugs are being given (commonly the first year after injury), once they are discontinued some patients begin to suffer from epilepsy. Consequently 2 years after injury trials show little difference between the epilepsy rate in patients with or without anticonvulsant treatment. This applies to phenytoin or carbamezapine, but there is always hope that new drugs may give better results.

It is in any event often difficult to maintain compliance in patients who have never had a fit, whilst a significant number do develop side-effects. For phenytoin these include rashes, hyperplasia of the gums, and nystagmus and ataxia.

Advice about driving

Regulations that were very restrictive for patients who had had even a single fit have been progressively relaxed in a number of countries. In the UK a person may be eligible to have a private driving licence restored when 2 years have passed without a seizure during waking hours. Earlier restoration may be allowed for so-called provoked seizures, and early traumatic epilepsy has sometimes been proposed for this category although the data indicate that patients with early epilepsy have a considerable risk of late epilepsy. In patients who have not had a fit but who are in high-risk categories it is usually advised that they should not drive for a year after injury. Regulations are understandably stricter for vocational drivers (heavy goods vehicles or public service vehicles carrying passengers). They are unlikely to be eligible to drive vocationally until their risk of epilepsy is less than 2%, and that will mean a considerably longer wait after injuries associated with high risk.

Fat embolism

Cerebral symptoms due to fat embolism may mistakenly lead to suspicion of an intracranial haematoma or other complication. Sometimes the accompanying features suggest the correct diagnosis, or it may be made only retrospectively when investigations have excluded cerebral compression.

Pulmonary fat embolism is an almost invariable finding in autopsies after fracture of a marrow bone; only a few have systemic emboli, concentrated in the brain and the renal glomeruli. Filtration of the fat globules by the pulmonary capillaries causes respiratory problems ranging from a mild reduction in the PaO_2 to acute respiratory distress syndrome (ARDS).

Cerebral symptoms consist of drowsiness, confusion, epilepsy and cerebral irritation. Pulmonary symptoms usually come on at the same time, suddenly, usually 1–3 days after injury. Dyspnoea with tachypnoea, tachycardia and pyrexia tend to suggest bronchopneumonia. The petechial rash is a later development on the second or third day, and appears over the base of the neck, front of the shoulders, upper chest, conjunctiva and retina.

Diagnosis is certain when the rash is recognized. Fat in the sputum indicates pulmonary embolism. Fat droplets in the urine are important evidence of systemic spread, though they may be found only in catheter specimens emptying the whole bladder, as the fat floats and remains with any residual urine. When severe, treatment includes ventilatory support, usually with positive end expiratory pressure (PEEP), diuretics and antibiotics.

Caroticocavernous fistula

This may follow relatively trivial blunt head injuries and is commonest in middle-aged women. Whether these patients already have an aneurysmal or arteriosclerotic weakness of the carotid artery in the cavernous sinus cannot be determined, but as a quarter of the patients develop a fistula spontaneously, without any remembered trauma, this is probably a factor in some cases.

It is usually a few days after the injury when the patient suddenly becomes aware of a noise in the head, a continuous to-and-fro murmur synchronous with the pulse. The clinician can readily hear it with a stethoscope placed over the eyeball, and usually from a much wider area in the frontal region; the bruit may be reduced or even abolished by compression of the carotid artery in the neck. Pain may accompany the onset of the bruit and proptosis develops after a delay which can vary from hours to months. This may be quite mild or so severe as to lead to corneal ulceration, because the lids cannot close over the protruded globe; it usually affects the ipsilateral eye only, but, because of variations in the pattern of the ophthalmic veins which drain into the cavernous sinus, both eyes may be affected or occasionally only the contralateral one. The protruding eye may pulsate and there is usually marked chemosis and congestion of conjunctival vessels; the oedematous conjunctival sacs may hang down over the cheek in severe cases. Eye movements may be restricted mechanically or because of ophthalmoplegia, giving rise to diplopia. The fundus may show haemorrhages and congested, pulsating veins, but it can remain normal.

Carotid angiography shows the escape of contrast from the carotid siphon into the cavernous sinus and its draining veins (Fig. 11.8); there may be poor filling of the intracranial branches if the fistula is a large one. The other causes of severe exophthalmos, cavernous sinus thrombosis, endocrine exophthalmos and carotid aneurysm, do not produce a bruit or this angiographic appearance.

The course is variable. Spontaneous cures do occur; the bruit abruptly stops and the proptosis subsequently subsides. In other cases, although the bruit persists the proptosis is not severe, equilibrium is reached and no treatment is called for. However, the bruit may be so loud and so annoying to the patient that he or she demands relief; or the proptosis is so severe that something has to be done either because of the unsightly appearance of the eye or of the threat to vision.

Carotid artery ligation in the neck was once the first line of attack; if the bruit persisted the aneurysm was then 'trapped' with a carotid clip above the cavernous sinus. This often proved ineffective and a more successful approach is direct occlusion of the fistula itself with fine detachable balloon catheters passed up the carotid artery under radiological control.

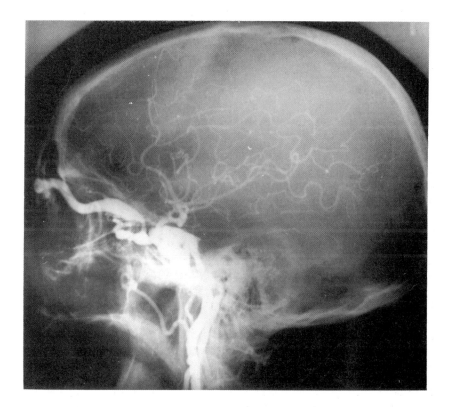

Fig. 11.8   Caroticocavernous fistula. Angiogram shows large ophthalmic vein draining the cavernous sinus filled whilst contrast is still in the intracranial arteries and in the carotid branches in the neck.

Repair of skull defects (cranioplasty)

Different materials are available. The most reliable, both for acceptance by the tissues and for a satisfactory cosmetic result, is the patient's own bone flap if this has been preserved. Metal plates (of tantalum) need careful working before operation to achieve a satisfactory contour. Screws make fitting easy, although they can work loose. They are radiopaque but non-ferrous, thus producing no artefact on MRI. If the plate slips, or is at all inexact or has a sharp edge, it may ulcerate through the skin and has then to be removed.

Plastic materials (such as acrylic) provide an alternative. These can either be premoulded or worked into shape at operation whilst they set rapidly in the bone defect. They are radiotranslucent and excite no tissue reaction.

Attempts at cranioplasty should not be made if there has been local infection until the wound has been completely healed and free of inflammation for 6–12 months. Young children should not have a defect repaired until after the age of 5 years because of skull growth. Small defects covered by thick scalp do not need to be repaired as there is very little risk of damage to the underlying brain; sometimes patients are worried about such defects, and it may then be reasonable to offer to close them. But no promise should be made that symptoms such as headache or other post-traumatic symptoms will resolve after cranioplasty, as patients sometimes expect.

Further reading

Frequency, causes, severity

Brookes M., MacMillan R., Cully S. *et al.* (1990). Head injuries in accident and emergency departments. How different are children from adults? *J. Epidemiol. Community Health*; **44:** 147–51.

Foulkes M.A., Eisenberg H.M., Jane J.A. *et al.* (1991). The trauma coma data bank: design, methods and baseline characteristics. *J. Neurosurg.*; **75:** S8–13.

Jennett B. (1976). Assessment of the severity of head injury. *J. Neurol. Neurosurg. Psychiatry*; **39:** 647–55.

Jennett B., Frankowski R. (1990). Epidemiology of head injury. In: Braakman R. (ed.) *Handbook of Clinical Neurology*; **13(57):** *Head Injury* 1–16 . Amsterdam: Elsevier.

Jennett B., MacMillan R. (1981). Epidemiology of head injury. *Br. Med. J.*; **282:** 191–4.

Levin H.S., Eisenberg H.M., Benton A.L. (eds.) (1989). *Mild Head Injury*. Oxford: Oxford University Press.

Marshall L.F., Marshall S.B., Klauber M.R. *et al.* (1991). A new classification of head injury based on computerised tomography. *J. Neurosurg.*; **75:** S14–20.

Sosin D.M., Sachs J.J., Schmidt S.M. (1989). Head injury associated deaths in the United States from 1979–86. *JAMA*; **262:** 2251–5.

Teasdale G., Teasdale E., Hadley D. (1992). CT and MRI classification of head injury. *J. Neurotrauma*; **9:** S249–57.

Turazzi S., Bricolo A., Pasut M.L. *et al.* (1987). Changes produced by CT scanning in the outlook of severe head injury. *Acta Neurochir. (Wien)*; **85:** 87–95.

Pathology

Adams J.H. (1990). Brain damage in non-missile head injury in man. In: Braakman R. (ed.) *Handbook of Clinical Neurology*; **13(57):** *Head Injury* 43–64. Amsterdam: Elsevier.

Adams J.H., Graham D.I., Gennarelli T.A. *et al.* (1991) Diffuse axonal injury in non-missile head injury. *J. Neurosurg. Neurol. Psychiatry*; **54:** 481–3.

Blumbergs P.C., Jones N.R., North J.B. (1989). Diffuse axonal injury in head trauma. *J. Neurol. Neurosurg. Psychiatry*; **52:** 838–41.

Graham D.I., Ford I., Adams J.H. *et al.* (1989). Ischaemic brain damage is still common in fatal non-missile head injury. *J. Neurol. Neurosurg. Psychiatry*; **52:** 346–50.

Outcome

Alberico A.M., Ward J.D., Choi S.C. *et al.* (1987). Outcome after severe head injury. Relationship to mass lesions, diffuse injury and ICP course in paediatric and adult patients. *J. Neurosurg.*; **67:** 648–56.

Brooks N. (ed.) (1984). *Closed Head Injury: Psychological, Social and Family Consequences*. Oxford: Oxford University Press.

Cope D.N., Cole J.R., Hall K.M. (1991). Brain injury: analysis of outcome in a post-acute rehabilitation system. *Brain Injury*; **5:** 111–25, 127–39.

Gennnarelli T. A., Spielman G. M., Langfitt T. W. *et al.* (1982). Influence of the type of intracranial lesion on outcome from severe head injury. *J. Neurosurg.*; **56:** 26–32.

Gronwall D., Wrightson P. (1975). Delayed recovery of intellectual function after minor head injury. *Lancet*; **ii:** 605–9.

Gronwall D., Wrightson P. (1975). Cumulative effect of concussion. *Lancet*; **ii:** 995–7.

Jennett B. (1993). Vegetative survival: the medical facts and ethical dilemmas. *Neuropsych. Rehab.*; **3:** 99–108.

Jennett B., Bond M. R. (1975) Assessment of outcome after severe brain damage. A practical scale. *Lancet*; **i:** 480–4.

Jennett B., Plum F. (1972). Persistent vegetative state after brain damage. *Lancet* i; 734–7.

Jennett B., Teasdale G., Braakman R. *et al.* (1979). Prognosis of patients with severe head injury. *Neurosurgery*; **4: 283–9.**

Jennett B., Snoek J., Bond M.R. *et al.* (1981). Disability after severe head injury: observations on the use of the Glasgow Outcome Scale. *J. Neurol. Neurosurg. Psychiatry*; **44:** 285–93.

Klauber M.R., Marshall L.F., Leurssen T.G. *et al.* (1989). Determinants of head injury mortality: importance of the low-risk patient. *Neurosurgery*; **24:** 31–6.

Langfitt T. W. (1978). Measuring outcome from head injuries. *J. Neurosurg.*; **48:** 673–8.

Levin H.S., Mattis S., Ruff R.M. *et al.* (1987). Neurobehavioural outcome following minor head injury: a three center study. *J. Neurosurg.*; **66:** 234–43.

Marshall L.F., Gautille T., Klauber M. R. *et al.* (1991). The outcome of severe closed head injury. *J. Neurosurg.*; **75:** S28–36.

Middelboe T., Andersen H.S., Birket-Smith M. *et al.* (1992). Minor head injury: impact on general health after 1 year. A prospective follow-up study. *Acta Neurol. Scand,*; **85:** 5–9.

Murray L., Teasdale G. M., Murray G. *et al.* (1993). Does prediction outcome alter the management of head injured patients? *Lancet*; **341:**1487–91.

Rosenthal M., Griffith E. R., Bond M. R. *et al.* (eds.) (1989). *Rehabilitation of the Adult and Child with Traumatic Brain Injury*, 2nd edn. Philadelphia: F. A. Davis.

Ruff R.M., Young D., Gautille T. *et al.* (1991). Verbal learning deficit following severe head injury: heterogeneity in recovery over one year. *J. Neurosurg.*; **75:** S50–8.

Sumner D. (1964). Post-traumatic anosmia. *Brain*; **87:** 107–20.

Vollmer D.G., Torner J.C., Jane J.A. *et al.* (1991). Age and outcome following traumatic coma: why do older patients fare worse? *J. Neurosurg.*; **75:** S37–49.

Management

Bullock R., Teasdale G.M. (1990). Head injuries (A, B, C of major trauma series). *Br. Med. J.*; **300:** 1515–18, 1576–9.

Group of Neurosurgeons. (1984). Guidelines for initial management after head injury in adults. *Br. Med. J.*; **288:** 283–85.

Jennett B. (1980). Skull X-rays after recent head injury. *Clin. Radiol.*; **31:** 463–9.

Jennett B. (1988). Treatment of severe head injury. *J. Int. Care Med.*; **3:** 284–6.

Jennett B. (1990). Providing services for head injured patients and auditing their effectiveness. In: Braakman R. (ed.) *Handbook of Clinical Neurology*; **13 (57):** *Head Injury* 429–39, Amsterdam: Elsevier.

Jennett B. (1992). Severe head injuries: ethical aspects of management. *Br. J. Hosp. Med.*; **47:** 354–7.

Jennett B., Macpherson P. (1990). Implications of scanning recently head injured patients in general hospitals. *Clin. Radiol.*; **42:** 88–90.

Jennett B., Teasdale G. (1981). *Management of Head Injuries*. Philadelphia: F.A. Davis.

Jennett B., Teasdale G., Fry J. *et al.* (1980). Treatment for severe head injury. *J. Neurol. Neurosurg. Psychiatry*; **43:** 289–95.

Marmarou A., Anderson R. L., Ward J. D. *et al.* (1991). NINDS Trauma Coma Data Bank; Intracranial pressure monitoring methodology. *J. Neurosurg.*; **75:** S21–7.

Marmarou A., Anderson R. L., Ward J. D. *et al.* (1991). Impact of ICP instability and hypotension on outcome in patients with severe head trauma. *J. Neurosurg.*; **75:** S59–66.

Miller J. D., Dearden N. M. (1992). Measurement, analysis and the management of raised intracranial pressure. In: Teasdale G.M., Miller J.D. (eds.) *Current Neurosurgery.* Edinburgh: Churchill Livingstone.

Miller J.D., Butterworth J.F., Gudeman S.K. *et al.* (1981). Further experience in the management of severe head injury. *J. Neurosurg.*; **54:** 289–99.

National Study by the Royal College of Radiologists. (1981). Cost and benefits of skull radiography for head injury. *Lancet*; **ii:** 719–95.

Stein S.C., Ross S. E. (1990). The value of computed tomographic scans in patients with low risk head injuries. *Neurosurgery*; **26:** 638–40.

Swann I.J., Yates D. W. (1989). *Management of Minor Head Injuries.* London: Chapman and Hall Medical.

Todd N.V., Teasdale G. M. (1989). Steroids in human head injury: clinical studies. In: Capildeo R. (ed.) *Steroids in Diseases of the Central Nervous System.* London: John Wiley.

Haematoma

Aoki N. (1990). Chronic subdural haematoma in infancy; clinical analysis of 30 cases in the CT era. *J. Neurosurg.*; **73:** 201–5.

Bartlett J., Byrne P. (1991). Chronic subdural haematoma. *Br. J. Neurosurg.*; **5:** 459–61.

Bullock R., Teasdale G. M. (1990). Surgical management of traumatic intracranial haematomas. In: Braakman R. (ed.) *Handbook of Clinical Neurology*; **13 (57):** *Head Injury* 249–98. Amsterdam: Elsevier.

Howard M. A., Gross A. S., Dacey R. G. *et al.* (1989). Acute subdural haematomas: an age-dependent clinical entity. *J. Neurosurg.*; **71:** 858–63.

Kwan-Hon C., Mann K. S., Yue C. P. *et al.* (1990). The significance of skull fracture in acute traumatic intracranial haematomas in adolescence: a prospective study. *J. Neurosurg.*; **72:** 189–94.

Miller J.D., Murray L. S., Teasdale G. M. (1990). Development of a traumatic intracranial haematoma after minor head injury. *Neurosurgery*; **27:** 669–73.

Nath F. P., Mendelow A. D., Wu C. *et al.* (1989). Chronic subdural haematoma in the CT scan era. *Scot. Med. J.*; **30:** 152–5.

Teasdale G., Galbraith S., Murray L. *et al.* (1982). Management of traumatic intracranial haematoma. *Br. Med. J.*; **285:** 1695–7.

Teasdale G. M., Murray G., Anderson E. *et al.* (1990). Risks of acute traumatic intracranial haematoma in children and adults: implications for managing head injury. *Br. Med. J.*; **300:** 363–7.

Wilberger J. E., Harris M., Diamond D. L. (1991). Acute subdural hematoma: mortality and operative timing. *J. Neurosurg.*; **74:** 212–18.

Open injuries

Benzel E. C., Day W. T., Kesterson L. *et al.* (1991). Civilian craniocerebral gunshot wounds. *Neurosurgery*; **29:** 67–72.

Caldicott W. J. H., North J. B., Simpson D. A. (1973). Traumatic cerebrospinal fluid fistulas in children. *J. Neurosurg.*; **38:** 1–9.

Eljemel M. S. M., Foy P. M. (1990). Posttraumatic CSF fistulae: the case for surgical repair. *Br. J. Neurosurg.*; **4:** 479–83.

Griffiths H. B. (1990). CSF fistula and the surgeon. *Br. J. Neurosurg.*; **4:** 369–71.

Kaufman H., Schwab K., Salazar A.M. (1991). A national survey of neurosurgical care for penetrating head injuries. *Surg. Neurol.*; **36:** 370–7.

Miner M. E., Ewing-Cobbs L., Kopaniky D. R. *et al.* (1990). The results of treatment of gunshot wounds to the brain in children. *Neurosurgery*; **26:** 20–5.

Sande G. M., Galbraith S. L., McLatchie G. (1980). Infection after depressed fracture in the West of Scotland. *Scot. Med. J.*; **25:** 227–9.

Van den Heever C. M., Van der Merwe D. J. (1989). Management of depressed skull fractures: selective conservative management of non-missile injuries. *J. Neurosurg.*; **71:** 186–90.

Epilepsy

Editorial (1980). Epilepsy after head trauma and fitness to drive. *Lancet*; **i:** 401.

Jennett B. (1975). *Epilepsy after Non-missile Head Injuries*, 2nd edn. London: Heinemann Medical Books.

Jennett B. (1983). Anticonvulsant drugs and advice about driving after head injury and intracranial surgery. *Br. Med. J.*; **286:** 627–8.

North J. B. (1989). Anticonvulsant prophylaxis in neurosurgery. *Br. J. Neurosurg.*; **3:** 425–8.

Temkin N. R., Dikmen S. S., Wilensky A. J. *et al.* (1990). A randomised double-blind study of phenytoin for the prevention of post-traumatic seizures. *N. Engl. J. Med.*; **323:** 497–502.

Other complications

Andrews P. J. D., Piper I. R., Dearden N. M. *et al.* (1990). Secondary insults during intrahospital transport of head injured patients. *Lancet*; **335:** 327–30.

Bouzarth W. F., Shenkin H. A. (1982). Is cerebral hyponatraemia iatrogenic? *Lancet*; **i:** 1061–2.

Bruce D. A. (1984). Delayed deterioration of consciousness after trivial head injury. *Br. Med. J.*; **289:** 715–16.

Gentleman D., Jennett B. (1981). Hazards of inter-hospital transfer of comatose head injured patients. *Lancet*; **ii:** 853–5.

Gentleman D., Jennett B. (1990). Audit of transfer of unconscious head injured patients to a neurosurgical unit. *Lancet:* **335:** 330–4.

Jackowski A. (1992). Disordered sodium and water in neurosurgery. *Br. J. Neurosurg.*; **6:** 173–6.

Lobato R. D., Rivas J. J., Gomez P. A. *et al.* (1991). Head injured patients who talk and deteriorate into coma. Analysis of 211 cases studied with computerised tomography. *J. Neurosurg.*; **75:** 256–61.

Marsh H., Maurice-Williams R. S., Hatfield R. (1989). Where does the delay occur in the process of transfer to neurosurgical care? *Br. J. Neurosurg.*; **3:** 21–30.

Marshall L. F., Toole B. M., Bowers S. A. (1983). The National Trauma Data Bank. Patients who talk and deteriorate: implications for treatment. *J. Neurosurg.*; **59:** 285–8.

Miller J. D., Becker D. P. (1982). Secondary insults to the injured brain. *J. R. Coll. Surg. Edinb.*; **27:** 292–8.

Reilly P. I., Graham D. I., Adams J. H. (1975). Patients with head injury who talk and die. *Lancet*; **ii:** 375–7.

Rose J., Valtonen S., Jennett B. (1977). Avoidable factors contributing to death after head injury. *Br. Med. J.*; **2:** 615–18.

Sharples P. M., Storey A., Aynsley-Green A. *et al.* (1990). Avoidable factors contributing to death of children with head injury. *Br. Med. J.*; **300:** 87–91.

Part IV:

Spinal Lesions

Chapter 12

Spinal compression and injuries

General features

    Causes of spinal compression

Spinal tumours

Vascular lesions of the cord

Epidural spinal abscess

    Pott's paraplegia

Spinal injuries

    Continued management of the paraplegic

General features

Spinal compression, whatever its cause, demands surgical relief. Even when the cord has been distorted and compressed for years function may return to a surprising degree if the compression is relieved.

    Many conditions can bring about compression of the spinal cord but, as with brain compression, the resulting clinical state is similar whether it is due to tumour or abscess or some other pathological process. It is important to recognize spinal compression itself rather than to try to diagnose the underlying pathology, the nature of which may be revealed only at operation. Unfortunately many of the features of compression can also be produced by much more common intrinsic diseases of the spinal cord such as disseminated sclerosis, motor neuron disease, and subacute combined degeneration. Because compression is readily relieved in many cases physicians are rightly anxious not to overlook it by accepting a diagnosis which condemns a patient to progressive paralysis without hope of cure.

Clinical
Spinal compression causes a transverse spinal lesion and affects to some extent all cord functions (motor, sensory and autonomic) below that level (Fig. 12.1), while involvement of roots at the level of compression may give rise to pain and loss of function in a radicular distribution (Fig. 12.2).

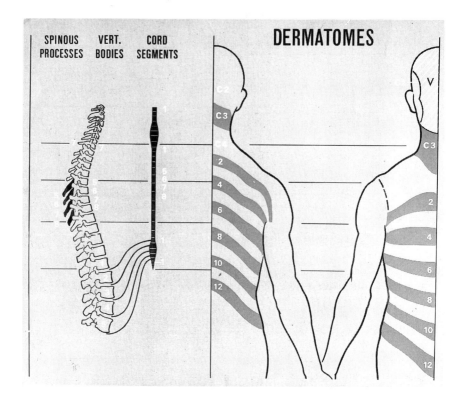

Fig. 12.1 Segmental innervation of the trunk. Lower thoracic dermatomes are very steep, with T12 running from the last rib behind to the symphysis pubis in front. Spinal cord segments do not correspond with vertebral bodies; and spinous processes correspond with neither; dermatomes are different again.

Cord lesions produce spastic weakness with increased tendon reflexes and an extensor plantar response, because the upper motor neuron is affected. Sensory loss from a partial lesion of the cord is 'dissociated', different modalities being affected in varying degrees because of the disposition of the long tracts in the cord. Compression on one side of the cord affects the pyramidal tract and posterior columns, giving spastic weakness and loss of vibration and joint position sense on the same side as the compression; involvement of the crossed spinothalamic tract causes loss of pain and temperature sense on the opposite side. Hemisection of the cord such as this is not to be expected in a pure form; it is sometimes termed the Brown-Séquard syndrome (Fig. 16.2).

Root lesions tend to affect motor and sensory functions to the same degree, and all sensory modalities are involved. Motor weakness is flaccid with loss or depression of tendon reflexes, a lower motor neuron lesion. If one root only is affected there may be severe radicular pain, but very little weakness or sensory loss may be detected because of the overlap between adjacent territories.

Cervical compression shows most clearly the combination of radicular and cord signs, because failure of function of the roots at this level is immediately

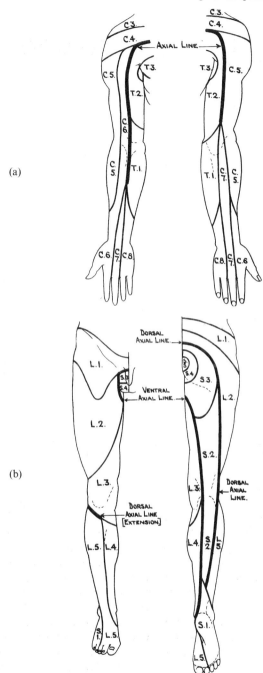

(a) The upper limb monopolizes segments C5–T1, leaving C4 and T2 adjoining on the trunk. Axial lines mark where non-consecutive segments meet in the limbs. (b) The lower limb monopolizes segments L3–S2, leaving L2 adjoining S2 and S3 on the buttock.

Fig. 12.2 Root dermatomes.

evident to the patient in the muscles of the arm and hand. The level of the sensory loss due to cord involvement is commonly several segments lower than expected, and sacral sensation may be spared although the lesion appears to be otherwise complete.

Thoracic compression presents as a cord lesion with a clear-cut sensory level in the expected situation; radicular involvement is limited to girdle pain.

Lumbar lesions are predominantly radicular because the cord ends about the interspace between vertebral bodies L1 and 2, below which only the roots of the cauda equina are affected. Flaccid paraplegia with absent reflexes is associated with radicular sensory loss and an atonic bladder. High lumbar lesions may affect also the upper motor neurons of the sacral segments in the conus medullaris, making for a mixed clinical syndrome with absent tendon reflexes and the plantar responses (if still active) extensor.

Neurogenic claudication is caused by compression of the cauda equina in a narrow lumbar spinal canal. It consists of paraesthesiae, numbness or weakness developing consecutively after a certain amount of exercise; there may also be some calf pain. In most instances a compressing lesion is found; this may be a central disc protrusion or a congenital or acquired narrowing of the bony canal; the mechanism is uncertain.

Investigation

Plain X-rays frequently show evidence of the underlying condition such as tumour or tuberculosis, but do not directly reveal spinal compression *per se*. Myelography or high-field-strength MRI (1.5 T) using surface coils permits examination of the whole length of the spinal canal and provides a screening method for patients with suspected cord compression. If the approximate level is known then CT scanning, ideally combined with intrathecal contrast, should clearly define the exact site and extent of the lesion in relation to the cord and the surrounding bone. Myelography, MRI or reconstructed CT scans produce a longitudinal view whereas axial views require CT or high-field-strength MRI.

Lumbar puncture is no longer recommended as an investigation for spinal cord compression, but still serves as a method for introducing intrathecal contrast. CSF stagnates below a block, the protein level rises and the fluid becomes xanthochromic. Only a few drops of syrupy yellow fluid, which coagulates on exposure to air in the collecting tube, may be obtained on puncture; the pressure is sometimes too low to measure. Protein levels of up to 5 g (5000 mg) per 10ml occur; a high protein level with xanthochromia but no cells (the Froin syndrome) is the result of a mechanical block and not of any particular condition. A dry tap may occur if the needle enters a tumour which is filling the lumbar sac.

Myelography involves a water-soluble contrast medium (Omnipaque/Niopam) being injected into the lumbar theca and run up and down the spine with the aid of a tilting table whilst the radiologist carries out continuous screening to observe irregularities of flow and any temporary block. Films are taken to be examined in detail later but are often less informative than the direct observation of the contrast moving on the image intensifier. Even with a complete block, the contrast can usually be coaxed around the obstruction by increasing the injecting pressure, to identify the upper limit of the compression. If this fails contrast can be introduced from above through a lateral cervical injection.

The outline of the spinal cord can be recognized as an area of diminished density. Appearances should enable distinction between extradural, intradural extramedullary and intradural intramedullary lesions p. 245 (Figs 12.7 and 12.8b pp. 251–2).

Low-pressure headache occasionally develops and is treated by bed rest and high fluid intake. Aggravation of CNS signs occurs rarely, probably due to a critically poised tumour changing position after CSF is removed. Now that water-based rather than the oil-based contrast Myodil is used, arachnoiditis no longer complicates myelography.

CT scanning requires some knowledge of the lesion site as it is impractical to scan more than a few levels at a time. A CT scan will demonstrate any bony or disc space abnormality and its effect on the spinal canal, but some intrathecal contrast is necessary to show up structures within the canal (Figs 12.5d and 12.6c pp. 249 and 251).

MRI is the optimal technique for investigating lesions within the spinal cord itself, differentiating intramedullary cysts or syrinx from tumour (Fig. 12.9 p. 253). In addition, in contrast to CT scanning, its ability to produce direct images in the sagittal plane make it the ideal method for imaging the cervicomedullary junction.

Causes of spinal compression

Tumour
 Extradural
  Primary
  Secondary
 Intradural
  Primary

Infection
 Extradural
  Staphylococcal (or other pyogenic organism)
  Tuberculosis (Pott's paraplegia)
 Intradural
  Infected dermoid
  Tuberculoma
  Staphylococcal (or other pyogenic organism)

Prolapsed intervertebral disc (central)

Spinal cord injury

Cyst
 Arachnoid
 Syringomyelia

Skeletal deformity
 Congenital
  Kyphoscoliosis
  Craniovertebral anomaly
  Achondroplasia
  Spondylolisthesis
  Diastematomyelia

Acquired
  Paget's disease
  Rheumatoid arthritis

Haemorrhage

Spinal tumours

This term includes all tumours encroaching on the bony spinal canal, and these account for most instances of spinal compression.

Pathology

Tumours are classified according to their relationship to the dura and the cord (medulla) (Fig. 12.3), and by histological types. Certain tumours favour particular situations and the following cross-classification results.

Extradural
  Secondary carcinoma
  Primary sarcoma
  Reticulosis (including myeloma)
  Chordoma
  Neurofibroma (some only)
  Meningioma (rarely)

Intradural
  Extramedullary
  Neurofibroma
  Meningioma
  Epidermoid
  Intramedullary
  Ependymoma
  Astrocytoma series

Malignant extradural tumours are the commonest spinal neoplasms encountered by the surgeon. They can arise either in the vertebrae, where they cause pathological fracture and collapse, or in the extradural tissue between theca and bone. The dura is seldom invaded even though tumour has completely encircled it like a cuff. Haematogenous spread of carcinoma is common from bronchus, breast or prostate. Myeloma forms a destructive vertebral lesion, but other reticuloses and sarcoma commonly affect soft tissue without bony involvement. Sometimes the spinal canal is directly invaded by a neighbouring tumour in the lung, chest wall or retroperitoneal tissues. Lateral X-rays may show vertebral collapse, the anteroposterior (AP) view erosion of a single pedicle (Fig. 12.4).

Neurofibroma is the commonest tumour, making up rather less than a third of all tumours. Any spinal level may be affected and most tumours are intradural; combined extradural and intradural forms occur in the cervical region, and thoracic neurofibromas are sometimes wholly extradural. Arising in relation to a nerve root, they form either a lozenge-shaped intraspinal mass or a dumb-bell tumour growing through an intervertebral foramen, partly intra- and partly extraspinal (Fig. 12.5 a and b). The intraspinal part may be

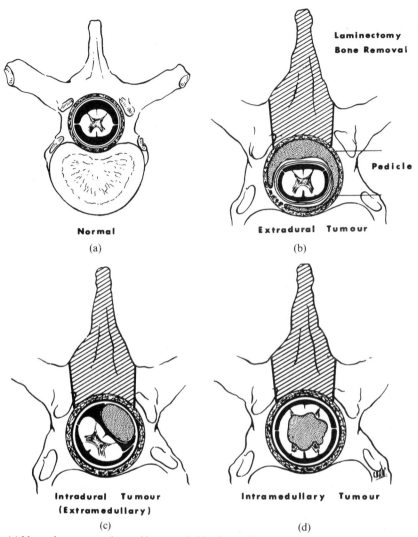

(a) Normal anatomy – the cord is suspended by dentate ligaments within the subarachnoid space (black), outside which is extradural space. (b) Extradural tumour surrounding the dural sac like a cuff. (c) Intradural (extramedullary) tumour displacing the cord. The bony removal may be extended to include the pedicle for extra exposure. (d) Intramedullary tumour expanding the cord.

Fig. 12.3   Approach to different anatomical types of spinal tumour.

extradural or intradural or both; the extraspinal may present as a lump in the neck or a shadow in the posterior mediastinum which is discovered when the chest is X-rayed for some other reason. If there is evidence of neurofibromatosis (café-au-lait skin marks or cutaneous polyps), the possibility of multiple tumours must be considered, some of which may be on cranial nerves. Radiological bone change is common; either pedicular erosion or expansion of an intervertebral foramen (Figs 12.5 c and d, 12.6 b and c). CT scan also shows the extraspinal extent of the tumour (Fig. 12.5d).

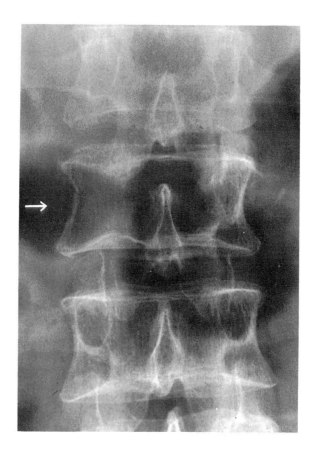

Fig. 12.4   Metastasis: missing pedicle due to destructive deposit.

Meningiomas are rather less common, and are almost confined to the thoracic spine and to middle-aged women. Rarely they occur at the foramen magnum where they lie anteriorly. An oval mass is formed which is adherent to the inner surface of the dura, but separates readily from the cord, although it may have deeply indented it and displaced it to one side of the spinal canal. Bone change is unusual.

Gliomas form tumours within the cord itself in 80% cases. About half of these are ependymomas, the remainder astrocytomas of varying grades of malignancy. The whole cord is swollen, and the bony spinal canal is expanded with narrowing of the pedicles over several segments. Glioma is the only common intradural tumour, but angiomas also occur in this situation (p. 255). Most of the other 20% of gliomas occur in the lumbosacral canal, arising from the filum terminale below the end of the cord. They displace the roots and cause scalloping of the posterior aspect of the vertebral bodies. Almost all are ependymomas, and are sometimes termed 'giant tumours of the cauda equina'. Sometimes an intracranial ependymoma or medulloblastoma seeds into the spinal subarachnoid space, and multiple deposits are found.

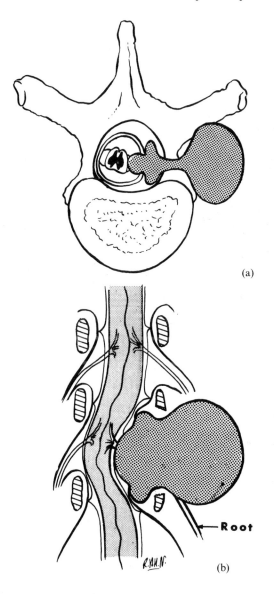

(a)

(b)

(a) The intraspinal part may be partly intradural. (b) Tumour originates on a root and escapes by enlarging the bony foramen of exit, eroding pedicles.

Fig. 12.5   Thoracic dumb-bell neurofibroma.

Epidermoids also occur in the lumbosacral canal; some appear to be the result of implanted skin tissue from the use of a lumbar puncture needle without a stilette.

Dermoids occur as intradural tumours, which may also be intramedullary; they are truly congenital tumours containing hair and sebaceous material, and may be connected with the skin by a sinus and thereby liable to infection.

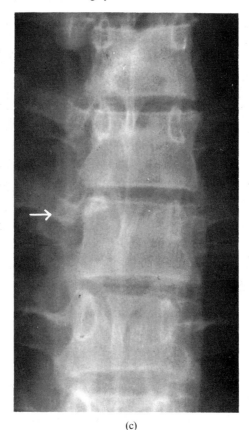

(c)

Fig. 12.5   (*cont*) (c) The lower part of one thoracic pedicle eroded by neurofibroma in the foramen.

Lipomas are also probably dermoids of a kind, because fat is not normally found within the theca; these are usually combined intramedullary and extramedullary tumours by the time they come to operation, and it is hard to determine in which situation the growth began.

Clinical

Tumour compression may be acute or chronic, producing two quite distinct syndromes.

Acute compression most often results from malignant extradural tumours, with paraplegia developing over hours or days, perhaps after a week or so of backache or root pain. If sudden vertebral collapse occurs, such as may happen with a carcinomatous deposit or myeloma, the onset of cord compression is associated with the most agonizing pain. Spinal tenderness and local kyphosis may be found. This clinical syndrome of rapidly developing flaccid paraplegia can also be produced by extradural staphylococcal abscess or by massive central protrusion of a disc. All three conditions demand urgent surgery, and the importance of distinguishing between them is to choose the correct route of access – in particular, avoiding laminectomy for thoracic disc. The distinction can be made either with myelography or CT or MRI.

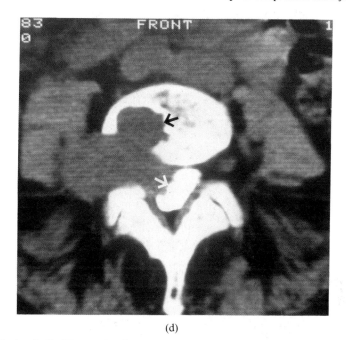

(d)

Fig. 12.5 (*cont*) (d) CT scan showing tumour eroding the vertebral body (black arrow) and displacing the contrast-filled dural sac (white arrow).

There are other causes of a sudden transverse lesion which do not call for operation. The commonest are acute demyelinating and vascular occlusions in the cord, but all are included in the term 'transverse myelitis,' which is no more than a label for rapidly developing paraplegia without evidence of compression. Although some mild prodromal root irritation does sometimes occur with these conditions, pain is usually much less common than with compression. If investigation reveals compression the spine should be explored.

Chronic compression is the mode of onset for the benign extradural and for intradural tumours, and presents an entirely different clinical appearance. There is no limit to the length of time over which a spinal tumour may give rise to symptoms, nor is there any combination of neurological signs which a tumour may not bring about.

Pain is the earliest feature as a rule; this may be either backache due to bone erosion or disturbance of spinal mechanics or root pain. This is an acute lancinating pain, referred along the length of a root, which in the thoracic region is described as girdle pain; movement or raising intrathecal pressure by coughing or sneezing may precipitate a spasm. Spinal tumour pain is often worse at night; the patient may walk the floor in an attempt to gain relief, in contrast to pain due to prolapsed disc which is almost always improved by bed rest.

Eventually most patients develop weakness, wasting, spasticity or sensory and sphincter disorders. But pain may persist for many years before CNS signs appear, in particular with lumbosacral tumours. The spinal canal is so capacious here that giant tumours can develop with bone erosion before the roots of the cauda equina are embarrassed. However, disorders of spinal movement

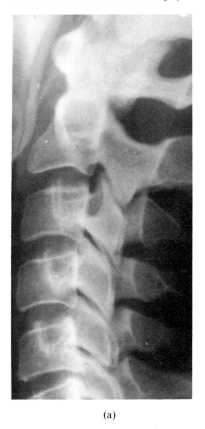
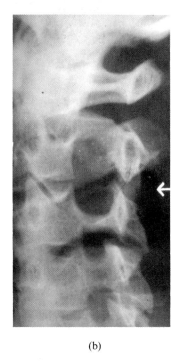

(a)   (b)

(a) Lateral view – bone erosion could be overlooked as foramina are largely hidden. (b) Oblique view – smoothly enlarged C2/3 foramen.

Fig. 12.6   Cervical dumb-bell tumour.

are usually produced, and these closely resemble those due to prolapsed disc – scoliosis, muscle spasm and restricted straight-leg raising. Tumours at the foramen magnum form another puzzling group, because the lower cranial nerves may be involved so that an intracranial tumour is suspected. Pain and sensory loss are restricted to a narrow collar distribution, whilst motor symptoms may involve any combination of the four limbs. Some investigations are difficult to interpret in this region but diagnosis is important because most tumours are meningiomas and can be removed.

Investigation
Plain X-rays are particularly important in suspected extradural compression where bone involvement is common. Lateral views may show altered bone density or collapse, AP views abnormalities of the pedicles (Figs 12.4 and 12.5c). Slowly growing tumours within the spinal canal cause thinning of the pedicles (Fig. 12.8a) and scalloping of the vertebral bodies. Oblique views may show a dilated intervertebral foramen, suggesting neurofibroma (Fig. 12.6b)

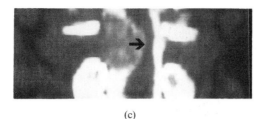

(c)

Fig. 12.6 (*cont*) (c) CT scan after intrathecal contrast reconstructed in the coronal plane showing intradural, extramedullary tumour compressing the spinal cord (arrow), and extruding through the C1/2 foramen (different case).

The use of myelography, CT scanning or MRI depends on availability and local preference.

Myelography may provide all the necessary information. Extradural masses produce an abrupt cut-off, and the displacement of the theca away from the bone may be observed in lateral projections. Intradural extramedullary tumours may cause a curved margin; they may displace the cord to one side, and produce a 'shoulder' of contrast (Fig. 12.7). Intramedullary tumours cause widening of the cord shadow and expansion of the root pockets (Fig. 12.8b), but allowance must be made for the normal lumbar and cervical enlargements. Tortuous filling defects represent dilated vessels and, although simulating arteriovenous malformation, are usually caused by venous congestion at the pole of a tumour.

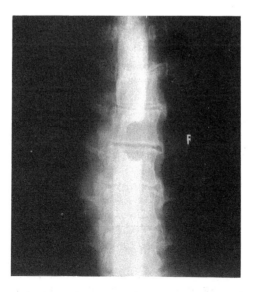

Fig. 12.7 Meningioma – myelographic appearance of intradural extramedullary tumour with spinal cord shadow deviated away from the lesion.

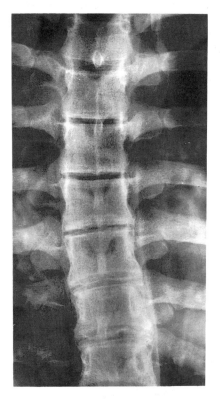
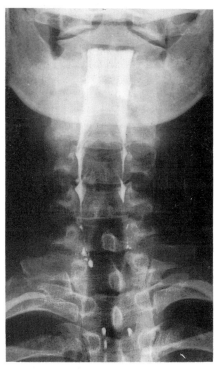

(a)   (b)

(a) Pedicles eroded over many segments. Normal pedicles can be seen in the uppermost vertebrae; in the two lowermost vertebrae the pedicles are visible but thinner on their medial aspects. (b) Myelogram (different case) – widening of spinal subarachnoid space; contrast trickles around the edge of the central tumour, filling the root pockets like rose thorns.

Fig. 12.8   Intramedullary tumour.

CT scanning provides an axial view at a preselected level and demonstrates tumour involvement of adjacent bone or extension through a foramen into paraspinous tissues (Fig. 12.5d). Intrathecal contrast is usually required to identify structures within the spinal canal (Figs 12.5d and 12.6c). CT scanning is seldom sufficiently sensitive to demonstrate lesions within the cord itself.

MRI is the method of choice for suspected intramedullary tumours. This will differentiate tumour from syringomyelia, and will show the tumour extent and the presence of any associated cysts (Fig. 12.9).

Differential diagnosis

Spinal tumour is a rarity compared with the many common conditions it can simulate during its clinical evolution. Lumbar backache and leg pain will suggest prolapsed disc, but when due to tumour these symptoms seldom settle with rest. Backache alone may lead to suspicion of ankylosing spondylitis, especially if muscle spasm leads to a frozen spine. The seeming anomaly of pain presumed of skeletal origin, which fails to respond to rest, sometimes leads to the suspicion that the patient's complaints have a psychosomatic explanation, and not infrequently the psychiatrist sees the patient before the surgeon does. Visceral disease may be simulated by lower thoracic radicular pain, so much so that the abdomen is opened. When retention of urine appears before other signs, CNS primary genitourinary disease may be suspected, whereas if motor signs predominate, intrinsic disease of the cord such as disseminated (multiple) sclerosis or motor neurone disease may be considered.

Few spinal tumours will be overlooked if all patients who have persistent backache or root pain, which does not respond as expected to adequate rest, undergo further investigation. A 'normal' CT scan of the lowest two or three disc levels fails to exclude a conus tumour and if symptoms persist, myelography (or MRI) is essential, particularly in the presence of neurological signs. With so uncommon a condition giving rise to such prosaic symptoms many patients will necessarily be investigated with negative results, but this is justified by the high likelihood of successful removal if a tumour is found.

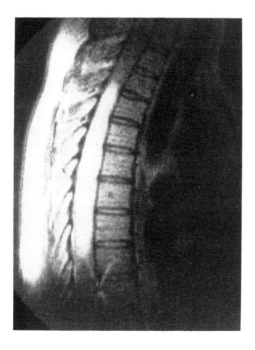

Fig. 12.9 T1-weighted MRI with gadopentetate enhacement showing intramedullary tumour extending over five thoracic segments.

Treatment

Decompression should be performed whenever a spinal tumour is diagnosed, unless it is an unquestionably malignant one in a patient already dying of cancer. The more rapidly paraplegia has developed, the greater the urgency for decompression of the cord by operation. There are a variety of routes from which to choose and selection depends upon the location of the compressing lesion. These include laminectomy with or without pediculectomy (posterior route), lateral approaches including costotransversectomy or an anterior route if necessary to any level of the spine. In general, posterior lesions are reached posteriorly, anterior lesions anteriorly, etc.

Meningiomas and neurofibromas can be removed completely in most instances, but the extraspinal part of a neurofibroma may require a second operation by a different approach. Sometimes this part of the tumour is doing little harm and can be left, although sarcomatous change is always a rare possibility.

If investigations suggest intramedullary tumour, surgery requires careful planning because there is a risk that manipulation within the cord will disturb whatever function remains. Sometimes such a tumour is cystic and improvement may follow release of the fluid contents through a small incision strictly in the posterior median raphe of the cord. Recurrence is seldom effectively delayed by attempting to encourage continuous drainage of the cyst via a tube led into the subarachnoid space. Much depends on whether there is a good plane of cleavage such as with ependymoma, as distinct from the poorly defined margin of an astrocytoma. An extensive laminectomy is required and then a myelotomy. With the use of the microscope, ultrasonic detector, and, for removal, laser and ultrasonic aspirator, it is often possible to effect macroscopic removal. However, when biopsy reveals a malignant intramedullary tumour no attempt should be made to undertake removal – a laminectomy and perhaps opening the dura should suffice before treatment with radiotherapy.

Ependymomas, alone of gliomas, have a fairly good outlook. They are radiosensitive so that even incompletely removed tumour growth can be controlled for a time. Many occur in the lumbosacral canal, where a total but piecemeal removal is often possible by teasing tumour away from the roots of the cauda equina.

Malignant extradural tumours cannot be extirpated completely, but laminectomy and removal of as much growth as possible, without opening the dura, may relieve root pain and backache satisfactorily. Some of the primary extradural tumours respond well to radiation postoperatively, and reticulosarcoma in particular may not recur for 10 years or more. When recurrence is long delayed there is always the possibility that the new symptoms are due to radiation effects on the cord. This diagnosis must also be thought of whenever a patient who has had radiation for other conditions in the neighbourhood of the cord begins to suffer from any kind of myelopathy; those at risk include cases of carcinoma of the larynx or oesophagus and ankylosing spondylitis. Secondary carcinoma has a poor outlook, with three-quarters of patients dead within 6 months of operation; prognosis is particularly poor when the primary is in the bronchus and the onset of paraplegia has been rapid, whilst the 5% or so who survive more than a year are mostly from breast or prostate. Unfortunately the presence of primary carcinoma is not recognized before operation in 40–50% of patients, and urgent surgery must be carried out lest the compression be due to one of the more favourable primary (though malignant) tumours; even when histology of the spinal mass is available, the site of the primary may remain a mystery, but most such cases prove to have small bronchial tumours.

Recovery of function after the removal of a benign extramedullary tumour can be dramatic, and patients who were bedridden may walk again in weeks. More often the final stages of improvement are slow, and active rehabilitation is vital if the most is to be made of the benefits of operation in patients already severely paralysed. Recovery of neurological function may continue for many months, and, in the case of regenerating cauda equina lesions, for as long as 2 years; both patient and physiotherapist may need to be reminded of this when morale flags.

Initially careful nursing is needed (p. 259) but the patient may get out of bed as soon as the sutures are removed, provided there is not gross vertebral body destruction. Even the most extensive laminectomy does not affect the weight-bearing components of the spine, and no special support or care is called for. However, in some patients removal of tumour may need bone removal beyond the laminae and the spine may then become unstable and require some form of fixation, such as internal metal mechanisms. In children the possibility of future spinal deformity as growth proceeds needs to be kept in mind. Splints and calipers may be needed as temporary measures, together with sticks or tripods.

Vascular lesions of the cord

Arteriovenous malformations probably affect cord function more often by deprivation of blood supply, aggravated by episodes of haemorrhage and thrombosis, than by compression. Occurring mostly below the mid thoracic level, these irregular collections of abnormal vessels lie partly on the cord substance and partly within the cord; however, a significant proportion are purely retromedullary, with a nidus lying outside the cord and often outside the dura. This type is perhaps better classified as an arteriovenous fistula rather than malformation.

Clinically there may be a steadily progressive neurological deficit, but more often the course is episodic and remitting, simulating multiple sclerosis. Moreover both conditions may be aggravated by pregnancy. Some relapses may be recognized as haemorrhagic, either because of symptoms of spinal subarachnoid haemorrhage, or because bloody or xanthochromic fluid is obtained on lumbar puncture. Myelography shows tortuous filling defects due to dilated vessels, but spinal angiography is required to show the precise position of the nidus and to identify the feeding vessels. Treatment involves removal of the fistula rather than the dilated cord veins. This is relatively straightforward when the lesion lies wholly outwith the spinal cord, but is far more hazardous when it is buried within the cord substance, even with such aids as the operating microscope and the laser.

Haemorrhage compressing the cord is a rare event. Extradural, subdural or intramedullary (haematomyelia) haemorrhages occur, as complications of trauma, arteriovenous malformations or haemophilia; some are associated with anticoagulant therapy, but many are idiopathic.

Thrombosis of the anterior spinal artery is an occasional cause of transverse myelitis, usually causing an incomplete transverse lesion affecting motor more than sensory function and always sparing joint position sense.

Epidural spinal abscess

This commonly takes the form of an acute infection and causes rapidly developing paraplegia.

Following a distant infection, usually a staphylococcal skin lesion such as a boil, epidural pus accumulates with or without vertebral osteomyelitis. Bone changes can seldom be detected on X-ray unless there is associated osteomyelitis. The diagnosis rests on a history of backache and root pain associated with pyrexia and malaise, followed after a few days by spreading numbness and later weakness of the legs. The spine is tender locally, and there may be muscle spasm and postural scoliosis. The white blood cell count is raised and also the sedimentation rate. Lumbar puncture and myelography can safely be carried out below the lesion, but a high puncture with a low lesion can result in the needle entering the abscess and draining pus, or even passing through the cavity, carrying infection into the theca. MRI avoids this risk.

Cord function is threatened by compression and urgent laminectomy is required; as much pus as possible is removed, but the dura is not opened. Maximal doses of systemic antibiotics are given on the presumption that the organisms are staphylococci, pending a bacteriological report. Provided surgery is expeditious the outlook is good. Delayed diagnosis risks permanent paraplegia or quadriplegia.

Pott's paraplegia

Spinal tuberculosis is still an occasional cause of cord compression. Initially infection is bony, an osteomyelitis affecting two or more adjacent vertebral bodies (rarely laminae) and destroying the intervening discs. Collapse and kyphosis develop, and a paravertebral abscess collects on one or both sides. Cord compression early in the illness is usually due to the abscess, but when occurring late in the healing or quiescent phase is due to bone deformity. At either time it may be ascribed to sequestrated bone or disc, or to accumulations of granulation tissue or caseous material.

Cord involvement complicates about 30% of cases of thoracic spinal tuberculosis, the part of the spine most often affected. All degrees of compression occur, from altered reflexes to total paraplegia. Before antituberculous chemotherapy was available only about 50% of patients with Pott's paraplegia recovered sufficiently to walk usefully, and 25% died. Operation did little to help, both because it was often complicated by meningitis or by chronic wound sinuses, and because laminectomy (the only procedure then performed) failed to deal with the compressing material which was situated anterior to the cord.

Chemotherapy has made surgery much less often necessary, and much safer when it is needed. Ambulant chemotherapy is now the common treatment, with frequent observation by clinical examination and X-rays. If signs progress in spite of this, or if a large paravertebral abscess develops, surgery may be needed – in the former case by anterolateral decompression and in the latter by drainage through the more limited approach of costotransversectomy.

Spinal injuries

The vast majority of closed spinal injuries leave the cord and roots unscathed. Most of those associated with cord damage have a fracture-dislocation in the cervical region (50%), or at the thoracolumbar junction (40%). Some cervical injuries follow hyperextension and may then be associated with a head injury (a frontal blow causing the hyperextension). A relatively trivial injury of this kind, without a fracture, may produce profound paralysis if the patient already suffers from cervical spondylosis (p. 273).

Clinical
Both the spinal cord and the roots at the level of the injury are usually damaged. There may be a transient loss of function from 'concussion' of the cord. Recovery from this may begin within 6 hours, and should be readily detected within 24 hours. When there is a complete lesion immediately after injury it is therefore impossible for some time to predict the chances of recovery, but if there is any evidence of conduction of impulses past the area of injury, a considerable degree of recovery can confidently be expected. If on the other hand no function at all has returned by 24 hours, it can safely be assumed that the lesion is complete and permanent, provided it is the cord itself which is involved.

With thoracolumbar injuries, however, it is the roots of the cauda equina which are damaged. It is vital to distinguish between root and cord lesions, because even though there is no sign of returning root activity some weeks after injury, recovery can still occur by a process of regeneration similar to that observed after peripheral nerve injuries. No such regeneration is possible in the spinal cord. When a mixed lesion of cauda equina and conus medullaris occurs, the root damage may give a false impression of the level of the lesion.

Management
As in the management of head injuries, little can be done to restore damage already done, and efforts are therefore directed to the prevention of complications and to providing the best conditions for natural recovery. As with head injuries, the success of treatment depends mainly on skilled nursing. Surgical intervention may rarely be needed to decompress the cord if there is an acute traumatic disc prolapse or a foreign body in the spinal canal. It is often carried out for stabilization of the spine to prevent further damage, or to ensure a stable vertebral column that will permit earlier rehabilitation.

Immediate management of spinal cord injury
In the majority of patients, damage to the spinal cord is maximal at the time of injury and that is why the emphasis in treatment is on preventing further damage, and then on starting early rehabilitation. Pathological studies have however shown that immediately after injury there may be little apparent cord damage; but within a few hours patchy necrosis develops and this eventually progresses to cavitation with gliosis and fibrosis. There is an associated

reduction in blood flow and oxygen tension. For this reason some have suggested that intervention by methods other than treatment of manifest cardiovascular or respiratory dysfunction may improve outcome by reducing ischaemia or oedema. These include steroids, mannitol, hyperbaric oxygen, catecholamine antagonists, dimethyl sulphoxide and cooling of the cord by hypothermic irrigation.

Only methylprednisolone given within 8 hours of injury improves the level of recovery in a proportion of cases. No other treatment has been shown to be effective.

It is also claimed that laminectomy increases spinal cord blood flow by relieving persisting compression, but there is no clinical evidence that after complete injury of the cord decompression improves function.

Spinal column injury

Until the stability of the fracture has been assessed, which should be done as soon as possible, the spine must be handled with great care. The danger of inflicting additional damage is greatest in the cervical region. A temporary collar, either of leather or improvised out of cardboard or newspaper, will prevent sudden flexion or extension. During turning in bed, positioning for X-rays or transferring the patient from the bed to a trolley, firm traction should be exerted manually. Patients with unstable cervical spine injuries must be placed as soon as possible on cervical traction, which is best achieved with the Gardner–Wells tongs.

Radiology is obviously crucial but it can be difficult both because of technical difficulties in visualizing certain important regions, particularly the lower cervical and upper thoracic regions. When there is doubt about the presence of a fracture, a CT scan will often show abnormalities not seen on plain X-ray. Especially with hyperextension injuries there may be no apparent bony damage, although the patient is totally paraplegic. Careful inspection may reveal small avulsion fractures of the spinous process, or of the anteroinferior margin of the body, and these indicate that there has been hyperflexion or hyperextension, although the spine now has normal alignment. It is vitally important to see all seven cervical vertebrae and many patients will need films taken in both flexion and extension. Myelography is rarely if ever needed for spinal injuries now that CT and MRI are available.

Occasionally in a patient with an incomplete lesion the signs increase during the first few hours or days. The most important cause is an unrecognized unstable spine; very rarely there is a traumatic intervertebral disc protrusion. Whether delayed deterioration is due to cord oedema or local ischaemia is uncertain, but such deterioration is often reversible.

Reduction of the fracture is necessary when there is persisting deformity at the site of injury. It is usually achieved by continuous skull traction to which graded increases in weight are added until there is reduction. During this, frequent radiological control is necessary and it is important to avoid over-distraction, since this may produce ischaemia in the cord. Skull calipers are the safest way of maintaining traction, and are easily put in under local anaesthesia; the patient need not be moved from the bed or trolley for this minor procedure. The Gardner–Wells tongs, which penetrate the outer table of the skull, are placed symmetrically 4 cm above the external auditory meati. About 2 kg traction is enough to keep the neck in a safe, neutral position, but much greater weights may be needed to reduce difficult fracture-dislocation. Using a variety of pulley holders the patient can assume almost any position in bed and nursing procedures are both easier and safer once calipers are in position. Muscle spasm rapidly subsides and the patient is soon much more comfortable. Occasionally manipulation under general anaesthesia will achieve reduction when traction has failed. Failure of the reduction is generally due to over-riding and locking of the facet joints and reduction can then only be achieved by open operation, usually followed by fixation and fusion.

Early stabilization by fixation reduces the incidence of complications from bed rest, such as pressure sores, pneumonia and thrombophlebitis, the patient has less pain and can participate in rehabilitation and mobilization at an earlier stage, thus reducing hospital time and costs. Depending on the type of instability, fixation can be achieved using either an external orthosis such as a halo device or by internal means. The latter can be achieved in a variety of ways according to the type of injury. These include metal wire, clamps, pedicle screws or anterior vertebral plates, in combination with bone grafting.

Thoracolumbar fracture-dislocations are usually relatively stable compared with cervical injuries, and, if the patient is moved with care, and nursed in slight hyperextension with a pillow in the small of the back, most remain reduced. When there is instability, and particularly if the lesion is incomplete and could therefore be made worse, decompression of the spinal canal followed by internal fixation and bone grafting to restore the normal thoracolumbar curve is advised. Several effective methods are available for anterior, lateral or posterior fixation.

Continued management of the paraplegic

General care
Active nursing of the paraplegic patient is the same whether the primary pathology is trauma, tumour or infection. It assumes particular importance after spinal injuries, because the problem presents itself suddenly in any hospital in the country where accidents are accepted. Failure to institute proper nursing care promptly can have disastrous effects; it can take months to heal sores or cure urinary tract infections which became established in the first weeks after injury. Yet no special skills are needed, only the conviction that active care is required, and that none of these complications need develop.

The skin
Pressure sores are quite simply the result of pressure on vulnerable areas of skin, where bone closely underlies it. The paraplegic patient has lost both the sensory urge and the motor power to shift position. But in addition to this, in the acute phase of spinal injury, the skin is exceptionally liable to pressure damage because of autonomic disturbance, and the patient needs to be turned every 2 hours, day and night. Special spinal beds that turn or are fitted with active mattresses preclude the need to nurse patients face-down. If these are unavailable, however, the patient must be turned regularly every 2 hours through lateral, supine and even prone positions.

The bladder
At first the bladder is without tone, and when it is full there is overflow incontinence. After a few weeks, if the lesion is above the conus, an automatic

(autonomic) bladder is established, because a reflex arc is left intact between the bladder and the isolated lower part of the spinal cord. Active voiding occurs in response to stimuli such as distension by a sufficient volume of urine, or by scratching the skin in the region of the genitalia. Some patients learn to use this reflex regularly before distension causes involuntary emptying of the bladder. However, unexpected stimuli are always liable to trigger this mechanism, and few patients can rely on keeping dry without wearing a urinal of some kind. Lesions involving the conus or roots leave a lower motor neuron bladder, atonic and needing to be emptied by external pressure on the abdomen. Often there is a combination of upper and lower motor neuron dysfunction, and these mixed bladders can have both disordered detrusor and sphincter function.

Urethral catheterization should be done immediately because it is now believed that even a brief period of distension beyond 800 ml may cause permanent detrusor damage. Multiple injuries are commonly present and catheterization makes hourly monitoring or output possible, which may be important. If infection is to be minimized then catheterization must be done with meticulous technique. Daily washouts of the bladder with 1:5000 chlorhexidene should be continued as long as a catheter remains in the bladder. The catheter is changed weekly, or sooner if it becomes blocked. If urethritis develops it may respond to local irrigation; a Foley catheter should be removed and a small Gibbon type passed twice a day until inflammation has settled.

Closed suprapubic drainage, using a small catheter introduced by a stab method, is good emergency treatment, especially if there is a perineal injury making it impossible to establish urethral drainage.

Open suprapubic drainage is now seldom employed. Even with suction the bladder is rarely completely emptied and it is impossible to prevent infection; because it is never distended the bladder may contract and it is then difficult to close the fistula and establish an automatic bladder.

The later management of the bladder cannot be discussed in detail. In principle it consists of maintaining adequate bladder drainage so as to prevent dilatation of the upper urinary tract, and of recognizing and treating infections. These are easily overlooked in a paraplegic patient who cannot complain of dysuria or frequency; the common signs are headache, pyrexia and an increase in spasticity and flexor spasms. If drainage is unsatisfactory, the risk of recurrent infection is higher; a residual urine of less than 50 ml should be the aim of treatment. Implanted electronic devices can be used in selected patients to trigger and to complete bladder emptying. These greatly reduce or eliminate urinary incontinence and infection.

The limbs

From the start all joints in the paralysed limbs should be put through their full range of movements daily. As tone returns and spasticity develops, physiotherapy becomes vital in preventing contractures. Carefully padded splints, tailored for the individual patient, may be required to prevent deformities developing. Flexor spasms, usually the most troublesome, are reduced in the prone position, and the patient should learn to sleep on his or her face; this will also tend to overcome the tendency to fixed hip flexion. Drugs may also help. Diazepam appears to have a general depressive effect on the reflex arc, and can give useful relief, although sometimes at the price of some dependence.

The drugs which reduce muscle spasm may act centrally (baclofen) or peripherally (Dantrium); for severe cases intrathecal microgram doses of baclofen may help. Attempts to deal with spasticity by cutting tendons, muscles or peripheral nerves are rarely successful, whilst intrathecal injections of phenol or alcohol are less selective and only suitable for occasional patients with complete spinal lesions, who cannot be made worse.

General condition

In the early weeks after injury patients frequently develop a negative nitrogen balance and become anaemic. If bed sores and urinary infections are allowed to develop they may aggravate these metabolic disorders, which in turn hinder the control of infection and the healing of sores. Due to lack of sympathetic tone following paraplegia, especially with cervical lesions, blood pressure commonly stabilizes at about 90/70 mmHg. There is no need to treat this either in the acute or later stages. Patients who have cervical cord damage lose their intercostal muscles for breathing and with lesions above the C5 segment diaphragmatic function may be lost. Early instruction and management by a physiotherapist are essential and measurement of forced vital capacity is a useful indicator, as is tidal volume. Tracheostomy may be required during the first few weeks.

Final rehabilitation

The paraplegic (except those with high cervical lesions) now has a reasonable expectation of leaving hospital within 6 months, and leading an independent life. This aim is most likely to be realized by rehabilitation in a special unit where there are no concessions to invalidism, and where the patient can be rigorously trained in the discipline necessary to avoid pressure sores and urinary infections – complications which remain threats even after the patient leaves hospital. A wheelchair life may call for special arrangements at home and at work, but with determination these adjustments can be made, provided the patient is willing and well-advised.

Further reading

Bloom H. J. G., Ellis H., Jennett W. B. (1955). The early diagnosis of spinal tumours. *Br. Med. J.*; **1,**: 10–16.

Bracken M. B., Sheperd M. J., Collins W. F. *et al.* (1992). Methylprednisolone or naloxone treatment after acute spinal cord injury: one year follow-up data. *J. Neurosurg.*; **76,**: 23–31.

Ekong C. E. U., Schwartz M. L., Tator C. H. *et al.* (1981). Odontoid fracture: management with early mobilisation using the halo device. *Neurosurgery*; **9,**: 631–7.

Findlay G. F. G. (1984). Adverse effects of the management of malignant spinal cord compression. *J. Neurol. Neurosurg. Psychiatry*; **47,**: 761–8.

Guidetti B., Mercuri S., Vagnozzi R. (1981). Longterm results of the surgical treatment of 129 intramedullary spinal gliomas. *J. Neurosurg.*; **54,**: 323–30.

Hardcastle P., Bedbrook G., Curtis K. (1987). Longterm results of conservative and operative management in complete paraplegics with spinal cord injuries between T10 and L2 with respect to function. *Clin. Orthop. Rel. Res.*; **224,**: 88–96.

Johnston R. A. (1991). Surgery of the spine. *J. Neurol. Neurosurg. Psychiatry*; **53,**: 1021–3.

Johnston R. A., Hadley D. M. (1991). Tuberculous infection of the thoracic spine. In: Tarlov E. (ed.) *Neurosurgical Treatment of Disorders of the Thoracic Spine*. Parkridge, Ill: American Association of Neurological Surgery.

McCormick P. C., Torres R., Post K. D. *et al.* (1990). Intramedullary ependymoma of the spinal cord. *J. Neurosurg.*; **72,:** 523–32.

Maurice-Williams R. S., Richardson P. L. (1988). Spinal cord decompression: delay in the diagnosis and referral of a common neurosurgical emergency. *Br. J. Neurosurg.*; **2,:** 55–60.

Meyer P. R. (ed.) (1989). *Surgery of Spinal Trauma.* Edinburgh: Churchill Livingstone.

Meyer P. R., Cybulski G. R., Rusin J. J. *et al.* (1991). Spinal cord injury. *Neurol. Clin.*; **9,:** 625–61.

Rosenblum B., Oldfield E. H., Dappman J. L. *et al.* (1987). Spinal arteriovenous malformations: a comparison of dural arteriovenous fistulas and intradural arteriovenous malformations in 81 patients. *J. Neurosurg.*; **67,:** 795–802.

Shephard R.H. (1992). Spinal arteriovenous malformations and subarachnoid haemorrhage. *Br. J. Neurosurg.*; **6,:** 5–12.

Siegal T., Siegal T. (1985). Surgical decompression of anterior and posterior malignant epidural tumours compressing the spinal cord: a prospective study. *Neurosurgery*; **17,:** 424–32.

Sundaresan N., Digiacinto G. V., Hughes J.E.O. *et al.* (1991). Treatment of neoplastic cord compression: results of a prospective study. *Neurosurgery*; **29,:** 645–50.

Chapter 13

Prolapsed intervertebral disc

Lumbar spine

Cervical spine

Acute disc prolapse
Cervical spondylosis
Cervical spondolytic radiculopathy
Cervical myelopathy

Thoracic spine

Degeneration and trauma combine to produce disc lesions; the two factors operate in varying proportions in different parts of the spine, and from one individual to another. Degeneration is a normal ageing process; the large fluid nucleus pulposus of childhood undergoes progressive dehydration and shrinkage throughout life. Trauma, in the form of a single major incident or of repeated minor stresses (sometimes occupational), may directly precipitate prolapse or it may accentuate degenerative changes which predispose to prolapse in the future.

The highly mobile cervical spine is more prone to degenerative changes, and most disc protrusions in this region occur at or past middle age. In the lumbar region trauma is more often predominant, and young persons in physically stressful occupations, such as miners or nurses, are common sufferers. A disc protrusion may be lateral (Fig. 13.1a) compressing a single nerve root, or central (Fig. 13.1b), causing pressure on the spinal cord or, in the lumbar region, the cauda equina.

Lumbar spine

Pathogenesis
Some 90–95% of prolapsed lumbar intervertebral discs occur at the L4/5 or L5/S1 levels. Only rarely do discs at two levels prolapse at the same time. Most lesions are lateral and affect either the L5 or S1 nerve root; but the few central protrusions that occur are important because they can produce paraplegia with sphincter involvement.

Often the onset is undramatic, sometimes following unaccustomed activity

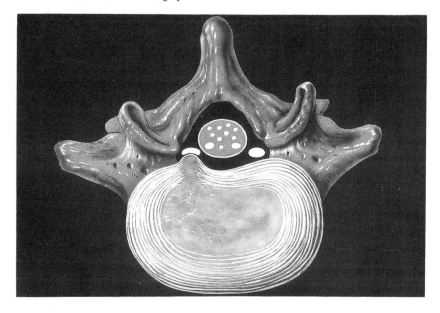

(a)

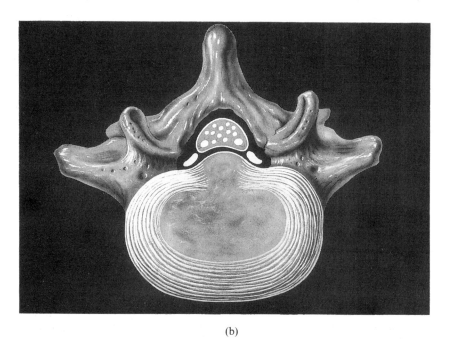

(b)

(a) Lateral lesions affect one, at most, two roots causing unilateral symptoms. (b) Central lesions may compress emerging roots (extradurally) on both sides, but can also affect all the roots of the cauda equina (intradurally) at that level.

Fig. 13.1   Lumbar disc prolapse.

such as digging the garden or playing games after a long interval. No immediate ill effect is felt, but the patient wakes next morning with severe backache and may be unable to get out of bed. After several days in bed the back pain usually subsides; further attacks follow similar strains, perhaps with years of freedom between episodes. Usually after one or more incidents of backache alone the pain begins to spread into the buttock and down the leg, but this can occur in the first attack.

A single sudden injury or strain is the obvious cause in some cases. As the incident occurs – often lifting a heavy weight – the patient is struck by severe pain in the back with or without leg pain. He or she may be unable to get up off the ground or be able only to hobble away bent double. A few cases develop during pregnancy, and may recur only in subsequent pregnancies; physiological laxity of ligaments may be a factor in these cases, and the protrusions are often central rather than lateral.

Some patients are unable to recall any unusual strain before their first attack, which may have been dismissed as muscle or ligamentous strain. Even patients who do claim some obvious cause for their condition may remember attacks of back pain years before, and it is likely that these were due to the early stages of their disc disease.

For so common a disease there is surprising ignorance of the aetiology, but clearly trauma is seldom the sole factor, even in the lumbar region. Operative findings are often difficult to relate to clinical manifestations; the removal of a small protrusion may afford dramatic relief from severe symptoms, whilst operation during an acute episode of pain may reveal a totally sequestrated fragment of disc so adherent to its surroundings that it must have been extruded months previously. Radiculitis is probably an important factor, and the dura around the nerve root is sometimes seen to be inflamed at operation during an acute attack. Resolution of symptoms with conservative treatment may be due to subsidence of this inflammation, or to the root changing position in relation to the disc, rather than to the protrusion reducing itself.

Clinical syndromes
Two components can be recognized in most instances – the spinal and the radicular – but either may occur alone.

Spinal pain probably results from the torn annulus fibrosus in the acute stage, but when the condition becomes chronic, secondary factors such as arthritis of the interarticular joints may contribute. The mechanics of the spine are disturbed, giving rise to characteristic signs – loss of lumbar lordosis (rare in any other condition), scoliosis and acute spasm of the erector spinae. This may result in a completely 'frozen' spine, attempts at toe-touching produce movement only at the hip joint whilst the lumbar spine remains rigid.

Radicular pain from the lower two disc spaces may spread only as far as the buttock but usually radiates to the calf and ankle. The rare upper disc protrusions cause anterior crural pain, affecting the front of the thigh. Root pain is aggravated by movement, by strains such as coughing and sneezing which increase intrathecal pressure, and by straight-leg raising. The sciatic nerve may be tender to palpation in the buttock. Paraesthesiae may affect dermatomes around the foot, and are often precipitated by the same factors as aggravate the pain.

Objective evidence of root compression may be found, but even with severe leg pain there may be no neurological signs. Sensory loss is usually limited to diminished appreciation of pin-prick in part of the L5 or S1 dermatome, according to the root affected (Fig. 12.2b). Weakness of the extensor hallucis

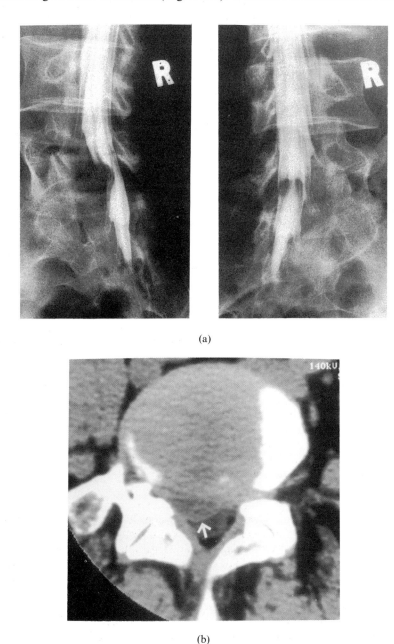

(a)

(b)

Fig. 13.2 Lumbar disc lesion (a) Lumbar radiculogram – filling defect opposite disc space. (b) Axial CT scan across the L5/S1 disc space showing lateral disc protrusion (arrow).

longus and wasting of extensor digitorum brevis (which normally forms a bulge on the dorsum of the foot) are frequent with L5 root lesions; occasionally severe footdrop develops and persists after the pain has subsided. Reduction or complete absence of the ankle jerk usually indicates compression of S1 root. However, neither this nor the distribution of motor and sensory signs and symptoms reliably localizes the level of the protrusion; there are variations in the distribution of the roots forming the lumbosacral plexus, whilst a disc at the upper level (L4/5) can compress both the lower roots at the same time (Fig. 13.1a); moreover both discs may be prolapsed.

With a central protrusion both ankle jerks may be absent and there may be perineal numbness. Sometimes urinary retention or bilateral footdrop, or both, come on insidiously without a great deal of pain. Occasionally a patient wakes up after manipulation under anaesthesia to find the pain gone but the legs weak. Clinical evidence of bilateral root or bladder involvement or perineal numbness requires immediate investigation; if a central disc is revealed, urgent operation should be recommended.

Investigation

Plain X-rays may show narrowing of the disc space but this only indicates degeneration within the disc substance and does not necessarily correlate with prolapse of the disc. Sometimes X-rays shows evidence of spinal tumour, ankylosing spondylitis or vertebral tuberculosis, but these are relatively rare.

Lumbar puncture for purposes of radiculography will usually be above the lesion but may show increased protein content as a result either of a central protrusion or of a block due to other causes, in particular tumour.

Contrast radiculography outlines the spinal canal from the sacrum up to the lumbar conus at T12/L1, using non-ionic water soluble medium. The AP and lateral diameter of the spinal canal can be assessed and any compromise by a bulging annulus fibrosis or prolapsed disc fragment is seen (Fig. 13.2a). The individual nerve roots are readily identified running down and laterally below their respective vertebral pedicles (i.e. L5 root runs below the pedicle of L5). If the root is compressed by a disc prolapse it will not fill out with contrast.

CT scanning gives the surgeon even more information, without requiring the need for intrathecal contrast. The axial view of the spinal canal shows the abnormal disc in relation to the nerve root (Fig. 13.2b). This has now largely replaced radiculography where it is available. MRI is also valuable but of much more restricted availability.

Conservative treatment

The majority of episodes diagnosed as disc protrusions settle in time without operative treatment. Complete bed rest, lying flat with only one pillow, accelerates resolution as well as affording immediate relief of pain in most cases. A firm mattress is better than a soft one, and this may be achieved with fracture boards or by putting the mattress on the floor. An unyielding mattress limits spinal flexion, which is painful, and it is much easier to turn over on a flat surface than in a hollow. A severe attack requires at least a fortnight strictly in bed, followed by gradual mobilization. Continuous pelvic traction may give relief from acute pain when bed rest alone has proved ineffective. Analgesia and occasionally a mild sedative such as Valium to relax muscle tone may also help. When pain recurs as soon as the patient gets up, some continuing help may be given by a three-point lumbar support (Neofract or moulded plastic lumbar jacket). This has the advantage that as improvement sets in it can be discarded for gradually increasing periods, yet is still available should a recurrence develop. These devices do not so much support the spine as prevent excessive movement which might aggravate the root lesion.

Manipulation is practised much more widely than many doctors imagine. Numerous patients find someone willing to give them local treatment of this kind when they feel they are receiving insufficient sympathy or attention from their ordinary medical attendants. Chronic recurring disc pain is very demoralizing, and it is small comfort to be assured that it is a common condition, that it will settle in time, and that is is unlikely to result in serious disability. Many patients report dramatic cures from manipulation and in skilled hands and with proper precautions it has a limited place in treatment. Whether its effects have an organic basis, or whether the benefits result from a powerful placebo effect, remains unknown.

When manipulations have to be repeated they tend to be of less value each time. It is unlikely that a prolapsed disc is ever restored to its rightful place; more likely a loose fragment is slipped away from the root or secondary non-articular adhesions are broken down. Excessive flexion, especially under anaesthesia, is dangerous, and no manipulation should be considered if a central lesion is suspected; patients have been made paraplegic by manipulation in these circumstances.

Operation
Surgery is necessary only when conservative measures fail, and, except when there is cauda equina compression, should not be offered to a patient who has not given bed rest a serious trial. Many patients diagnosed as having a disc lesion enjoy long remissions or suffer only one attack. The indications for surgery are:

1. Recurrent episodes of pain, especially when root pain predominates over backache.
2. An unrelieved acute attack of root pain, even when it is the first episode. A few patients, most of whom prove to have extruded a massive fragment of disc, continue to experience excruciating pain even in bed and on traction; no one should under-estimate the severity of this pain, which can reduce the toughest stoic to tears. In such instances early operation is indicated even if there are no neurological signs.
3. Progressive CNS involvement, either extending sensory loss or rapidly worsening paralysis of the dorsiflexors. The place of surgery is disputed when the patient presents with an established footdrop of some weeks duration but is quite free of pain. Nerve conduction tests are of value, in that if the root is shown to be completely 'dead', surgery is unlikely to restore any function. Otherwise surgical and conservative management tend to produce equally good results in terms of return of dorsiflexion.
4. Suspected central protrusion, as indicated by bilateral root pain or bilateral root signs, even though limited to absent ankle jerks or sensory loss. Once paraplegia is established recovery is extremely slow and usually incomplete, and operation in these cases should be urged whether or not pain is severe.

The best surgical results are in patients who present with a good clinical history of root pain, clinical evidence of nerve root compression, and a confirmatory CT or radiculogram. In many the decision is not clear-cut and experience proves an asset in patient selection for surgery.

Technique

Neurosurgeons usually perform this operation in the prone position, in which case the hips should be supported so that the abdomen is free of the table; this greatly reduces congestion in the extradural veins and makes for an easier exposure. Alternatively the lateral position may be used, or the patient may crouch on the table over bent knees and hips with the object of opening up the interlaminar spaces.

Although loosely referred to as laminectomy, such a complete exposure is usually reserved for large central protrusions. The optimal surgical procedure is microdiscectomy. The incision is 4 cm long and made 1 cm lateral to the midline at the affected level, as confirmed by X-ray on the operating table. The actual procedure is very similar to that when a microscope is not used, but soft tissue damage is less, visualization of important structures clearer, and post-operative pain reduced. For the usual lateral lesions the muscles need to be stripped from the spinous processes on the affected side only. The margins of the laminae above and below the space are nibbled away, and the ligamentum flavum removed to expose the root and the disc beyond it. The annulus fibrosus is usually intact over the disc, and must be incised before disc material can be removed, but sometimes it has already ruptured and disc fragments are found free in the spinal canal; they may then migrate some distance from the level of the disc from which they sequestrated.

It is not enough to remove only the sequestrated fragment because more may prolapse later; the disc space should be gently emptied as far as possible, using a curette, but the end-plates must be left intact in order to reduce the risk of postoperative discitis. Disc material is lifted out using 2–3 mm disc rongeurs Great care is taken not to penetrate the anterior annulus, with the risk of damage to the major blood vessels in front of the vertebrae.

Free movement in bed may be permitted immediately after operation, and the patient can get up in 24 hours if comfortable in bed. Fairly rapid mobilization under the supervision of a physiotherapist is valuable. With microdiscectomy, patients may be fit for discharge within 48 hours, although the average stay is 4–5 days. It is unwise to send a patient home until his or her confidence is fully restored, and this takes longer in some patients than in others. Normal activities should be resumed gradually; an individual might return to office work within a month, but heavy work or strenuous games should not be considered until 2 or 3 months after operation. After this no restriction is necessary, and there is no reason for wearing any form of support.

Complications

There is a 2.5% risk of wound infection, and a 1% risk of root damage causing footdrop or weak plantar flexion. Bacterial infection of the disc space is reported in about 1%, but should be less if the end-plates are left intact. If it develops it is treated by bed rest and antibiotics.

Results

With judicious selection there is a 90–95% chance of good relief of root pain but only a 60% chance of permanent relief of spinal pain. In 5% disc prolapse recurs at the same level. As soon as the patient recovers from the anaesthetic, he or she may remark that his or her leg or back feels free again and that the pain has gone. However, the continuation or the reappearance of root pain during the first fortnight after operation is common and is no reason for anxiety. It is probably due to inflammatory changes in the compressed root which may have been temporarily aggravated by retraction at operation. Neurological signs recover variably, and some degree of sensory loss and a depressed ankle jerk may persist indefinitely. Root pain is more reliably relieved than backache and the patients who rate the success of operation as only 'fair' mostly suffer from continuing backache or stiffness; a few patients claim to be no better after operation and continue to suffer from episodic root pain but no patient should be worse. Sometimes persisting symptoms are due to a migrated fragment missed at operation or to a second protrusion not discovered at operation. Apart from these obvious causes for failure, results tend to be less favourable in patients with heavy manual occupations and when leg pain has persisted for more than a year before operation. Results are less good for juvenile (<16 years) disc disease. Patients with occupations or leisure activities which inevitably put strain on the back should be strongly advised to seek an alternative job or sport, even though pain has satisfactorily subsided either with conservative measures or after operation.

After major cauda equina compression motor recovery continues slowly over 18 months or more; control of the bladder is regained only slowly and often incompletely. Perineal sensory loss may persist and interfere with sexual function in the female.

Recurrence

Reappearance of pain, or of a complete disc syndrome, occurs in up to 10% of patients after successful operation, sometimes after several years of complete freedom from symptoms. The usual explanations are:

1.   Recurrent protrusion at the operated site.
2.   Protrusion of a previously unaffected disc.
3.   Adhesions between the root and the operated disc.
4.   Arachnoiditis related to contrast medium – now uncommon with water-soluble materials.

Cervical spine

Disc disease in the cervical region seldom takes the form of the protrusion of a single nucleus pulposus. Degenerative changes affecting several discs are more usual, giving rise to the radiological appearance of cervical spondylosis – although this may be accompanied by no signs or symptoms whatever.

Acute disc prolapse

This can occur at any age, and in a spine showing no radiological evidence of spondylosis, although it may be superimposed on this degenerative condition. Often a single incident of trauma is remembered, which was followed at first by only neck stiffness but later by signs of CNS disorder. Acute prolapse may be central or lateral. Central protrusions cause myelopathy, weakness and spasticity of the legs, sometimes associated with root symptoms and signs in the upper limbs. A lateral protrusion causes acute root pain in one arm and muscle wasting may develop in the appropriate innervations. Sometimes such a relatively acute syndrome may occur days or weeks after an episode of trauma; symptoms may steadily progress, and therefore simulate a spinal tumour. CT or MRI is the best way of confirming the pathological cause and the exact position in relation to the cord and roots (Figs 13.3 and 13.4). If they are not available a myelogram will show a filling defect or even a complete block.

For acute central disc protrusion early surgical decompression is recommended. This requires an anterior approach, using a microsurgical procedure with or without fusion. Acute lateral disc lesions may settle with conservative treatment (collar and analgesics). If symptoms persist or progress then surgical excision may be through a posterior foraminotomy or by anterior access; occasionally the lateral approach of Verbiest is used.

During the induction of anaesthesia and positioning on the table the head should be handled with great care, preferably with a collar in position. After operation most recommend the use of a soft collar for a month or so.

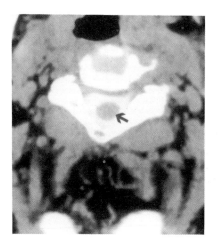

(a)

Fig. 13.3 Axial CT of the cervical spine with intrathecal contrast. (a) Scan across the C3/4 disc space, showing a spinal canal of normal diameter, with the spinal cord outlined by CSF contrast medium (arrow).

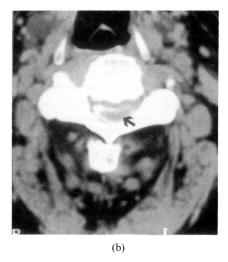

(b)

Fig. 13.3 (*cont*) (b) Scan in the same patient across the C4/5 disc space, showing marked canal narrowing and cord compression (arrow) by osteophytes.

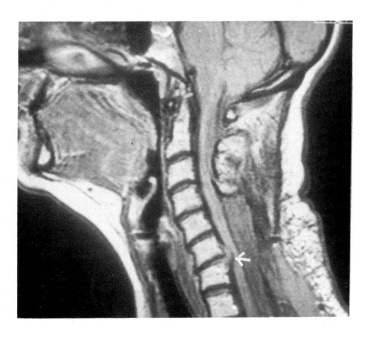

Fig. 13.4   Proton density sagittal MRI – showing soft disc protusion at C6/7 (arrow).

Cervical spondylosis

This results from an ageing process. Radiological changes are found in 75% of patients over 50 years of age who have no spontaneous complaints referable to the neck. Because these changes appear earlier in men than in women they are presumed to be related in part to occupational trauma, but seldom is any direct association demonstrated. However, trauma may clearly be the factor precipitating symptoms in a patient afflicted with spondylosis.

Pathology

The primary lesion is probably collapse of the disc with annular protrusion around its whole circumference. As ligaments are pulled away from their attachment to the margins of the vertebral bodies, reactive osteophytosis develops, and the ligaments themselves thicken. Together with the annular protrusion, osteophytes and ligaments reduce the anteroposterior diameter of the spinal canal. Osteoarthritic changes of the neurocentral joints, which abut on the foramina from C3 to C7, lead to further bony proliferation, which encroaches on the intervertebral foramina already narrowed by disc protrusion and osteophytes. The mobility of the spine itself is also impaired, restricted where disc changes are advanced and excessive at unaffected levels above and below.

Many factors contribute to the production of symptoms and signs when these do appear. The spinal cord, lying tethered in a narrowed spinal canal, is liable to suffer additional compression during even normal neck movements. In extension, for example, the ligamenta flava wrinkle and can form a posterior compressing agent. When extremes of movement are reached the cord is in great jeopardy, and sudden symptoms may follow excessive flexion or extension due to accidental trauma or to seemingly uneventful endoscopy under anaesthesia.

Radiological signs

1. *Narrowing of the disc space*, affects one space only in 40%, two spaces in 40%, and more than two in the rest. In rather more than a third, C5/6 is affected, and in rather less than a third, C6/7 or C4/5; less often, C3/4 is involved and C7/T1 only rarely.
2. *Change in the normal curve*, commonly a loss of the natural lordosis, may be restricted to two adjacent vertebrae, and limited mobility between them is best demonstrated by comparing films taken in flexion and extension.
3. *Osteophytes* are more obvious anteriorly but posterior overgrowth is more important; foraminal narrowing is seen only in oblique views.
4. *Myelographic indentations* of the anterior dura do not always conform to the levels of maximum disc collapse and osteophytosis. Posterior indentations due to ligamenta flava are seen when films are taken in extension. A complete block is unusual, but when it occurs may indicate acute disc prolapse.
5. *A CT scan* performed within a few hours of the myelogram may more accurately delineate the site and extent of the compression (Fig. 13.3). Similar changes can also be seen on sagittal MRI scans (Fig. 13.4).

Clinical syndromes

Advanced radiological changes can occur without any clinical accompaniments; but a number of asymptomatic patients, in whom spondylosis is a chance finding, prove on careful examination to have evidence of mild cord compression (spasticity, increased reflexes or sensory changes). When there are florid symptoms and signs they do not always correspond to the level of maximum radiological change. Even when both radicular and cord involvement occur, one or other is usually predominant. In consequence two main syndromes, cervical radiculopathy and cervical myelopathy, are recognized.

Cervical spondolytic radiculopathy

Pain is the principal complaint – dull and aching in the neck and shoulder with shooting pain down the arm to the elbow or wrist. Although only one root is affected, the pain spreads beyond the dermatome distribution, probably because it develops also within muscles supplied by that root. Pain may also arise from the disc itself, causing referred pain in the neck, trapezius region and scapular region.

Muscle spasm and tenderness may give rise to secondary spread of pain, especially to the occipital region, where it is complained of as headache.

Paraesthesiae are frequently experienced in the arm and the tip of the thumb (C6 root from C5/6 lesion) or the middle finger (C7 from C6/7 lesion). Sensory loss, weakness, wasting and reflex changes are usually slight.

These complaints may appear relatively suddenly, sometimes precipitated by trauma, or they can develop insidiously; repeated attacks of acute pain occur in some patients. Occasionally the pain is related to movement and position. This condition must be distinguished from postviral brachial neuritis, thoracic outlet compression of the brachial plexus and peripheral entrapment of the median or ulnar nerves. The latter is sometimes seen in conjunction with spondylosis, the double-crush syndrome.

Treatment of cervical spondolytic radiculopathy

Providing rest for the affected part is the basis of all methods. Aggravating movements must be avoided, whatever these are in the individual case. The arm may be supported from the unaffected shoulder with a sling, and this together with analgesics, and local heat and short-wave diathermy may be sufficient to give relief. Active physiotherapy is contraindicated, apart from shoulder girdle strengthening exercises. Non-steroidal anti-inflammatory medication may be helpful.

A collar provides more effective immobilization, the best being a Philadelphia-style collar with occipital and mental support. Simple ring collars are acceptable, but soft collars are a waste of time. To be effective the collar must be worn properly and consistently. When improvement occurs the collar can be discontinued gradually. Patients can often be induced to return to work whilst still wearing a collar, and this is advantageous because immobilization should be continued for 3 or 4 weeks after pain has subsided; relapse often follows premature return to normal free movement.

Skull traction, using Gardner–Wells cervical traction calipers and 2–2.5 kg weight, is reserved for those who fail to respond to simpler methods. Manual traction in various directions is first tried until the right one is found. Traction often relieves acute pain rapidly, and can be replaced by a collar after 2 or 3 weeks. Manipulation may be of value in skilled hands, and always provided there is no evidence of cord compression.

Surgical decompression by posterior foraminotomy or by anterior cervical decompression, with or without fusion, are effective means of relieving persistent pain from this condition. In properly selected patients there is a greater than 80 % likelihood of benefit by either method.

Cervical spondolytic myelopathy

Insidious development of spasticity in the legs is the most frequent mode of onset, noticed first either as slowness or clumsiness in walking. Weakness is less striking than increased tone and exaggerated deep reflexes. Rather more than two-thirds have some sensory loss, but unless the myelopathy is advanced, there is rarely a definite sensory level, and then it is often upper thoracic rather than cervical; in the rest the deficit is radicular in pattern or, occasionally, a suspended area of loss over the thorax such as accompanies syringomyelia is evident. Many complain of neck pain and stiffness, and have clumsy hands and paraesthesiae with a C3/4 osteophyte.

Sudden aggravation of cervical myelopathy, or even the abrupt appearance of spinal cord symptoms for the first time, may follow trauma. Hyperextension injuries insufficient to cause fracture or dislocation are particularly liable to precipitate a transverse spinal lesion in a patient with cervical spondylosis, even when this has hitherto been asymptomatic. Tripping and falling on the head (with resulting frontal abrasions) is a common mechanism, but another is hyperextension during surgical procedures such as tonsillectomy, bronchoscopy or oesophagoscopy; even the manipulations required to pass an endotracheal tube by an anaesthetist can jeopardize the cord, especially when all protective muscle spasm has been abolished by relaxant drugs. The resulting central cord syndrome causes lower motor neuron lesions in the hands and spasticity in the legs. Over a course of 18 months some 50 % improve.

Before accepting spinal cord symptoms as due to spondylosis, it is vital to exclude other treatable conditions such as spinal cord tumour, subacute combined degeneration and neurosyphilis; also to distinguish primary degenerations such as motor neurone disease and multiple sclerosis, which have a less favourable prognosis than spondylotic myelopathy and are not helped by operation. Considering the frequency with which radiological changes occur there is a danger of attributing to spondylosis any cervical cord disorder first appearing in middle age.

Treatment of myelopathy

The natural history is of unpredictable progression, usually slow. Once symptoms appear, surgical decompression should be considered, either by an anterior or posterior route. The anterior approach consists of the removal of the relevant disc along with the osteophytic bar. Decompression must be extended laterally to the proximal root canals. A peg of allograft bone or lyophilized radiation-sterilized xenograft bone replaces a core of tissue of the same size, consisting of parts of the opposing vertebral bodies and the intervening degenerated disc (Cloward's operation). This may be done at two or three levels if necessary. Occasionally additional anterior fixation is required with a metal plate. With careful selection, 70–80 % of patients should improve.

Laminectomy is reserved for multiple-level involvement or when a thickened ligamentum flavum causes posterior cord compression. The results are less satisfactory, usually because such patients have a more advanced myelopathy.

Thoracic spine

Less than 1 % of disc lesions are thoracic, and all these occur below the fifth thoracic vertebra. Most patients are between 40 and 50 years old, and a number recall an injury before the onset of symptoms. Radicular pain is abdominal in distribution and is readily mistaken for visceral disease. Spinal cord compression can develop without any pain at all, and may then resemble primary degenerative disease of the cord. Paraplegia may develop rapidly over a few days or increase gradually over many months, or even years. An anterior lesion is produced, akin to anterior spinal artery thrombosis, with spastic weakness of the legs and spinothalamic rather than posterior column sensory loss.

Radiological evidence of degeneration in the thoracic spine takes the form of calcification in the disc spaces, not narrowing or osteophytic lipping. Calcified discs are an occasional incidental finding in the middle-aged, and when a clinical disc syndrome does develop, this may not correspond to one of the calcified interspaces. Myelography may demonstrate a filling defect but CT or MRI are better methods of investigation.

Operation is difficult because the thoracic spinal canal is naturally narrow and largely filled by the spinal cord. The disc lesion is central and anterior to the cord, which is even less tolerant to retraction when already stretched over a hump than in the cervical region. Posterior laminectomy is therefore always avoided in view of the extremely high risk of producing permanent cord damage. A careful approach from the side is necessary and the disc is removed either by a transthoracic anterolateral approach or by a costotransversectomy.

Further reading

Benjamin V. (1983). Diagnosis and management of thoracic disc disease. *Clin. Neurosurg.*; **30**: 577–605.

Caspar W., Campbell B., Barbier D.D. *et al.* (1991). The Caspar microsurgical discectomy and comparison with conventional standard lumbar disc procedure. *Neurosurgery*; **28**: 78–87.

Ciric I., Mikhael M.A., Tarkington J.A. *et al.* (1980). The lateral recess syndrome. *J. Neurosurg.*; **53**: 433–43.

Cloward R. (1958). The anterior approach for the removal of ruptured cervical discs. *J. Neurosurg.*; **15**: 602–17.

Epstein J.A., Lavine L.S. (1964). Herniated lumbar intervertebral discs in teenage children. *J. Neurosurg.*; **21**: 1070–5.

Jacobson I. (1992). Lumbar spinal stenosis. In: Teasdale G.M., Miller J.D. (eds.) *Current Neurosurgery*. Edinburgh: Churchill Livingstone.

Jeffreys R.V. (1986). The surgical treatment of cervical myelopathy due to spondylosis and disc degeneration. *J. Neurol. Neurosurg. Psychiatry.*; **49**: 353–61.

Jennett W.B. (1958). A study of 25 cases of compression of the cauda equina by prolapsed intervertebral discs. *J. Neurol. Neurosurg. Psychiatry.*; **19**: 109–16.

Lunsford L.D., Bissonette D.J., Jannetta P.J. *et al.* (1980). Anterior surgery for cervical disc disease. Part I: treatment of lateral cervical disc herniation in 253 cases. *J. Neurosurg.*; **53:** 1–11.

Lunsford L.D., Bissonette D.J., Zorub D.S. (1980). Anterior surgery for cervical disc disease. Part 2: treatment of cervical spondylotic myelopathy in 32 cases. *J. Neurosurg.*; **53:** 12–19.

O'Laoire S.A., Crockard H.A., Thomas D.G. (1981). Prognosis of sphincter recovery after operation for cauda equina compression owing to lumbar disc prolapse. *Br. Med. J.*; **282:** 1852–4.

Onik G., Maroon J., Davis G.W. (1989). Automated percutaneous discectomy at the L5–S1 level. *Clin. Orthop. Rel. Res.*; **238:** 71–6.

Pappas C.T.E., Harrington T., Sonntag V.K.H. (1992). Outcome analysis in 654 surgically treated lumbar disc herniations. *Neurosurgery*; **30:** 862–6.

Pearce J., Moll M.H. (1967). Conservative treatment and natural history of acute lumbar disc lesions. *J. Neurol. Neurosurg. Psychiatry*; **30:** 13–17.

Russell T. (1989). Thoracic intervertebral disc protrusion: experience of 67 cases and review of the literature. *Br. J. Neurosurg.*; **3:** 153–60.

Shaw M.D.M., Russell J.A., Grossart K.W. (1978). The changing pattern of spinal arachnoiditis. *J. Neurol. Neurosurg. Psychiatry*; **41:** 97–107.

Shields C.B., Reiss S.J., Garveston H.D. (1987). Chemonucleolysis with chymopapain: results in 150 patients. *J. Neurosurg.*; **67:** 187–91.

Waddell G., Kummel E.G., Lotto W.N. *et al.* (1979). Failed lumbar disc surgery and repeat surgery following industrial injuries. *J. Bone Joint Surg.*; **61-A:** 201–7.

Weinstein P.R. (1983). Diagnosis and management of lumbar spinal stenosis. *Neurosurgery*; **30:** 677–97.

Part V:

Congenital Conditions

Chapter 14

Hydrocephalus and other cranial abnormalities

Infantile hydrocephalus

Juvenile and adult hydrocephalus

Aqueduct stenosis (iter stricture)
Normal-pressure hydrocephalus

Abnormalities of the skull

Craniostenosis
Cranium bifidum
Hypertelorism

Infantile hydrocephalus

Pathology
Obstructive (non-communicating) hydrocephalus is due to a block within the
ventricular system which prevents the escape of CSF into the subarachnoid
space. The block is normally at one of the narrows: foramen of Monro,
aqueduct of Sylvius or the foramina of exit from the fourth ventricle
(Fig. 2.3).

In communicating hydrocephalus the ventricles and the subarachnoid space
are in communication; the cause is still most often an obstruction but placed
more distally, around the basal cisterns or at the arachnoid villi. Although
CSF can escape into the cisterna magna and the lumbar theca it may fail to
reach, or to be absorbed through, the arachnoid villi which lie over the surface
of the cerebral hemispheres in the supratentorial compartment.

Very occasionally it may develop due to obstruction in the superior longitudinal sinus (causing reduced absorption of CSF). Rarely cases of communicating hydrocephalus are due to overproduction of CSF, such as when there
is a papilloma of the choroid plexus.

Communicating and non-communicating forms of hydrocephalus are
about equally common in infancy; sometimes secondary block develops,
converting one form into the other. It is seldom easy, even at postmortem
examination, to determine with certainty the primary cause of hydrocephalus.
The commonest factors appear to be birth trauma and meningitis, each of

which excites a meningeal reaction with subsequent adhesions at several sites. The commonest site is the cisterna ambiens, the narrow space between the midbrain and the tentorial edge (Fig. 2.4); the arachnoid villi related to the superior longitudinal sinus may also be involved in adhesions. Premature babies who have had intraventricular bleeding are now another frequent group with hydrocephalus. Congenital malformations are found in about a quarter, most commonly a narrowed aqueduct, atresia of the exit foramina of the fourth ventricle, or an Arnold–Chiari malformation. This last is almost always found when hydrocephalus is associated with spina bifida (p. 293).

Occasional cases of infantile hydrocephalus are due to tumour. In almost a quarter no obvious cause can be found, but as both birth trauma and neonatal infections are readily overlooked it is quite likely that these account for most of the remaining cases.

Clinical

In the first 6 months of life raised pressure produces an enlarging head and bulging fontanelle rather than headaches and papilloedema. The parents may have noticed the big head since birth, or it may only have been obvious recently. The head circumference can be compared with a chart showing the normal limits (Fig. 14.1). The rate of growth can be assessed by repeating the measurement in 2 or 3 weeks, if the circumference is not already very abnormal. Doubt may arise in families who tend to have big heads, but the top of the head is then usually rather flat, and the face is large in proportion to the skull vault rather then dwarfed by it as in hydrocephalus.

A bulging fontanelle is a more reliable sign of raised pressure if the head is not very big, but it must be felt while the child is quiet. Dehydration due to vomiting or poor feeding, not uncommon in hydrocephalus, may cause the fontanelle to feel soft in spite of expanding ventricles.

Less constant features are epilepsy of some kind, major convulsions being less common than minor twitchings, or sudden head sagging, or eye rolling; mental retardation evidenced by slowness in passing the normal milestones; blindness with pale optic discs; and spasticity of one or more limbs. Many of these signs are probably due to underlying brain damage (e.g. birth trauma or congenital malformation) rather than to the effects of the dilated ventricles.

Investigations

Plain X-rays may show separation of the sutures. If there is a blocked aqueduct the posterior fossa may be small because the cisterna magna has never developed. Craniovertebral or other bony anomalies may suggest the possibility of a malformation of the brain.

CT scanning confirms the diagnosis of hydrocephalus and, because it can be repeated, the progress of this condition can be followed. However, the accumulated radiation of very often repeated scans makes it important to remember the value of observing head circumference as a means of monitoring. Ultrasound is also of value in infants, indicating ventricular size. MRI gives much more information than CT about the underlying lesion.

Ventriculography, the injection of air into the ventricles, is much less informative and can cause complications, and is now seldom used.

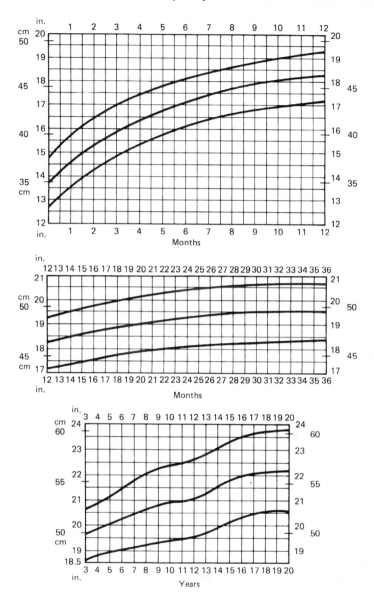

Fig. 14.1 Normal head circumference in infancy. The chart shows the upper limit for 90% of normal infants: average values are 1.25 cm less.

Natural history

The natural outcome of hydrocephalus is uncertain, but recent studies suggest that only 25 % of those diagnosed within the first 3 months of life will attain adult life. Two-thirds of the deaths are in the first 18 months, and more than half are ascribed to hydrocephalus itself without an obvious complication. Meningitis and chest infection are frequently recognized as the cause of death, but these infants readily succumb to intercurrent infection of all kinds.

If a child lives for 1 or 2 years, his or her chances of surviving without treatment rise to about 50 %, although he or she may remain handicapped. The survivors include those whose hydrocephalus has undergone natural arrest, which most often occurs between 9 months and 2 years of age. The head never gets smaller, but resumes growth when the normal head – body ratio is restored by development of the rest of the body.

About a third of cases which arrest naturally, or are controlled by treatment, have normal intelligence and a third have no physical abnormality; but less than a fifth are free of both mental and physical handicap. Physical disabilities include blindness and spasticity, and the latter may be severe enough to render a child bedridden. Severe mental and physical handicaps tend to be associated, but neither appears to be related to the duration of head enlargement, to the thickness of cortex, or to head size, except when this is extreme. Hydrocephalus with spina bifida rarely survives without disability. It seems likely that continuing disabilities are more often related to underlying brain damage than solely to ventricular dilatation.

Treatment

Progressive hydrocephalus demands treatment unless brain damage or malformation is obviously so severe as to make useful survival unlikely. Even though some cases do become arrested this may not occur before irreparable damage has been done. If the head is still actively enlarging, operation should not be postponed in the hope of spontaneous cure.

Three different types of operation are available, but some patients require more than one procedure before the hydrocephalus is controlled.

1. Shunts (drains)

CSF can be diverted to other body cavities from which it is absorbed. Shunts from the lumbar theca are effective only for communicating hydrocephalus and are now seldom used. But all types can be treated by ventricular shunts, which are also effective when there are multiple obstructions in the CSF pathways (Fig. 14.2). The simplest to perform is ventriculoperitoneal drainage. An occipital burr hole enables the tube to be placed in the lateral ventricle, and it is then led subcutaneously down the neck and trunk, making subcutaneous incisions where needed. If it works, this type of operation is probably the best. It is applicable to all types of hydrocephalus, and is simple and safe to perform and to adjust if necessary when blockage occurs. A flushing device can be placed in the burr hole to help keep the system clear and to allow access to the CSF. A valve is put in the system to prevent drainage being too rapid and altering with changing posture. Evolving technology is making it possible to replace valves set at high, medium or low pressure by ones that can have their pressure altered in situ, and a flow-sensitive device that will ensure steady flow has also been developed.

Ventriculoatrial shunt is an alternative, but because of its complication rate is seldom the first procedure of choice. A one-way valve is essential to prevent reflex of blood and it is placed subcutaneously behind the right ear, and connected by fine plastic tubing to the lateral ventricle above and, via the internal jugular vein, to the superior vena cava below; some surgeons prefer the tip to be in the atrium.

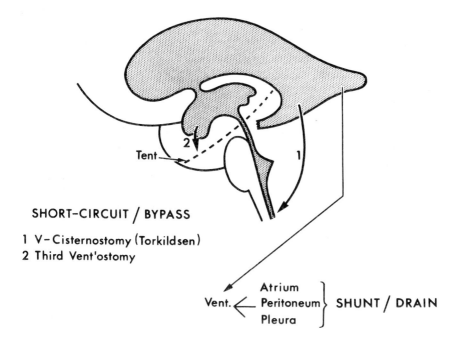

SHORT-CIRCUIT / BYPASS

1 V-Cisternostomy (Torkildsen)
2 Third Vent'ostomy

$$\begin{array}{l} \text{Atrium} \\ \text{Vent.} \longleftarrow \text{Peritoneum} \\ \text{Pleura} \end{array} \Big\} \text{ SHUNT / DRAIN}$$

Fig. 14.2 Operations for hydrocephalus.

Complications of shunting

Blockage of the tube is the commonest complication and revision operations are usually effective and can often be limited to the lower end of a ventriculo-peritoneal shunt. Occasionally valve resistance increases with time and a replacement is needed. With ventriculoatrial shunts jugular thrombosis may be the cause of malfunction, requiring transfer to the other side or replacement by ventriculoperitoneal shunt.

Infection is not uncommon, associated with colonization of the tube or valve by low-grade organisms; occasionally the skin over the valve insert ulcerates. Treatment depends on replacement of the system after a period of external drainage. With ventriculoatrial shunting infection carries the risk of chronic bacteraemia with anaemia and splenomegaly – another reason why this method is now seldom used.

Over-drainage can occur even with a valve and result in a slit ventricle picture on CT or MRI, with recurrent or persistent headache; acute or chronic subdural haematoma may develop. Treatment is by use of a variable-pressure or steady-flow valve, perhaps combined with an antisiphon device.

How long these various shunts continue to function is uncertain, because even if they cease to drain on account of blockage of the tube, or growth of the child, hydrocephalus does not necessarily recur. Other channels may have opened up by this time, or the active phase of the hydrocephalus may have passed. In either event a temporary diversion of CSF may effect a permanent cure. On the other hand some children develop raised pressure again after many years, indicating that they require continued drainage. Such late relapse may follow interference with the lower end of the system by an unsuspecting general surgeon in the abdomen.

2. Short circuits (bypassing the block)

These are attempts to re-establish the circulation of CSF by providing a bypass around the block, the level of which must be known before the appropriate procedure can be done (Fig. 14.2). Torkildsen's operation (ventriculo-cisternostomy), in which one or both lateral ventricles are put in communication with the cisterna magna, is less effective for infantile hydrocephalus than it is for pure aqueduct blockage in older children and adults. Third ventriculostomy consists of making a hole in the lamina terminalis to allow CSF to escape from the ventricle into the chiasmatic cistern and this may be done endoscopically. The ventriculoscope can also be used to ablate the choroid plexus, thereby reducing production of CSF, and this may alter the balance of CSF flow enough to prevent decompensation, usually after other treatment.

3. Direct attack on the block

Obstruction at the foramen magnum due to Arnold–Chiari malformation may be relieved by posterior fossa decompression. If the outlets from the fourth ventricle are blocked but the subarachnoid space is patent, relief may follow opening the ventricle. Both these procedures are more successful in mild cases in older children; in infancy the posterior fossa is difficult to explore – large venous sinuses in the dura make access difficult and the cisterna magna is often very small.

Juvenile and adult hydrocephalus

Most obstructive hydrocephalus after infancy is secondary to a tumour in the posterior fossa, midbrain or third ventricle. However, some are due to primary aqueduct blocks which failed to produce a markedly enlarged head in infancy, perhaps because they were incomplete.

Aqueduct stenosis (iter stricture)

Pathology

Stenosis consists of simple narrowing of the iter without any other surrounding abnormality or any associated development defect.

Gliosis, said by some to be the commonest type when hydrocephalus develops late, consists of a narrow iter surrounded by dense gliotic proliferation in the periaqueductal grey matter. Neurofibromatosis is a frequent accompaniment.

Forking of the aqueduct is more often found in infancy, associated with Arnold–Chiari malformation. A relatively large dorsal channel and several tiny ventral ones do not together comprise a sufficient cross-section to deal adequately with the CSF flow.

When hydrocephalus develops slowly over the years many secondary changes are found within the cranium. Constant pulsatile pressure of the convolutions of the brain against the bone of the skull erodes the inner table, causing irregular recesses filled by small herniae of brain. In places the skull sometimes gives way completely; if this is over one of the paranasal air sinuses and the dura is breached, spontaneous (i.e. non-traumatic) CSF rhinorrhoea develops. Diverticula of the ventricles may push out into the subarachnoid space, especially from the region of the trigone of the lateral ventricle into the cisterns in the pineal region. If a diverticulum ruptures, the tension of the hydrocephalus is relieved, and this self-cure may account for the long survival of some patients with advanced dilatation. Such a diverticulum can act as a local 'tumour' and compress the midbrain, producing local signs and displacement. It has been suggested that aqueduct stenosis may sometimes be secondary to communicating hydrocephalus, the dilated temporal horns of the ventricle compressing the aqueduct in a pincer grip, and initiating permanent damage.

Clinical

Most patients are first seen in late childhood and are rather plump, with a somewhat large head; a mild degree of infantilism may be observed, probably the result of pressure from the dilated third ventricle on the suprasellar region. Some present with headache, vomiting and signs of raised pressure. These may have been precipitated by a recent mild head injury or one of the infectious diseases of childhood, which have disturbed the delicate equilibrium so far maintained. Sometimes this condition is discovered by chance when the fundi are examined or the skull X-rayed for some other reason.

Chronic papilloedema with commencing atrophy is usually found on examination. Midbrain compression frequently results in loss of upward gaze of the eyes, and the pupils react sluggishly to light. A mild tremor is common and may suggest a cerebellar lesion; a number of these patients are investigated in the expectation of finding a posterior fossa tumour.

X-ray of skull may show the beaten silver appearance (digital markings) of the vault together with other signs of long-standing raised pressure – the sutures are widened and the pituitary fossa enlarged with erosion of the dorsum sellae (Fig. 4.1). A shallow posterior fossa, as judged by the position of the grooves for the transverse sinus and the low-lying torcula, is also characteristic.

CT scanning will show a large third ventricle and small fourth, whilst MRI gives much better visualization of the aqueduct itself and of CSF flow/voids, and may indicate that what was thought to be gliosis is in fact a hamartoma or other lesion.

Treatment

A single ventriculoperitoneal shunt should produce favourable results and in adults does not require revision due to growth. Torkildsen's ventriculocisternostomy was designed for treating this condition but is less easy to perform. The arch of the atlas is taken off, and the posterior rim of the foramen magnum nibbled away. An occipital burr hole is made and a catheter passed through it into the lateral ventricle; the outer end is led subcutaneously to the midline exposure, and the end placed in the cisterna magna, or the subarachnoid space of the cervical spine (Fig. 14.2). The tube may not drain immediately, but lumbar punctures for a few days may encourage it to start. There may be a cellular reaction for the first week. Many patients have now had these tubes in place for 15 years, and those seen at postmortem usually look as clean as the day they were put in, with no ventricular reaction.

Normal-pressure hydrocephalus

Certain patients with presenile dementia associated with marked disorder of gait, and often incontinence, have been shown to have enlarged ventricles associated with relatively little cortical atrophy. Because some of these patients improve markedly after ventricular shunting operations it has been suggested that their neurological dysfunction may be due to a pressure effect on the brain from the increased internal surface of the ventricles. ICP monitoring indicates that pressure is normal, or subject to only minor peaks (usually at night). Isotope encephalography suggests that the hydrocephalus may be due to failure of normal processing of absorptive CSF to the supratentorial subarachnoid space; tests show isotope still in the ventricles at a time when it should have disappeared. Artificial CSF infusions have demonstrated reduced absorptive capacity. No investigations so far devised can reliably predict which patients will benefit from shunting operations, although the presence of B waves during 24-hours ICP pressure monitoring and the absence of periventricular density change and deep white matter lesions on CT scan or MRI are favourable indicants. Only about a third of patients do benefit from surgery, and many of these have a history of a preceding event, such as subarachnoid haemorrhage, head injury or meningitis which might have reduced absorptive capacity.

Abnormalities of the skull

There are three main types of abnormalities of the skull: craniostenosis, cranium bifidum and hypertelorism.

Craniostenosis

This results from early closure of one or more sutures, but the primary abnormality is now believed to be in the skull base with secondary tensions transmitted to the skull vault through its dural and fascial attachments. It is occasionally associated with facial dysostoses, sometimes with limb abnormalities, giving rise to a variety of syndromes such as Crouzon's and Apert's.

The incidence of all varieties is at least 1 in 20 000. What happens depends on which suture is affected, which part of it and how fast the closure occurs. The sagittal suture is most often affected, giving the long, narrow skull of scaphocephaly. Unilateral coronal closure flattens the frontal bone and orbit (plagiocephaly) with which is associated a high sweeping rise of the sphenoidal ridge on the affected side. Bilateral coronal suture craniosynostosis gives a short high head – brachycephaly or turricephaly. Without treatment pansynostosis causes a small but normally shaped head presenting with raised ICP at the age of 5–7 years. With only one or two sutures involved deformity is maximal, but the risk of associated pressure problems rises as more sutures are involved. Surgery is needed by 3–6 months to correct the deformity, and this will also serve to prevent pressure problems.

While strip craniectomy, with formation of an artificial suture, is still used with success in sagittal and lambdoid synostosis, effective surgery for coronal and metopic sutural involvement must involve cuts in the skull base anteriorly with orbital ridge advancement. Premature sutural reclosure with bone produced from the dura is prevented by Silastic bone edging or extensive bony resection. These surgical procedures gives good long-term results. Complications and mortality are very low except when multiple sutural closure is associated with hydrocephalus. In Crouzon's syndrome and similar combined craniofacial dysostoses, the associated lower facial deformities require maxillofacial surgery, which should be delayed until the early teens, when growth is completed.

Cranium bifidum

This may present as an occipital or frontal cephalocele. The occipital lesion may be either a meningocele or an encephalocele, and is often associated with hydrocephalus from aqueduct stenosis or Chiari malformations. When repairing an occipital defect it can be difficult to find room within the abnormal cranium for the contents of an encephalocele and major cranial reconstructive surgery may be necessary. Whether these children will go on to develop normally is difficult to predict.

Frontal lesions are almost all encephaloceles, and usually involve the base of the anterior fossa and/or the nasal and facial bones. Adequate repair can involve extensive craniofacial surgery, but the outlook is good both for neurological and intellectual development.

Hypertelorism

This reflects an abnormal distance between the medial orbital walls, normally measured on X-rays as 2–3 cm at the age of 12 years. Hypertelorism may be a primary defect but is more commonly due to craniofacial deformities associated with cleft palate or hare-lip. The cosmetic defect produced by these abnormalities can be horrendous, precluding any possibility of the individual integrating successfully into modern society. The complicated and demanding craniofacial reconstructive surgery required to treat such children is well worthwhile, and the mortality acceptably low. These operations require close teamwork between neurosurgeon, plastic surgeon and the maxillofacial surgeons experienced in the field of craniofacial surgery.

Further reading

Amaches A.L., Wellington J. (1984). Infantile hydrocephalus: longterm results of surgical therapy. *Childs Brain*; **11:** 217–19.

Black P. McL., Ojemann R. G., Tzouras A. (1985). CSF shunts for dementia, incontinence and gait disturbance. *Clin. Neurosurg.*; **32:** 632–56.

Cohen M. M. (ed.) (1986). *Craniosynostosis: Diagnosis, Evaluation and Management.* New York: Raven Press.

Hockley A. D., Wake M. J., Goldin H. (1988). Surgical management of craniosynostosis. *Br. J. Neurosurg.*; **2:** 307–14.

Olds M. V., Storrs B., Walker M. L. (1986). Surgical treatment of sagittal synostosis. *Neurosurgery*; **18:** 345–7.

Persing J. A., Jane J. A., Delashaw J. B. (1990). Treatment of bilateral coronal synostosis in infancy: a holistic approach. *J. Neurosurg.*; **72:** 171–5.

Pickard J. D. (1982). Adult communicating hydrocephalus. *Br. Med. J.*; **1:** 35–43.

Pudenz R. H. (1981). Treatment of hydrocephalus: an historical review. *Surg. Neurol.*; **15:** 15–26.

Pudenz R. H., Foltz E. L. (1991). Hydrocephalus: overdrainage by ventricular shunts. A review and recommendations. *Surg. Neurol.*; **35:** 200–12.

Raimondi A. J., Samuelson G., Yarzagaray L. *et al.* (1969). Atresia of the foramina of Luschka and Magendie: the Dandy-Walker cyst. *J. Neurosurg.*; **31:** 202–16.

Robertson I. J. A., Leggate J. R. S., Miller J. D. *et al.* (1990). Aqueduct stenosis – presentation and prognosis. *Br. J. Neurosurg.*; **4:** 101–6.

Chapter 15

Congenital spinal abnormalities

Spinal dysraphism

    Spina bifida cystica (aperta)
    Spina bifida occulta

Neural anomalies

    Cerebellar ectopia
    Syringomyelia

Vertebral anomalies

    Craniovertebral anomalies
    Fusion of adjacent cervical vertebrae
    Basilar impression
    Spondylolisthesis

Anomalies of development in the spine most commonly derive from failure of fusion of the neural tube and adjacent cutaneous, muscular and osseous structures; these are embraced by the term spinal dysraphism which includes defects which may affect neural tissues only indirectly, such as lumbosacral lipomas. Clearly different are anomalies which primarily affect the neural tube and need not be associated with any bony abnormality, although in practice such an association is very common (e.g. cerebellar ectopia with lumbosacral spina bifida). Separate again are anomalies primarily of the vertebrae which may affect the neural contents of the canal only after many years as a result of the deformity produced.

Spinal dysraphism

Spina bifida cystica (aperta)

This major abnormality is much less common than it was due both to reduced incidence and to detection by prenatal screening soon enough to allow abortion. It affects the lumbosacral region in 80% of cases. Simple meningocele accounts for only 5% and consists of a herniation of the subarachnoid space only, without any nervous tissue. Survival without disability is the rule, and hydrocephalus seldom develops; when it does it usually undergoes natural arrest. The swelling may already be covered with skin at birth, but if not the membrane soon epithelializes and thickens to form a firm covering. Excision is simple and free from risk.

Myelomeningocele is much more serious, consisting of abnormal spinal cord and roots exposed by a skin defect. Some degree of paralysis of the legs and bladder is common, and in severe cases the anal sphincter is lax. Three-quarters develop hydrocephalus, usually related to associated cerebellar ectopia (see below), and this makes for a less favourable prognosis; indeed hydrocephalus and infection were largely responsible for the 90% mortality which was usual in the first year of life until the last decade. Since the introduction of effective operations for hydrocephalus, the availability of antibiotics, and the practice of early closure of the skin defect, over 50% of those who survive the first 24 hours now reach school age. Even with the spinal lesion healed and the hydrocephalus controlled, some persisting handicap is usual, but the frequency and severity of this vary considerably in different series: the combination of urinary incontinence, some degree of paraplegia (perhaps with talipes or congenital dislocation of the hip) and possibly mental retardation presents formidable social and educational problems, as well as the need for continuing medical supervision by a team of experts. Because of this there is now increasing acceptance of the view that surgical closure should be carried out only on those babies with a restricted lesion, good sphincter tone, reasonable limb movements and in whom there are no other associated congenital anomalies. For the best results in those chosen for surgery the skin closure should be done in the first 24–48 hours, in order to prevent infection and scabbing of the exposed neural tube. A decision must therefore be reached quickly, which is best done by a team of surgeons and paediatricians, having decided on criteria beforehand, and then applying these in individual cases as they occur.

Operation in the first 48 hours causes very little upset and can be done under local or general anaesthesia. Elaborate flaps of skin, fascia or muscle are unwise. The head is kept low for a few days to minimize the risk of CSF leakage, and care is taken to avoid faecal contamination of the wound. The head circumference is regularly checked for evidence of hydrocephalus; orthopaedic and urological assessment and follow-up are arranged.

Spina bifida occulta

A bony defect in the lamina of the first sacral vertebra is frequently seen on X-ray, and is of no significance. When a more extensive laminar defect is found, often with widening of the interpedicular distances, one of a number of other lesions may be discovered which can lead to progressive neurological deficit in the lower limbs. The clinical syndrome is similar for all lesions, consisting of disordered gait and a deformed foot (usually cavovarus); these are progressive and may be associated with an obvious neurological deficit or a neurogenic bladder disorder. MRI or myelography shows a low conus medullaris (below the body of L3), or a mass (lipoma or dermoid) or spinal cord deformity (diastematomyelia). The latter consists of duplication of the spinal cord over a few segments, sometimes with separate dural tubes, separated by an intervening bony spur which can stretch neural structures. Intraspinal lipoma may be connected with a subcutaneous lipoma over the sacrum, whilst patients with any of these lesions may have a tuft of long hairs or a sinus over the lumbosacral region. Although the disability caused by these lesions may be slowly progressive there is a good case for exploration in order to prevent further damage by ascent of a tethered cord with the growth of the child, or by growth of a mass (lipoma or dermoid) which impinges on the roots and cord. The decision to operate can be difficult because the procedure may aggravate the disability, but if there is definite progression surgery is justified.

Neural anomalies

Cerebellar ectopia

Cerebellar ectopia or encephalocranial disproportion is an invariable finding when meningomyelocele is associated with hydrocephalus. The most obvious abnormality is elongation of the cerebellar vermis which may reach the lower cervical vertebrae; it is bound by vascular adhesions to the herniated medulla, and the lower cranial nerves and upper cervical nerve roots have to travel upwards to their exit foramina. This component of the abnormality, which may be associated with obstruction of CSF flow, is sometimes termed the Arnold–Chiari malformation. In fact the cerebral hemispheres are usually enlarged and the tentorium low, resulting in a small posterior fossa with crowding of structures through the foramen magnum. A third of brains with this abnormality also have aqueduct stenosis. Hydromyelia and syringomyelia are also common (see below). Milder degrees of ectopia may be symptomless and may be identified by MRI without any abnormality in the spinal column. If symptoms progress, a posterior fossa decompression should produce improvement in a third of patients and halt progression in another third.

Syringomyelia

Syringomyelia consists of the syndrome of central cord dysfunction associated with a cystic cavitation; the cyst fluid often has the composition of normal CSF and it is now believed that the condition is in fact hydromyelia. Dilatation of the central canal is believed to result from CSF being forced into this situation by a valvular action due to a hindbrain anomaly. Certainly in many patients with syringomyelia, who are subjected to posterior fossa exploration, cerebella ectopia is found; if not, there are usually numerous adhesions.

The clinical features consist of gradually developing wasting of the small muscles of the hand and loss of spinothalamic sensation (pain and temperature). This may lead to inadvertent burns, and to trophic joint changes. Spasticity of the legs may develop, and if the medulla is involved, nystagmus and bulbar palsy. Progress may be very gradual, but sudden or steady worsening can occur. MRI is now the investigation of choice.

If an associated Arnold–Chiari malformation exists, then posterior fossa decompression may also benefit the symptoms from the syringomyelia. Otherwise treatment depends on the insertion of tubing to maintain drainage, but benefits may be limited and may only be temporary.

Vertebral anomalies

Craniovertebral anomalies

Development defects of the bony spine are particularly common in the cervical region. The consequences for the cord are largely similar to those associated with cervical spondylosis, which may indeed develop due to the abnormalities of intervertebral movement. Chronic myelopathy and the liability to profound paralysis following minor trauma are shared by both conditions.

Fusion of adjacent cervical vertebrae

This is commonest at the C2/3 interspace, but the atlas is often occipitalized in addition. This anomaly is particularly likely to be followed by spondylosis at joints below the fusion, and to be associated with a short neck recognizable clinically (the Klippel–Feil syndrome).

Basilar impression

This is the commonest anomaly, consisting of invagination of part of the rim of the foramen magnum into the skull so that it is higher than the occipital squama immediately lateral to it. Basilar impression is often associated with other anomalies, in particular, vertical translocation of the odontoid peg. It may also develop as an acquired rather than congenital disease secondary to Paget's disease, rickets or other diseases causing softening of bone.

Hydrocephalus results from blockage of the outlet of the fourth ventricle by the rim of the foramen magnum, an abnormally high odontoid process, secondary dural bands and arachnoid adhesions, or abnormally low tonsils.

All degrees of clinical abnormality are encountered. Certain signs are probably due to associated maldevelopment within the nervous system (vertical nystagmus, mirror movements in the limbs, and loss of postural sense in the arms and legs). A chronic myelopathy can develop with basilar impression alone or from an associated vertical shift of the odontoid. Spastic quadriparesis is the most obvious feature, but cerebellar ataxia, dysarthria and lateral nystagmus also occur, and there may be hydrocephalus with papilloedema in addition. MRI, reconstructed CT or myelography can each demonstrate the extent of the medullary compression. Neurological deterioration indicates the need for an anterior decompression through the transoral route, combined with posterior fixation to provide stability

Spondylolisthesis

This is a forward displacement of one vertebral body over another, either at the L4/5 level due to degeneration of the joints, or at the L5/S1 level due to a developmental defect of the pars articularis. It is doubtful whether this in itself ever causes nerve root pressure, although it may produce backache and accentuate the effects of a disc lesion or joint disease on the nerve root. Whether such a disc lesion should be treated in the usual way, or the removal of the disc should be followed by an interbody fusion, is a matter of controversy.

Further reading

Dale A. J. D. (1969). Diastematomyelia. *Arch. Neurol.*; **20:** 309–17.

Evans R. C., Tew B., Thomas M.D. *et al.* (1985). Selective surgical management of neural tube malformations. *Arch. Dis. Child.*; **60:** 415–19.

Hoffman H. J., Taechobarn C., Hendrick E.B. *et al.* (1985). Management of lipomyelo-meningoceles. Experience in the Hospital for Sick Children, Toronto. *J. Neurosurg.*; **62:** 1–8.

Hubballah M. Y., Hoffman H. J. (1987). Early repair of myelomeningocele and simultaneous insertion of VP shunt: technique and results. *Neurosurgery*; **20:** 21–3.

McLone D. G. (1986). Treatment of myelomeningocele: arguments against selection. *Clin. Neurosurg.*; **33:** 359–70.

Rekate H. R. (1985). To shunt or not to shunt: hydrocephalus and dysraphism. *Clin. Neurosurg.*; **32:** 593–607.

Rothman R.H., Simone S.A. (eds.) (1992). *The Spine: Congenital Malformations Section II.* Philadelphia: W. B. Saunders, pp. 229–501.

Schlesinger E. B., Antunes J. L., Michelsen W. J. *et al.* (1981). Hydromyelia: clinical presentation and modalities of treatment. *Neurosurgery*; **9:** 356–65.

Schut L., Bruce D. A., Sutton L. N. (1983). The management of the child with lipomyelo-meningoceles. *Clin. Neurosurg.*; **30:** 464–76.

Surana R. H., Quinn F. M. J., Guiney E. J. *et al.* (1991). Are the selection criteria for the conservative management in spina bifida still applicable? *Eur. J. Paediatr. Surg.*; **1:** (suppl 1): 35–7.

Sutton L. N., Charney E. B., Bruce D. A. *et al.* (1986). Myelomeningocele – the question of selection. *Clin. Neurosurg.*; **33:** 371–81.

Williams B. (1992). Syringomyelia. In: Teasdale G. M., Miller J. D. (eds.) *Current Neurosurgery.* Edinburgh: Churchill Livingstone.

Part VI:

Lesion-Making in the Nervous System

Chapter 16

Functional and stereotactic surgery

Principles of stereotactic surgery

Methods of lesion-making

Movement disorders

Epilepsy

Psychosurgery

Surgical relief of pain

Pathophysiology of pain

Treatment of pain from inoperable cancer

Sites of operative intervention for pain relief

    Posterior nerve roots
    The spinal cord

Neuralgia

    Trigeminal neuralgia
    Glossopharyngeal neuralgia
    Atypical facial pain
    Other neuralgias

Planned destruction of certain structures in the brain, spinal cord or nerves now forms an integral part of neurosurgery. The functional purpose may be to influence the care of epilepsy, to relieve intractable pain, to improve extrapyramidal movement disorders, or to alter behaviour in occasional cases of mental disorder resistant to all other treatment. Some structures can be exposed and dealt with under direct vision. Other targets are deeply situated and can be reached only by needles and probes directed from outside, using stereotactic techniques to ensure accurate placement in relation to radiological images. Stereotactic techniques are now more commonly used to reach deeply placed lesions that are inaccessible to open surgery in order to verify their nature by biopsy, to evacuate cysts or abscesses, or to insert therapeutic agents (p. 104).

Principles of stereotactic surgery (Fig. 16.1)

Three main manoeuvres are involved. First a rigid frame carrying an adjustable probe holder has to be fixed to the skull. There are several varieties of these, as surgeons have a tendency to develop their own modification of more standard instruments. Next the pathological lesion or anatomical reference points have to be identified on CT or MRI images, and related to measured points on the frame which show up on the same image. On the basis of these measurements the probe holder is adjusted to guide its end to the desired target area. When function is to be modified by operation it is the functional rather

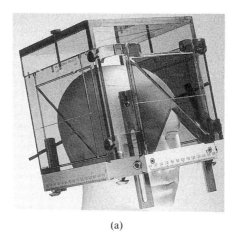

(a)

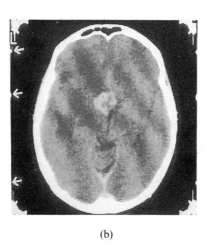

(b)

(a) The frame is fixed to the skull with four pins and CT indicator panels are attached to the frame. (b) CT imaging identifies fiducial points (arrowed) which appear on all slices of the examination. These permit calculation of the X, Y and Z coordinates of the target. Reproduced with permission from Elekta Instruments.

Fig. 16.1   The Leksell stereotactic system.

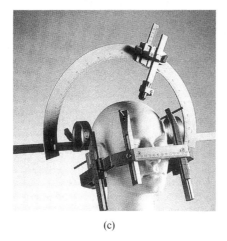

(c)

Fig. 16.1 (*cont*) (c) The indicator panels are removed and replaced with the stereotactic arc adjusted to the appropriate settings so that the centre of the arc matches the target. Reproduced with permission from Elekta Instruments.

than the anatomical localization which is important. However accurate the instruments, individual anatomical variations will always limit the accuracy of placement. For that reason verification is essential, usually by observing the effect of electrical stimulation or of a temporary lesion on function in the conscious patient.

Methods of lesion-making

Thermal lesions are the most commonly used, produced by passing a radiofrequency current of megacycle frequency through a fine monopolar electrode bared for the last few millimetres of its shaft. The size of the lesion is determined by the size of the probe, by the extent of the temperature change and its duration. The basic shape of the lesion is ovoid but this can be somewhat modified by varying the amount of probe that is left uninsulated. A degree of control of lesion size is possible using a thermostat in the probe to monitor the temperature. If only a limited deviation from normal is allowed (up to 40°C), a temporary lesion may be produced and its effects observed.

Chemical lesions have been used for many years, notably phenol, now replaced with glycerol, injections into the trigeminal ganglion, and a range of substances intrathecally for the treatment of pain in the limbs.

Mechanical lesions are employed when direct exposure of the target is possible, as in epilepsy surgery, decompression of the trigeminal root or cordotomy in the cervical spine.

Radiation can be employed either externally or internally. Multiple stereotactically focused beams of radiation produce a very precise lesion. The most useful application of this technique is in treating small arteriovenous malformations (p. 162). The limitations are the availability and expense of the equipment; only one centre provides this service in the UK. Radiation can also be applied locally to a target by stereotactically implanting radioactive seeds within the brain substance (brachytherapy; p. 96).

Movement disorders

Surgery for dyskinesias began with treating parkinsonism but since the intro-duction of L-dopa, surgery is more often used for certain cases of torsion dystonia, hemiballismus, choreoathetosis and spasmodic torticollis (now widely regarded as a restricted form of torsion dystonia). It is still used for parkinsonism when drugs are ineffective, too toxic or are not available. A similar lesion is made by most surgeons for all these conditions, in the ventrolateral nucleus of the thalamus; sometimes an additional or alternative lesion is made in the globus pallidus; this is believed by some to be more effective in relieving rigidity or spasticity, whilst the thalamic lesion relieves tremor.

The size as well as the site of the lesion may be important in determining the outcome; as a principle, the smallest lesion which is effective is usually made, because the unknown factor in every case is the amount of damage already suffered by the brain as the result of the primary disease process. If this is appreciable the additional therapeutic lesion may cause new deficits in motor control, higher sensory function or in subtle features such as motor initiative or sensory awareness. As a result a patient whose tremor or rigidity is relieved may fail to use his or her improved limb or may have added disabilities related to the motor function of the body as a whole.

The sole objective of surgery for movement disorders is to improve the overall motor function of the patient: not necessarily to eliminate the last remnant of abnormal movement, which in any event often worries the relatives more than the patient, but rather to increase the ease with which the hand or leg can be used: not necessarily to eliminate the dystonia in severe athetosis but to prevent the wild excursions of the limbs and trunk which tend to throw the patient off balance. Much good can be achieved by aiming for a less than perfect elimination of all signs and symptoms in order to avoid any increase in functional impairment in other ways.

Epilepsy

Epilepsy is a presenting feature of many intracranial conditions treated by surgery but in the present context operations specifically designed to relieve epilepsy are considered. These are mostly directed towards removal of an area of abnormally functioning brain. Only patients with intractable seizures, resistant to anticonvulsant medication pushed to its highest tolerable dose, become candidates for epilepsy surgery. The majority of such patients suffer from temporal lobe epilepsy (i.e. complex partial seizures); temporal lobe resections account for about 75% of operations performed for epilepsy. Other techniques include extratemporal resections, hemispherectomy and corpus callosotomy.

The success of such surgery depends on the identification of that part of the brain which is functioning abnormally. This is less easy than might appear, because secondary epileptic activity may be induced in areas adjacent to, or even remote from, the primary lesion. Both EEG and imaging techniques play an important part in planning surgery. *Videotelemetric monitoring* enables accurate observation of the seizure and localization of the simultaneous electrical activity. If necessary, percutaneously sited sphenoidal electrodes, foramen ovale electrodes or, in some cases, stereotactically placed depth electrodes give additional information on the site of origin of seizure activity.

Imaging techniques now play an important role, not just by demonstrating the presence of lesions such as indolent glioma, hamartoma or arteriovenous malformation (one or other of which is found in about one-third of patients), but also in detecting mesial temporal sclerosis present in up to a half of those with temporal lobe epilepsy. *MRI* has superseded CT scanning for this purpose; the highest-field-strength scanners are readily capable of detecting the hippocampal atrophy seen in mesial sclerosis. *SPECT* is also proving valuable by demonstrating hyperperfusion at the site of the focus during seizure activity, followed by hypoperfusion during the interictal period.

Temporal lobectomy

Temporal seizures usually begin with discharges in the hippocampus or amygdala (i.e. in the most medial temporal structures). Operative measures consist of either removing the anterior 4–5cm of temporal lobe along with these important medial structures or alternatively selectively removing the amygdala and anterior hippocampus. This latter procedure, although seemingly less destructive, does not appear to improve results or reduce the mild postoperative cognitive changes sometimes seen. Up to 60% of patients become seizure-free after operation and a further 20–30% show a significant improvement in seizure frequency (90% benefit overall). In about 75% of resected specimens, some pathological abnormality is found and outcome in terms of seizure control is best in this group. This may take the form of a very low-grade glioma or an angioma or other vascular malformation which may have partly calcified; in some an active glioma is discovered. The commonest lesion, however, is an atrophic one consisting of sclerosis and loss of neurons in the region of the hippocampus, uncus and Ammon's horn. The frequency of this medial sclerosis of the temporal lobe naturally raises the question of aetiology. One hypothesis is that this is a sequel of birth trauma, which has caused tentorial herniation and subsequent scarring. A more widely accepted explanation is that medial sclerosis results from one or more bouts of prolonged seizures (lasting 30 minutes or more) occurring in the first 3 years of life. Certainly children who have died from uncontrolled status consistently have neuronal necrosis in these structures, which is believed to be ischaemic in origin. Moreover many patients with temporal lobe epilepsy give a history of prolonged seizures in childhood.

Local cortical excisions are less often performed, but intractable seizures originating from a focal lesion outwith the temporal lobe may be worth resecting. Such lesions include scars left by a penetrating wound or an abscess, an indolent glioma, cavernous angioma or a patch of cortical dysplasia. It is in such cases that operative electrocorticography can be of most help to the surgeon in indicating the exact location and extent of abnormally functioning cortex. The surgeon may test the activity in the remaining brain after the initial excision. It may also help him or her avoid excision of functionally vital areas such as the motor strip which can be identified by stimulation. When such electrical exploration is called for at operation the anaesthesia must not interfere with cortical activity. Local anaesthesia is the most reliable and has stood the test of time, but the neuroleptanalgesic drugs form a very useful supplement. The success of local cortical excision depends on the successful removal of the focal pathology. At least two-thirds should benefit, but results do not match those for temporal lobe resections.

Hemispherectomy can benefit children contracting severe hemiplegia in the first 2 years of life and who are subject to insistent epilepsy. Such children usually appear retarded in addition to suffering from hemiplegia and epilepsy. Although the operation either removes or disconnects all of the cortex of one hemisphere, leaving the basal ganglia intact, crude movement and sensation are usually preserved in the contralateral limbs and may indeed improve after operation so that walking becomes possible. Over 80% become seizure-free. Relieved of the burden of frequent fits, patients may improve greatly in behaviour and apparently in intellectual performance. The improvement may enable attendance at a special school and aid social integration.

Callosotomy

Division of the corpus callosum may help patients with intractable generalized (atonic, tonic or myoclonic) seizures, theoretically by preventing generalization and reverberation from one hemisphere to the other. Problems associated with disconnection are minimized by performing the procedure in two stages. Few patients become seizure-free, but up to two-thirds may obtain improved control.

Psychosurgery

It is 100 years since a survivor of severe frontal lobe damage was observed to have alteration of his personality, becoming uninhibited and emotionally unrestrained. Only in 1933 did Moniz propose a surgical assault on the frontal lobe as a means of treating patients with mental illness. The original procedure, standard leucotomy, cut most fibres to and from the frontal poles and produced marked personality change and intellectual damage as byproducts of its beneficial effects in diminishing tension and aggression. Because of this, and because recently introduced drugs have made it possible to produce reversible control of behaviour, this original operation is now rarely performed. However, more restrictive procedures have been devised, which are beneficial without producing permanent adverse effects on the personality. These are directed at various parts of the limbic system, of which the frontothalamic fibres cut in the standard leukotomy are also a part; they include orbital undercutting, limited frontothalamic lesions, cingulectomy and amygdalotomy. Most mental conditions originally treated surgically (schizophrenia and depressive psychosis) are now more satisfactorily controlled by drugs, and the indications for these new procedures are limited. Patients suffering from obsessional neuroses or chronic endogenous depression with agitation, who show marked tension, are most likely to benefit, providing there has been a reasonably stable premorbid personality.

Operation calls for only a few days in a surgical unit and can be carried out through a burr hole which needs only a very limited shaving of the head. The effect is seldom immediate and the patient should always return to the care of a psychiatrist, who should continue both drugs and supportive therapy, at least for a time. Organic complications of leucotomy are rare, but postoperative haemorrhage may occur and epilepsy occasionally develops even after many months.

Surgical relief of pain

The development of pain clinics and pain services, largely by anaesthetists, has reduced the role of the neurosurgeon in the management of pain to a limited group of specific conditions, and to a small set of patients unsuitable for or resistant to treatment by drugs or injections.

Pain is a complex sensory experience; in most instances it is useful and everyone must experience pain in infancy in order to learn to avoid the circumstances which provoke it. To be without the sensation of pain is a severe and often fatal handicap in children born with congenital insensitivity to tissue damage. As with other sensory experiences, there is no single brain centre for pain, although operations on the sensory system appear to modify the sensation. Only the patient can describe the sensation of pain and only he or she can say whether it is better or worse after operations designed to relieve pain.

Both the experience of pain and the patient's reaction to it may be modified by psychological factors which include the patient's normal personality and the attitude of those around him or her. The significance of the pain for the patient may determine the amount of anxiety it causes, whilst basic personality traits may affect the way in which the patient's pain is communicated to those near him or her. In some the discomfort and anxiety are apparently exaggerated; in others they are suppressed. Whilst pain is normally a warning reaction to noxious stimuli it may also form an expression of distress, a cry for help, a form of communication. These complex factors warrant serious attention when major procedures are proposed for the relief of pain which is considered overwhelming, because adjustments in certain factors forming the psychological background may make the situation much more tolerable and the need for surgery may then be less pressing. This is particularly the case with pain from advanced cancer, and to a lesser extent with the traumatic neuralgias.

Pathophysiology of pain

Recent concepts of pain include the recognition of pain-suppressor mechanisms, in the form of opiate or non-opiate receptors. A new approach to treatment is to activate these natural suppressors by electrical stimulation or chemical binding. Two main categories of chronic pain are now recognized. *Somatic* pain appears to result from prolonged activation of nociceptors by pathological processes, but this may produce some central imprint on the CNS. This would be the mechanism for trigeminal neuralgia and for most cancer pain. The other type is *central, dysaesthetic* or *deafferentation* pain.

This results from changes in the signal-elaborating mechanism secondary to injury to the nervous system, but independent of activation of peripheral nociceptors. This appears to account for pain after brachial plexus root avulsion, herpes zoster, cordotomy, surgical nerve section (anaesthesia dolorosa); phantom and thalamic pain are also deafferentation syndromes. While cancer usually causes pain by nociceptor activation, in the later stages destruction of nerves and ganglia may produce deafferentation.

Treatment of pain from inoperable cancer

Not all cancer is painful, even in the terminal stages. But sometimes when growths invade the bones of the spine or face, or extend into the sacral or brachial plexus, or into the posterior root ganglia, pain can surpass all other symptoms by its severity, its persistence and its devastating effect on morale. But care must be taken to confirm that it is in fact pain which is the real cause of distress, and that it is not being used as a distress signal, due to inability to cope with other aspects of progressive disease.

The increasing interest in palliative care, sometimes associated with services of the hospice movement, ensures that more patients have access to adequate treatment. Skilled use of analgesics in adequate doses (sometimes using motorized pump delivery) combined with antidepressants, steroids, anticonvulsants or non-steroidal anti-inflammatories can control the pain in many patients in whom it seemed that drugs were not initially helpful. Some cancers respond to hormonal drugs (breast and prostate).

Transcutaneous electrical nerve stimulation often provides some relief, either by activating large fibres and 'closing the gate' at the spinal level or by influencing higher centres.

Operative relief

A short expectancy of life is not necessarily an adequate criterion for withholding a neurosurgical operation for the relief of pain. With only a month to live, the pain from an operation wound may be more bearable than that due to malignant invasion of nerves, and everyone's morale will be higher if the patient dies free from distressing pain and from the feeling that everyone has given up.

But treatment must not compound the patient's sufferings, nothing adds more to the suffering than a useless operation. There are many risks and difficulties in the surgery of ill and dying patients, but there is no room for complacency over results. The appropriate procedure must be carefully selected and planned. It must be consistent with the patient's strength, and aim at permanent relief of pain for the rest of the patient's life. In few other instances in surgery is there such a premium on experience and judgement.

Sites of operative intervention for pain relief

Posterior nerve roots.
  Partial block of posterior nerve roots by intrathecal injection.
  Posterior rhizotomy in the spinal canal, or posterior fossa.

Spinal cord.
  Anterolateral cordotomy.
  Dorsal root entry zone (DREZ) lesions.
  Dorsal column stimulation.
  Anterior commissurotomy.
Brainstem.
Thalamus.
  Stereotactic thalamotomy.
  Deep brain stimulation.

Posterior nerve roots

Partial block of posterior roots by intrathecal chemicals was introduced in 1956 using phenol injected into the spinal canal with the aim of selectively and permanently damaging the posterior nerve roots from a specific dermatome distribution. But the ease with which this small procedure can be attempted bears little relation to the skill needed for its safe performance; the risk of the phenol spreading to involve the sacral roots and impairing sphincter control is high and restricts its use to patients with terminal malignancy. Injection of hypertonic saline (7%) into the lumbar theca provides an alternative method of producing selective root damage with less risk of serious complications.

Posterior rhizotomy implies section of the whole posterior root and this abolishes all sensation. This technique has been largely abandoned. Difficulty in ensuring destruction of all the sensory supply from a specific region probably accounts for the poor results. In some areas such as the face, posterior rhizotomy leaves an irritating numbness at times as painful as the original symptom (anaesthesia dolorosa).

The spinal cord

The spinal cord is not merely a cable carrying fibres upwards and downwards for the brain; it is part of the CNS and shares with it a multiplicity of collateral connections – many of the nerve fibres which enter synapse within the cord and contribute to the extensive integration of activity present at all spinal levels. A large number of the small-diameter fibres believed to carry pain sensation enter the cord from the sensory roots and cross to the opposite side within three to four segments of entering to form the spinothalamic tracts (Fig. 16.2).

Anterolateral cordotomy divides these smaller fibres in the anterolateral quadrant and raises the threshold to pain on the opposite side. It is a safer and more reliable method than intrathecal phenol for pain in the lower leg or pelvis. *Percutaneous cordotomy* has now replaced open operation; it avoids a major procedure under general anaesthesia, and the lesion can be accurately titrated because the patient is fully awake and cooperative. A needle is introduced into the cord under radiographic control, usually by a lateral approach between C1 and C2 vertebrae. The site can be verified by observing the effects of electrical stimulation and thermal lesion is then made.

Bilateral cordotomy may be necessary for bilateral pain. It can sometimes be judged that pain on the other side will be manageable with drugs once it is the only pain left. At other times bilateral cordotomy is clearly going to be

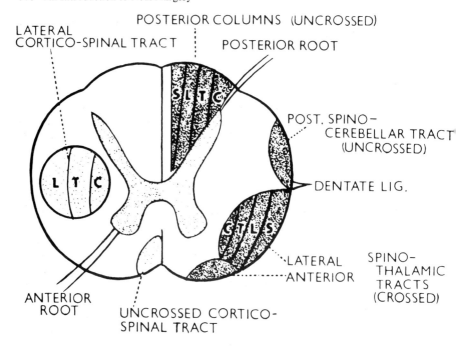

LATERAL
CORTICO-SPINAL TRACT

POSTERIOR COLUMNS (UNCROSSED)

POSTERIOR ROOT

POST. SPINO-
CEREBELLAR TRACT
(UNCROSSED)

DENTATE LIG.

LATERAL
ANTERIOR

SPINO-
THALAMIC
TRACTS
(CROSSED)

ANTERIOR
ROOT

UNCROSSED CORTICO-
SPINAL TRACT

DESCENDING   ASCENDING

c = cervical, t = thoracic, l = lumbar, s = sacral.

Fig. 16.2 Spinal cord tracts descending on the left and ascending on the right. c = cervical; l = lumbar; s = sacral; t = thoracic.

needed and the value of pain relief must be weighed against the increased risks of the bilateral operation.

As many as two-thirds of the patients will have bladder difficulty after bilateral cordotomy, and in half of these it will be permanent. One-fifth will have noticeable loss of power in the legs. To try to minimize these dangers the two cordotomies should be performed at different levels, one at C6 or 7, the other at C1, and in two stages. Cordotomy is rarely justified for non-fatal conditions.

DREZ lesions
After cord exposure, multiple radiofrequency lesions sited at the dorsal root entry zone have produced encouraging results in the treatment of deafferentation pain, particularly that following brachial plexus avulsion and postherpetic neuralgia. Despite recent modifications, the technique still carries some risk of producing ipsilateral leg weakness.

Dorsal column stimulation
Stimulation of electrodes inserted percutaneously to lie on the posterior aspect of the spinal cord provides pain relief in a proportion of patients with chronic

pain. If successful, a radiocontrolled receiver can be implanted subcutaneously for long-term treatment.

Anterior commissurotomy

The thin fibres which enter the cord from the posterior roots and cross over to the opposite side are the only group of fibres that do cross in any number. They may be cut by splitting the cord down the midline. This may relieve pain on both sides in the segmental area corresponding to the incision, but benefits are often short-lived and use of the techniques is restricted to a few centres.

The **brainstem** has been a disappointing site for surgery. After selective tractotomy either the pain relief is too incomplete and too brief, or sensory loss and ataxia are too extensive and too profound to make this a reliable method.

The **thalamus** can only be operated upon stereotactically but little reliance can be placed on these operations for pain at the present time. Small lesions in the posterior thalamus might give poorly localized sensory loss, even to pin-prick, but there will not necessarily be any relief of pain. The altered sensation, if it persists, may even make the pain seem worse and give an uncomfortable hypersensitivity to the skin. On the other hand some small lesions near the midline and in the region of the centre median and parafascicular nuclei may give relief of pain without any detectable sensory loss. With the development of other techniques, few now resort to stereotactic thalamotomy except perhaps for the treatment of intractable head and neck pain. *Deep brain stimulation* provides an alternative non-destructive method of treating pain from those sites. Implanted electrodes in the sensory relay nucleus of the thalamus, in the periventricular grey matter or in the internal capsule can lead to good pain relief in some patients, often persisting for prolonged periods beyond the duration of stimulation.

Neuralgia

Changes in the sensory system due to trauma, disease or degeneration can alter the conducting mechanism and thereby change the impulse patterns at any level. It appears that non-painful impulse patterns may be changed into painful impulse patterns *en route*. This probably plays some part in the genesis of the altered sensation in causalgia, postherpetic neuralgia, the thalamic syndrome and painful phantom limb. When certain types of neuralgia have been established for some time they become almost impossible to eradicate. It is as though the mechanism for learning has associated pain, and nothing but pain, with the one area for so long that it eventually interprets all stimuli as pain.

Neurosurgical operations aimed at relieving neuralgias may not only be ineffective but may even initiate a new pain or unpleasant sensation which is worse than the old. One misfortune is the appearance of anaesthesia dolorosa where severe and continuous pain is felt in a denervated area which is quite insensitive to all external stimulation. Nowadays it is common to start treatment with stimulation, either percutaneously or of the dorsal column with implanted electrodes; good relief is usual, but not in all patients.

Trigeminal neuralgia

Trigeminal neuralgia is the term applied to a particular facial pain which is unique amongst the neuralgias in that the pain can nearly always be completely controlled by treatment. If the same treatment is mistakenly given to patients with other forms of facial pain, they are unlikely to be improved and may be made worse.

The *age of onset* is usually over 50 years, and many patients are in the eighth or ninth decades; but it may start in patients as young as 25. Its occurrence in younger patients should arouse suspicion of associated disseminated sclerosis, a cerebellopontine angle tumour or a vascular lesion. It is commoner in women.

The main *clinical feature* is the sudden and severe pain that only lasts a moment and then goes, leaving nothing behind – except the fear of its return. Shaving, talking, washing or even a cold wind may disturb the skin of the upper lip and trigger a paroxysm of pain which is so severe that the patient is immobilized in agony. It is initially localized to one division of the trigeminal nerve, usually the second, but with time tends to spread to other divisions and increase in severity. Its course is interrupted by remissions of months or years of complete freedom from pain, and an elderly patient may die of an unrelated cause without it returning. It may become bilateral, either soon after its onset or after years of unilateral pain.

The trigger area may be in the gums or teeth. Some patients are given dental treatment for what is in fact trigeminal neuralgia; others seem to develop trigeminal neuralgia after prolonged and painful treatment for dental disease. Rarely does the first paroxysm of pain occur in the ophthalmic division, but it may spread to the forehead from the cheek and later appear to start from behind the eye.

Physical signs are few. The patient may present with a scarf around the head, and talk very little and out of the corner of the mouth. Thinness and dehydration from not eating, a dirty face from not washing or shaving, all from fear of precipitating an attack of pain, may be the only signs. Sometimes a slight subjective loss to pin-prick is found over one side – when it can be tested for – but the corneal reflexes, which are rarely brisk in old age, are usually equal.

Carbamazepine (Tegretol) has transformed the treatment of trigeminal neuralgia; injections and operations are much less frequently required since its introduction. In doses of 200 mg tablets up to 4 or 5 times daily it usually controls pain within 24 hours; the dose should be the smallest needed for the relief of pain, because some ataxia and blurring of vision may occur. Indeed most patients now coming to surgery are those who require such a high dosage to control their pain that toxic effects are troublesome; virtually all patients respond with adequate dosage, and the drug may be given as a therapeutic test when the diagnosis is in doubt. Long-term treatment with carbamazepine is best avoided as very occasionally it may cause marrow suppression; after 2–3 weeks of freedom from pain the dosage is reduced to ascertain if a natural remission has occurred, and if it has, the drug is discontinued. Analgesic drugs are virtually useless for this sudden type of pain and should not be used.

A variety of operative procedures are available; selection depends on the patient's age and general condition and on the experience and preference of the individual centre.

Percutaneous glycerol injection into the trigeminal ganglion has replaced the use of phenol which tended to produce widespread facial sensory loss with a risk of neuropathic keratitis. Glycerol appears to have a more selective action. Using radiological control a needle is inserted through the foramen ovale into the trigeminal cave. The needle enters the cheek just above the lateral to the angle of the mouth and passes upwards and backwards between the maxilla and the vertical ramus of the mandible to the foramen ovale; after advancing the needle through to the cave, CSF usually flows from the tip. An injection of water-soluble contrast confirms the needle position before injecting the glycerol. This technique carries a 70–80% success rate with minimal risk of unpleasant sensory side-effects.

Thermocoagulation of the retrogasserian rootlets or the ganglion of the trigeminal nerve can bring about analgesia in a selected area of the trigeminal distribution and a differential loss of pain sensation with retention of light touch. An electrode is inserted under radiological control through the foramen ovale. The tip position is adjusted until electrical stimulation produces sensations (usually paraesthesia, occasionally pain) in the region of the original pain. A radiofrequency lesion is made until analgesia, without anaesthesia, is produced in the appropriate area of the face. Thermocoagulation also carries a success rate of above 70% but it tends to produce larger areas of altered sensation. Sometimes this is of an unpleasant nature, occasionally as troublesome as the original symptoms.

Microvascular decompression involves direct exposure of the trigeminal nerve rootlets in the cerbellopontine angle. In a high proportion of patients an artery is seen to indent or abut the trigeminal roots, usually adjacent to the dorsal root entry zone. Interposing a small piece of sponge between artery and nerve gives pain relief in over 80% of patients. Although some question the mechanism involved, there is no doubt that this method produces excellent results whilst avoiding unpleasant sensory side-effects. The more major procedure however carries a 1% mortality risk and a threat of serious morbidity. For this reason it is best reserved for patients under the age of 70 years in good general health.

Trigeminal root section, either through an extradural approach in the middle fossa or through an intradural approach through the posterior fossa, inevitably results in facial anaesthesia; its use is best restricted to those patients in whom other techniques have failed.

Glossopharyngeal neuralgia

The one feature that most cases of glossopharyngeal neuralgia have in common is pain triggered by swallowing. There are two main sites of the pain – the throat or tongue and the ear. If the pain appears in the one it commonly radiates to the other. The patient usually indicates the site of the pain in the throat by pointing a finger to the tip of the hyoid bone below the angle of the jaw. Long remissions of pain are common; in some patients the pain never becomes unbearable. Rarely it occurs on both sides and very occasionally it is associated with trigeminal neuralgia. When pain on swallowing is severe there is soon a temptation to stop eating and old patients may become alarmingly cachectic. In many cases the diagnosis is difficult because the pain is diffuse and only inconstantly related to swallowing. There are no abnormal physical signs. The trigger spot can occasionally be identified on the back of the tongue and the pain briefly relieved by a lignocaine spray. When paroxysmal throat pain on swallowing is associated with transient syncope it certainly incriminates the ninth nerve: the innervation of the carotid sinus in the neck is responsible for the reflex bradycardia and hypotension. It is not uncommon to find some unexpected pathology associated with the lower cranial nerves which undoubtedly bears responsibility for the pain. Glossopharyngeal and vagal neuromas are the commonest findings in what is, however, a rare presentation.

In the absence of local pathology, carbamazepine often produces some benefit. Microvascular decompression of the ninth cranial nerve has been reported, but most surgeons section the ninth nerve roots, often along with the upper one or two rootlets of the adjacent tenth nerve which carries sensory fibres from areas close to those from which the pain arises.

Atypical facial pain

Facial pain which does not have the features of trigeminal or glossopharyngeal neuralgia, and does not appear to be associated with any other detectable pathology, presents a problem in diagnosis and often defies treatment.

The initial stage of trigeminal neuralgia may present as an atypical facial pain. The possibility always exists, too, that pain in the face is due to inflammation or neoplasia. It is feasible for either, in the early stages, to produce pain and yet avoid detection by even the most rigorous clinical and radiological examinations. Dental malocclusion may cause pain which appropriate mechanical adjustments will relieve.

Some patients complain of long-standing facial pain with none of the acute exacerbation or triggering qualities of the true neuralgias. The diagnosis remains provisional until sufficient time has elapsed to allow any other pathology to manifest itself. Facial pain in these patients, many of whom are middle-aged women, may be the presenting feature of an endogenous depression. These atypical facial neuralgias unassociated with any demonstrable pathology, do not respond to neurosurgical operation. Carbamazepine may help, but often antidepressant medication is the only useful treatment. Although sympathy should be offered, all requests for surgery must be refused.

Other neuralgias

Causalgia usually follows injury to a small nerve trunk in the arm or hand. Following incomplete repair of the nerve the scar overlying it, or the incompletely reinnervated skin beyond, becomes exquisitely tender and this may render the whole arm useless. Cervical sympathectomy, either pharmacological or surgical, may cure the condition if performed early, but it is not unknown for it to be treated by serial amputations up to the shoulder with the pain persisting in either the phantom or the stump after each operation. Posterior rhizotomy, cordotomy and thalamotomy may result in a severely disabled patient with unrelieved pain who eventually commits suicide in despair.

In *postherpetic neuralgia* the nervous tissue is damaged by infection. Again touch tends to exacerbate the pain. Transcutaneous stimulation and carbamazepine may provide some benefit, but in many only antidepressants help to alleviate the symptoms.

In the *thalamic syndrome* the damage arises usually from ischaemia or haemorrhage. The minor stroke, which is the usual cause, may give an initial hemiparesis with a profound hemianaesthesia and sensory ataxia. Most of the power eventually returns to the side but there may be some altered posture of the limbs at rest and some athetoid movements. Most of the feeling returns to the side also, but with it a distressing hypersensitivity to the slightest stimulus. The sensation may appear to be one of almost spontaneous pain, although it is usually precipitated by light contact with clothing, or exposure to a light draught of air. A stereotactic thalamotomy may bring effective relief but results are usually disappointing.

Further reading

Functional and stereotactic surgery

Miles J., Redfern R.M. (1987). The place of thalamotomy in the treatment of Parkinsonism. *Br. J. Neurosurg.*; **1**: 311–15.

Perry J.H., Rosenbaum A.E., Lunsford L.D. *et al.* (1980). Computed tomography/guided stereotactic surgery: conception and development of a new stereotactic methodology. *Neurosurgery*; **7**: 376–81.

Poynton A., Bridges P.K., Bartlett J.R. (1988). Psychosurgery in Britain now. *Br. J. Neurosurg.*; **2**: 297–306.

Epilepsy

Elwes R.D.C., Dunn G., Binnie C.D. *et al.* (1991). Outcome following resective surgery for temporal lobe epilepsy; a prospective study of 102 consecutive cases. *J. Neurol. Neurosurg. Psychiatry*; **54**: 949–52.

Luders H.O. (ed.) (1992). *Epilepsy Surgery.* New York: Raven Press.

Ojemann G. (1987). Surgical therapy for medically intractable epilepsy. *J. Neurosurg.*; **66**: 48–99.

Oxbury J.M., Adams C.B.T. (1989). Neurosurgery for epilepsy. *Br. J. Hosp. Med.*; **41**: 372–7.

Polkey C.E. (1990). Surgical treatment of epilepsy. *Lancet*; **ii**: 553–5.

Pain

Adams C.B.T. (1989). Miscrovascular decompression: an alternative view and hypothesis. *J. Neurosurg.*; **70**: 1–12.

Bates J.A., Nathan P.W. (1980). Transcutaneous electrical nerve stimulation for chronic pain. *Anaesthesia*; **35**: 817–22.

Bond M.R. (1984). *Pain: Its Nature, Analysis and Treatment*, 2nd edn. Edinburgh: Churchill Livingstone.

Burchiel K.J., Steege T.D., Howe J.F. *et al.* (1981). Comparison of percutaneous radiofrequency gangliolysis and microvascular decompression for the surgical management of tic doloreux. *Neurosurgery*; **9**: 111–19.

Gildenberg P.L. (1974). Percutaneous cervical cordotomy. *Clin. Neurosurg.*; **21**: 246–56.

Gybels J., Sweet W.H. (eds.) (1989). *Neurosurgical Treatment of Persistent Pain.* Basel: Kager.

Hakanson S. (1981). Trigeminal neuralgia treatment by the injection of glycerol into the trigeminal cistern. *Neurosurgery*; **9**: 638–46.

Hitchcock E.R. (1970). Hypothermic-saline subarachnoid irrigation. *Lancet*; **i**: 843.

Jannetta P.J. (1976). Microsurgical approach to the trigeminal nerve for tic doloreux. *Progn. Neurol. Surg.*; **7**: 180–200.

Kumar K., Nath R., Wyant G. (1991). Treatment of chronic pain by epidural spinal cord stimulation: a ten year experience. *J. Neurosurg.*; **75**: 402–7.

North R.B., Kidd D.H., Piantadosi S. *et al.* (1990). Percutaneous retrogasserian glycerol rhizot-omy. Predictions of success or failure in treatment of trigeminal neuralgia. *J. Neurosurg.*; **72:** 851–6.

Rawlings C.E., El-Naggar A.O., Nashold B.S. (1989). The DREZ procedure: an update on technique. *Br. J. Neurosurg.*; **3:** 633–42.

Sweet W.H. (1986). The treatment of trigeminal neuralgia. *N. Engl. J. Med.*; **315:** 174–7.

Young R. (1990). Clinical experience with radiofrequency and laser DREZ lesions. *J. Neurosurg.*; **72:** 715–20.

Index